Health Research Methods

a Canadian Perspective

Edited by

Kate Bassil

Denise Zabkiewicz

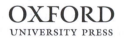

OXFORD

UNIVERSITY PRESS

OXFORD
UNIVERSITY PRESS

Oxford University Press is a department of the University of Oxford.
It furthers the University's objective of excellence in research, scholarship,
and education by publishing worldwide. Oxford is a registered trade mark of
Oxford University Press in the UK and in certain other countries.

Published in Canada by
Oxford University Press
8 Sampson Mews, Suite 204,
Don Mills, Ontario M3C 0H5 Canada

www.oupcanada.com

Library and Archives Canada Cataloguing in Publication

Health research methods : a Canadian perspective / edited by
Kate Bassil and Denise Zabkiewicz.

Includes bibliographical references.
ISBN 978-0-19-544716-3 (pbk.)

1. Health--Research--Methodology. 2. Health--Research--Canada.
I. Bassil, Kate, editor of compilation II. Zabkiewicz, Denise, editor of
compilation

R850.H42 2014   610.72   C2013-902374-7

Cover image: Joe Biafore/Getty Images

Oxford University Press is committed to our environment.
This book is printed on Forest Stewardship Council® certified paper
and comes from responsible sources.

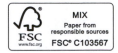

Printed and bound in Canada

1 2 3 4 — 17 16 15 14

Contents

CHAPTER 6   Overview of Study Designs in Health   101

Martin Tammemägi

CHAPTER 7   Measurement   119

David L. Streiner

CHAPTER 8   Sampling   143

Jean Dumais

CHAPTER 9   Qualitative Health Research   165

Rachelle Hole

CHAPTER 10   Measures of Frequency, Effect, and Outcome   191

David L. Streiner

CHAPTER 11   Quantitative Methods: Analysis   211

Charles H. Goldsmith

CHAPTER 12   Reporting Health Research 233

Donald C. Cole

CHAPTER 13   Knowledge Translation   247

Elliot M. Goldner

Preface

The idea for this book emerged from our own experience teaching health research methods. We struggled to find a textbook that met the needs of our students—one that provided an introductory and comprehensive overview of health research methods while showcasing the breadth and diversity of Canadian research. After teaching the methods course for several terms using various combinations of textbooks and peer-reviewed manuscripts, we felt it was time to develop a book that would meet the needs of students and our colleagues teaching similar courses. The initial proposal for the book was largely based on the structure and content of our course. Over time, as the chapter contributors joined the project, the book developed and now encompasses much more breadth, particularly with the inclusion of many research examples embedded throughout the chapters.

This book is comprised of contributions from experts in epidemiology, nursing, kinesiology, biostatistics, global health, medical sociology, social work, and public health, resulting in a multidisciplinary perspective of research methods. Additionally, each of the chapter contributors have presented a diversity of research examples that encompass some of their own original work as well as selected key milestones in Canadian health research. We hope this will provide the reader with an understanding of the range of methodologies applied across health disciplines.

We have attempted to present an introduction to health research methods in as clear and concise a manner as possible. We believe this book will appeal to anyone interested in an introduction to research methodology. We hope that you, the reader, not only gain substantive and fundamental knowledge of health related research practices and procedures from this book, but that you are enlightened and inspired by the breadth and diversity of the research presented here to further advance your learning and pursue your own research interests.

Acknowledgements

We are thankful to our colleagues who have contributed individual chapters to this book. Their efforts and commitment have enabled us to complete this project in a timely fashion. We have learned from their expertise as well as their collaboration, both of which have been highlights of this process.

At Oxford University Press we thank Mark Thompson, acquisitions editor, who assisted us during the proposal and initial peer-review stage. Lisa Peterson, our developmental editor for most of the project, provided ongoing feedback and advice for which we are very grateful. Serene Ong, copyeditor, assisted in preparing the final version. Jodi Lewchuk, developmental editor, provided guidance during the final stages of development.

We also appreciate the reviewers who provided valuable feedback on both the original book proposal and also the complete manuscript. We thank the following reviewers, as well as those who wish to remain anonymous for their suggestions: Debbie Brennick, Cape Breton University; Julie Brown, Fanshawe College; Murray Holtby, Mount Royal University; Donna Martin, University of Manitoba; Martin Tammemägi, Brock University.

We are blessed with dear friends and family that love and support us. During the last three years, they have provided encouragement to buoy our spirits when lagging and joyous cheers as we reached our milestones, even when the significant time devoted to the book often meant time away from them. Our deepest acknowledgements and appreciation go to our families, particularly Brian, Liam, and Ella Eaton and Jeff West. They have been our strongest advocates, most loyal supporters and trusted confidantes. Their love and commitment have sustained us and made this journey possible. For that and so much more, we are eternally grateful.

About the Contributors

Christine Allen, Ph.D., has an MA in the theory and practice of human rights and a Ph.D. in sociology, both from the University of Essex. She has taught ethnography and qualitative research methods at Simon Fraser University and in the sociology department at DePaul University. Her work appears in *Open Fire: Understanding Global Gun Cultures* (Berg Press), based on her ethnography of the gun rights movement in the United States.

Solomon R. Benatar, M.B.Ch.B., DSc (Med) was head of the Department of Medicine at the University of Cape Town and Chief Physician at Groote Schuur Hospital from 1980–1999, and founding director of the University of Cape Town's Centre for Bioethics (1992–2012). Dr Benatar has served as the international member of the CIHR's Standing Committee on Ethics (2007–2013), an ethics advisor to several national and international HIV/AIDS organizations and was president of the International Association of Bioethics from 2001–2003. He has taught research ethics for many years in Fogarty Center International-funded programs at the Joint Centre for Bioethics, University of Toronto and at the University of Cape Town.

Donald Cole, MD, M.Sc., is Associate Professor at the Dalla Lana School of Public Health, University of Toronto. Trained as a physician

(1978), he has practised primary care, public health, occupational health, and environmental health in Canada and in lower- and middle-income countries. A Tri-Council Eco-Research fellowship in environmental epidemiology (1993–1997) led to research on environmental contaminants, ecosystems, nutrition, agriculture, and human health. At the University of Toronto (2001), he has taught epidemiology and research methods, supervised masters and doctoral students, and started the Collaborative Ph.D. Program in Global Health (2008, Founding Director). He enjoys writing with colleagues and students, and has written over 170 peer reviewed papers, 37 book chapters, and one edited book.

Fernando De Maio, Ph.D., Associate Professor in the Department of Sociology, DePaul University. He obtained his Ph.D. in sociology from the University of Essex and is the author of two books: *Health & Social Theory* (2010) and *Global Health Inequities* (forthcoming), both published with Palgrave Macmillan. His work has also appeared in a wide range of academic journals, including *Journal of Epidemiology and Community Health, Global Public Health, Critical Public Health,* and *Salud Colectiva.*

Maureen Dobbins, RN, Ph.D., is Professor in the School of Nursing at McMaster University. Her research efforts seek to understand knowledge translation among public health decision makers in Canada. Since 2001, she has been the Director of Health Evidence (www.health-evidence.ca), a single source of high quality effectiveness evidence and one component of a comprehensive knowledge translation strategy for public health decision makers worldwide. On January 1, 2012, she also assumed the role of Scientific Director for the National Collaborating Centre Methods and Tools, one of six National Collaborating Centres for Public Health in Canada.

Jean Dumais, M.Sc., is chief of the Statistical Consultation Group and a survey methodologist at Statistics Canada. Upon completion of his M.Sc. from Université du Québec à Montréal in 1982, he joined Statistics Canada where he has worked on census, business (agriculture, transportation, prices), and social (education, health) surveys, mixing applied work and teaching.

Elliot Goldner, MD, M.H.Sc., FRCPC, is Professor in the Faculty of Health Sciences at Simon Fraser University and a fully qualified psychiatrist with specific expertise in health services and health policy. He founded the Centre for Applied Research in Mental Health & Addiction (CARMHA), a research unit designed to provide research support to government ministries, health authorities, and community agencies in their efforts to advance the quality of mental health and addiction services. He has authored more than 100 peer-reviewed publications and various government reports and studies, and is lead author of a textbook on mental health in Canada. He has served as the Chair of the Scientific Advisory Committee of the Mental Health Commission of Canada and Scientific Lead of the Knowledge Exchange Centre.

Charles Goldsmith, Ph.D., is a biostatistician with interests in evaluating therapies for musculoskeletal conditions. He currently holds an endowed Chair in Statistics for Arthritis and Musculoskeletal Conditions at the Arthritis Research Centre of Canada and is Professor in the Faculty of Health Sciences at Simon Fraser University. He is also Professor Emeritus of Biostatistics in the Department of Clinical Epidemiology & Biostatistics at McMaster University. He has published over 290 articles and 320 abstracts, is a member of several editorial boards of health related journals, and has interests in quality improvement, experimental design, study design, and analysis.

Rachelle Hole, Ph.D., is Associate Professor at the University of British Columbia (UBC), Okanagan, School of Social Work. Her research has focused on the areas of intellectual disabilities and critical disability studies. She currently serves as co-Director of the Centre for Inclusion and Citizenship (CIC), a partnership between UBC's School of Social Work and the community living sector (self-advocates, families, organizations) that seeks to further the inclusion and full citizenship of individuals with intellectual disabilities and their families locally, nationally, and globally through learning, research, and knowledge exchange.

Dario Kuzmanović is a research ethics manager at the Office of Research Ethics at the University of Toronto. He manages a unique, community-based HIV/AIDS research ethics board. He has an undergraduate degree from Western University and a graduate degree in Bioethics from U of T's Joint Centre for Bioethics. In 2011 he was awarded the Universities Without Walls Fellowship and in 2012 he received the CIHR-Social Research Centre's Fellowship for HIV research.

Renee MacPhee, Ph.D., is Assistant Professor in the Department of Kinesiology and Physical Education with a cross-appointment in the newly founded Health Sciences Program, both at Wilfrid Laurier University. Renee received her undergraduate degree in psychology from Carleton University, and her graduate and post-graduate degrees in health and gerontology from the University of Waterloo. Her research interests focus on health and wellness in the field of Emergency Medical Services, with a specific emphasis on physical injury, physical demands analyses, and the development of bona fide occupational requirements for paramedics.

Jennifer Robertson-Wilson, Ph.D., is Associate Professor in the Department of Kinesiology and Physical Education at Wilfrid Laurier University where she regularly teaches a second-year undergraduate course introducing research methods. Jennifer's research focuses on the implementation and evaluation of school-based physical activity policies. She also has an interest in how the built environment affects physical activity and behaviour.

David L. Streiner, Ph.D., C. Psych., is a clinical psychologist by training. He currently serves as Professor of psychiatry at the University of Toronto and Professor Emeritus in the Department of Clinical Epidemiology & Biostatistics and in the Department of Psychiatry & Behavioural Neurosciences, both at McMaster University. He is the senior scientific editor of *Health Reports*, and he sits on the editorial boards of four other journals. He has written and edited nine books in the areas of statistics, epidemiology, public health, and measurement theory, and has published over 350 articles in these and other areas.

Martin Tammemägi, DVM, Ph.D., is a professor in applied health sciences in the Department of Community Health Sciences at Brock University. After completing his DVM from the University of Guelph, Dr Tammemägi practised veterinary medicine for several years before he returned to the University of Toronto to supplement his training in epidemiology. Upon completion of his Ph.D., he served as the senior epidemiologist at the Henry Ford Health System in Detroit, Michigan for seven years before joining the Department of Community Health Sciences at Brock University in 2005. His research interests revolve around cancer epidemiology, lung cancer screening, and cancer risk prediction modelling.

About the Editors

Kate Bassil, Ph.D., is a manager in the Healthy Public Policy Directorate at Toronto Public Health and Assistant Professor at the Dalla Lana School of Public Health at the University of Toronto. Prior to this she was an epidemiologist in the Maternal-Infant Care Research Centre at Mount Sinai Hospital and before then, Assistant Professor in the Faculty of Health Sciences at Simon Fraser University, where she taught an introductory course in health research methods. She holds a Ph.D. in epidemiology from the Dalla Lana School of Public Health at the University of Toronto. Her areas of expertise include geospatial applications to public health issues, and the health impacts associated with climate change, particularly those due to extreme heat. She also co-led the development of the *Canadian Environmental Health Atlas,* an online resource for researchers and practitioners that illustrates the many ways the environment affects human health.

Denise Zabkiewicz, Ph.D., is Assistant Professor in the Faculty of Health Sciences at Simon Fraser University. She obtained her Ph.D. in epidemiology from the University of California, Berkeley. During the last decade, she has acquired considerable experience conducting longitudinal mixed methods research and data analyses examining issues surrounding employment, homelessness, welfare receipt, and substance abuse and mental health problems. While her areas of expertise include mental health and substance abuse epidemiology, and welfare and employment policy, her long term research interests include the investigation of policy, economic and social factors that influence the public health of disadvantaged populations in the community. She currently serves as a co-investigator on the Vancouver research team for the Mental Health Commission of Canada's Demonstration Project examining issues of homelessness among individuals with serious mental illness.

1 Introduction

Kate Bassil and Denise Zabkiewicz

CHAPTER OUTLINE

Defining Health Research

The purpose of this book is to provide a comprehensive introduction to health research methods. While there is no universal definition of "health" it is important to consider the meaning of this term before embarking on a more detailed discussion of the various methods that can be used to improve our understanding of human health. Perhaps the most famous and enduring definition of health is the one proposed by the World Health Organization in 1948 (WHO, 1948):

> Health is a state of complete physical, mental and social well-being and not merely the absence of disease or infirmity.

This definition is one of the most commonly used and cited, and is appealing as it speaks to the breadth of health beyond the physical sense, incorporating mental and social domains. However, it has received some criticism because of the difficulty in defining "well-being" and because it includes the concept of "complete," which makes it highly unlikely that anyone would be healthy for a reasonable period of time (Huber, 2011). Additionally, it speaks to health as a state of being, rather than recognizing it as a capacity or resource. Health is also intimately tied to personal circumstances that, in turn, are tied to social, cultural, economic, and environmental influences (Frankish, 1999). A more holistic definition of health that speaks to this concept is "the capacity of people to adapt to, respond to, or control life's challenges and changes" (Frankish et al., 1996). The WHO definition has since been updated to incorporate these kinds of concepts (WHO, 1984):

> . . . the extent to which an individual or group is able to realize aspirations and satisfy needs, and to change or cope with the environment. Health is a resource for everyday life, not the objective of living; it is a positive concept, emphasizing social and personal resources, as well as physical capacities.

This broad perspective of health is one that is used throughout this text, which takes a multidisciplinary approach to research methods.

The notion of "health research" can generally be thought of as any research that is relevant to health and incorporates a diverse number of methodologies. Research describes the systematic process of enquiry that aims to generate new scientific knowledge. The spectrum of health research is very broad. The Canadian Institute of Health Research (CIHR), the major federal agency responsible for funding health research in Canada, categorizes health research into four main themes that they refer to as the "four pillars of health research" (CIHR, 2007):

- biomedical research (investigating mechanisms of health or disease at the cellular, body system, or whole body level);
- clinical research (on, or for, patients, and includes diagnosis and intervention);
- health services and policy research (investigating health services themselves, how they are delivered, quality and costs, and how they are received), and
- social, cultural, environmental, and population health research (investigating populations and broader health determinants).

Clearly there are thousands of different health topics that fall into each of these themes. This text will illustrate how research methods can be applied to advance our understanding and generate new knowledge about human health.

The Purpose of Health Research

Research is a central component of improving health. There is a constant and ongoing need to generate new knowledge about health so that this information can be translated into effective actions that will ultimately improve the health of individuals.

There are several purposes of health research. Young (2004) describes four main categories: to describe, to explain, to predict, and to control. For example, some research aims to describe the state of health of a population, the incidence of a disease, the ways a disease manifests, and its signs and symptoms. This kind of research may make comparisons between people or groups to illustrate differences in health. There are numerous examples of this kind of health research; in reviewing recent issues of the *Canadian Journal of Public Health* we found several. For example, one study describes the rate of influenza vaccination uptake in pregnant women during the 2009 H1N1 pandemic (Liu, 2012). The vaccination rate for influenza in pregnant women is typically low. However, health authorities are encouraging pregnant women to get the vaccine and during the 2009 H1N1 influenza pandemic, pregnant women were identified as a priority group. This study described the vaccination rate of pregnant women in Ontario during this time and found that only 43 per cent received the vaccine. Women of younger age, lower socioeconomic status, those without an antenatal provider, and who smoked during pregnancy were less likely to receive the vaccine than other women in the study. By describing this population, the study identified a prenatal population that may benefit from targeted public health interventions to improve vaccination rates and prevent influenza.

Many health researchers aim to explain why a certain health problem occurs, and the differences among sub-populations of interest. A common research design that is used for this purpose is a cohort study, where a group of people are followed over a period of time with repeated monitoring of the health risks and outcomes of interest (this design is described in more detail in Chapter 6). There are several examples of this in the Canadian health research community. The Canadian Longitudinal Study on Aging is a large, national, long-term study that is following approximately 50,000 Canadian men and women between the ages of 45 and 85 for a period of at least 20 years to help improve our understanding of the aging process. A second example is the Ontario Health Study that aims to understand risk factors for a number of diseases including cancer, diabetes, heart disease, asthma, depression, and Alzheimer's. Nearly a quarter of a million adults in Ontario have been recruited to participate in this study that includes a combination of questionnaire and physical data collection methods. There are also Canadian cohort studies that focus on specific populations. The Maternal-Infant Research on Environmental Chemicals (MIREC) is a national five-year study that has recruited 2000 women during their first trimester of pregnancy to assess the health risks associated with exposure to various environmental chemicals, especially lead and mercury. All of these cohort studies aim to improve our understanding of the etiology of different diseases so that interventions can be designed and implemented to reduce their effects. This leads to the next purpose of health research—prediction and control.

Prediction and control speak to using the findings from research that describe and explain health phenomena to research that develops and evaluates strategies that mitigate these health problems. These may be clinical or public health interventions, but health research evidence can also offer a range of findings that inform the development of effective services and policy responses that seek to improve health outcomes.

Health services research seeks to measure and improve the safety, quality, accessibility, affordability, and organization of health care services, and the outcomes of health services for individuals and populations. In 2002, the professional organization for the field of health services research, AcademyHealth, described the scope of health services research as:

> . . . the multidisciplinary field of scientific investigation that studies how social factors, financing systems, organizational structures and processes, health technologies, and personal behaviors affect access to health care, the quality and cost of health care, and ultimately our health and well-being. Its research domains are individuals, families, organizations, institutions, communities, and populations (Lohr and Steinwachs, 2002).

Within this scope, health services research not only examines services as they relate to the health and well-being of individuals and the population, but also the process of care and the interactions of patients and providers as well as new diagnostic and treatment technologies, their impact on patient outcomes and health care costs. The At Home/Chez Soi study is a recent four-year project in five Canadian cities that provides an illustrative example of the broad scope of health services research. Funded by the government of Canada, the At Home/Chez Soi study has sought to not only identify the best housing and support services for individuals who are homeless and living with mental illness, but to better understand the costs associated with those services. (See Health Research in Action box 1.1 for more details.) Health services research is thus fundamental to the information government officials, insurers, providers, consumers, and others making decisions about health-related issues attend to (Steinwachs and Hughes, 2008).

With regard to the role and influence of health research on the development of public health policy, another illustrative example is presented in

1.1   Health Research in Action

The At Home/Chez Soi Project: Homelessness and Mental Health

(Goering et al., 2011; Zabkiewicz et al., 2012)

Over the past 30 years, a steady increase in the rate of homelessness has been documented and consequently, homelessness has become a major health and social problem across Canada. This increase has been accompanied by a more diverse homeless population, including a large and rapidly rising number of families, youth, and Aboriginal individuals, as well as disproportionately high rates of mental health problems. These trends have coincided with the deinstitutionalization of long stay psychiatric institutions, have been accompanied by reductions in government-supported health and social services, and have contributed to circumstances where many individuals with serious mental illness do not receive the health and social services they need to function adequately in the community. As a result, in many cities across Canada there has been a significant increase in the number of individuals with serious mental illness that are

inadequately housed and underserved by the current system.

In an effort to address these issues, Canada's federal government allocated CAD 110 million to the Mental Health Commission of Canada (MHCC) to conduct a national demonstration project to identify the best housing and support services for individuals who are homeless and living with mental illness. The project, entitled "At Home/Chez Soi," was conducted in five sites across Canada including: Moncton, Montreal, Toronto, Vancouver, and Winnipeg. While the five sites share a common underlying study design, each site had the option to incorporate an additional intervention arm that would best address the unique characteristics of their local context. Growing evidence indicates that patterns of social, health, and substance use characteristics among disadvantaged populations vary considerably across urban locations in Canada. This geographic variation in housing and health problems highlights the importance of considering the local context.

The At Home/Chez Soi study, the largest demonstration project of its kind in the world, was launched in November 2009, and is a four-

the research surrounding tobacco control policy (see Health Research in Action box 1.2). While the importance of policy development based on research evidence is recognized (Global Forum for Health Research, 2002), the existence of research alone is not sufficient to achieve evidence-based policy. Further, it is widely agreed that health policies do not reflect the extent of the evidence (Babor et al., 2010; COHRED, 2000; Lavis et al., 2002). These findings point to significant obstacles in the evidence-based policy-making process.

The wide range of health research and the various policy levels at which the research findings could be applied are two important factors that contribute to research utilization (Hanney et al.,

2003). Given the diversity in types of research (e.g., basic, clinical, applied) and the multiple levels of policy-making (e.g., governance, service, and practice), the uptake of research findings by policy-makers needs to be understood within a context that also includes the diverse values and philosophies of knowledge production as well as the practical considerations surrounding policy-making. In light of these issues, the evidence-based policy literature speaks to the importance of collaboration between policy-makers and researchers not only as it relates to setting priorities, but also in increasing the likelihood that the research will be noticed and utilized (Davis and Howden-Chapman, 1996).

year randomized controlled trial designed to provide evidence about what service and system interventions achieve improved housing stability, health, and well-being for the target population of adults who are homeless and mentally ill. The study draws from a Housing First model that takes into account individual needs and choices. Participants are first provided with a place to live and are then assisted in community integration through the provision of client-centred services. Unlike other programs, the Housing First model does not require sobriety or active treatment services as a condition for participation.

The study design was structured to assess the effectiveness of different models of care based on the participants' level of need. Individuals identified with high levels of need were randomized to either treatment as usual or to housing and support interventions: Housing First with Assertive Community Treatment (ACT). Individuals identified with moderate levels of need were randomized to treatment as usual or to Housing First with Intensive Case Management (ICM). Given that the interventions were selected to meet the needs of individuals within each need level, ACT was not compared directly with

ICM. Outcomes were assessed through direct comparison of the two high needs interventions and through a separate comparison involving the two moderate needs interventions.

Over 2000 homeless people participated across the country. Approximately half of them received housing and support services, and approximately half had access to the regular support and services available in their communities.

Given high rates of mental illness among homeless individuals, there is a growing need for effective approaches that integrate housing with intensive treatment and support. Obtaining a better understanding of how supported housing and services influence the health and well-being of homeless individuals is critical for the development of long-term, community-based solutions, and effective health and social policy. The At Home/Chez Soi study's randomized trial design is the gold standard approach for evaluation of service provider interventions and provides a powerful opportunity to help policy-makers better understand what needs to be done to solve chronic homelessness in Canada for people who experience mental illness.

1.2   Health Research in Action

Tobacco Control Policy

In the early 1950s, British researchers Doll and Hill published results from several studies that implicated the use of tobacco as a major risk factor for disease. In particular, they found that the risk of lung cancer was greatly increased among smokers relative to the risk among comparable non-smokers. By the early 1960s, both the UK Royal College of Physicians and the US Surgeon General had published authoritative reviews of the scientific evidence identifying smoking as a cause of lung cancer. A central factor in the evidence was the remarkably consistent findings across other epidemiologic research conducted

in the UK, the US, and Canada. The evidence was strong and clear.

Over the following decades, tobacco control policies have been implemented in Canada at the federal, provincial, and municipal levels with the aim to protect Canadians from the health risks associated with tobacco use. Regulations surrounding the production, taxation, pricing, labeling, and marketing of tobacco-based products have been implemented as have smoke-free regulations in a variety of settings, including workplaces, bars, and restaurants. Policies such as these, along with health education, have contributed to a dramatic decrease in the prevalence of smoking- and tobacco-related morbidity and mortality.

To summarize, health research is a tool for generating knowledge for education, disease prevention, and practice and policy development, as outlined in the examples above. There is often overlap between the various purposes discussed, however the overall purpose is the same—to improve health.

Health Research Milestones in Canada

There are numerous examples of how research has affected our health positively over the last several decades. Recognizing some of the groundbreaking and key health research that has been conducted in Canada is one of the important aims of this text. In addition to the many examples of Canadian studies that can be found throughout the chapters, the current section will showcase some Canadian health research milestones. While there are far too many to describe in detail, we have hand-picked a few examples from a variety of fields to show the breadth and diversity of Canadian health research.

Canadian scientists have made major contributions to gene discovery and genetic research that are related to hundreds of diseases including muscular dystrophy, dyslexia, Huntington's disease, Alzheimer's disease, breast cancer, and epilepsy. However, one of the most famous is the discovery of the gene for cystic fibrosis in 1989 by Drs. Lap-Chee Tsui, Manual Buchwald, and Jack Riordan at the Hospital for Sick Children in Toronto, Ontario. Cystic fibrosis is an inherited disease that mainly affects the lungs and the digestive system where mucus builds up, making it difficult to digest and absorb nutrients, and also causes severe respiratory problems. There is no known cure and ultimately most cystic fibrosis-related deaths are due to lung disease. Dr. Tsui and colleagues identified the defective gene that causes this disease, the cystic fibrosis transmembrane conductance regulator (Kerem

et al., 1989, Riordan et al., 1989, Rommens et al., 1989). The discovery of this gene has improved our understanding of how cystic fibrosis develops and manifests, and led to newborn screening for early detection, and new research targeting the root cause of the disease in hopes of finding more effective therapies.

There has also been landmark Canadian health research in disease prevention. An example of this is the development of vaccines. One of the most famous vaccine success stories is of the polio vaccine, where Canadian researchers played a pivotal role in its development. Polio, or poliomyelitis, is a disease that damages the nerve cells in the spinal cord and can lead to paralysis, deformed limbs, and death by asphyxiation. In 1952, Dr. Jonas Salk and his research team at the University of Pittsburgh developed a polio vaccine, however they had no way of producing the vaccine or developing a large study to assess its effectiveness. Researchers at the Connaught Medical Research Laboratories at the University of Toronto helped to further cultivate the polio vaccine. In particular, Dr. Leone Farrell developed the "Toronto technique" to cultivate bulk quantities which ultimately made it possible to conduct a large field study of the polio vaccine (Barreto, 2006). The Salk field trial took place in 1954 and was the largest medical experiment ever conducted, with nearly two million children in Canada, Finland, and the United States receiving the vaccine. Following the positive study findings that the vaccine was deemed to be effective, it continued to be manufactured and distributed by the Connaught Laboratories. Since the introduction of the vaccine polio has been eradicated from most parts of the world.

Other contributions in health research have focused on the treatment of disease. The discovery and production of insulin was a breakthrough development for the treatment of diabetes mellitus. Type 1 diabetes mellitus is a disease that can occur at most any age. However, it is most frequently diagnosed among children and adolescents. It is a condition that has been known to physicians since ancient times although it wasn't until the early part of the twentieth century that a treatment was found. Prior to the discovery of

insulin, type 1 diabetes was uniformly fatal and it was only with careful attention to diet, essentially a highly restricted starvation diet, that individuals with diabetes could expect to survive several years beyond the onset of disease before their inevitable death due to starvation, ketoacidosis,

1.3   Health Research in Action

The Discovery of Insulin

The story of the discovery of insulin begins in the early 1920s with Frederick Banting, a physician from London, Ontario. While preparing for a lecture at the University of Western Ontario, Banting came across a manuscript that inspired an idea that the ligation of the pancreatic duct would allow the internal secretion of the pancreas to be isolated without contamination from digestive enzymes. He shared this idea with a colleague at the University of Western Ontario and was referred to J.J.R. Macleod, a professor of physiology at the University of Toronto and a highly recognized authority on carbohydrate metabolism with a first-rate laboratory. Macleod was skeptical of Banting's idea. However, prior to departing for the summer, Macleod assisted Banting by providing him with laboratory space and introducing him to Charles Best, a physiology student who went on to become Banting's assistant, and J. Bertram Collip, a professor of physiology at the University of Alberta and an expert in tissue extraction.

Banting and Best began their research during the summer of 1921 with experiments on dogs. By the fall, they had isolated material from pancreatic extracts that dramatically prolonged the lives of diabetic dogs. On January 11, 1922, less than one year after the start of their research, they treated their first human patient, 14-year-old Leonard Thompson. While Thompson's blood sugar fell, he developed sterile abscesses at the site of the injection caused by the impurities in the extract. The trial was considered a failure. Shortly thereafter, Collip announced that he had identified a procedure to produce a purified

extract. Less than two weeks after the first trial, treatment of Leonard Thompson resumed with a purified extract called insulin. This preparation showed immediate and remarkable results with a significant drop in blood sugars and no toxic side effects. Further, with daily injections, acetone bodies disappeared from Thompson's urine and he felt better, looked better, and became more active. Six more patients were treated in February followed by a series of studies establishing guidelines for clinical use. By 1923, insulin was available in sufficient quantities for widespread distribution and treatment of diabetes.

While the success of the project was remarkable, it was not without elements of jealousy and contentiousness. In 1923, the Nobel Prize in Physiology or Medicine was awarded to Banting and Macleod, aggravating the already antagonistic relationship that had developed during the course of the research. Banting was angered by the omission of Best. There was also a perception that Macleod did not deserve to receive the prize as it was felt that he had done little during the early stages of the work. Thus, Banting not only publicly acknowledged Best's contribution, but announced that he would share his prize with Best. Macleod followed by sharing his prize with Collip in recognition of Collip's contributions. Years later, the Nobel Committee acknowledged that Best should have been awarded a share of the prize (Rosenfeld, 2002).

Despite the professional rivalry, all four investigators made significant contributions to the discovery of insulin. For a more detailed history of the discovery of insulin, see *The Discovery of Insulin* by Bliss (1982).

or infection. The discovery of insulin has been hailed as one of the most important advances in modern medicine. Further, not only was insulin discovered, but it was put into mass production in a very short time period, thereby rescuing starved young people, waiting at death's door (Roth et al., 2012). (See Health Research in Action box 1.3, for more details.)

The implementation of public health policies to reduce the incidence of disease is another important contribution resulting from Canadian health research. A good example of this is the addition of Vitamin D to milk to reduce the incidence of rickets, a childhood bone disorder where bones are prone to deformity and fracture. Dr. Charles Scriver, a physician and researcher at the Montreal Children's Hospital, realized that there was an important link between rickets and vitamin D deficiency through his research in the early 1960s. He successfully lobbied the government to add Vitamin D to all milk sold in Quebec and the incidence of rickets dropped dramatically from one in 200 newborns to one in 20,000. Vitamin D is now added to all milk products in Canada.

About This Textbook

Background

The idea for writing this textbook began in the classroom during our own teaching experiences in research methods at Simon Fraser University. Despite the need and demand for training in research methods, we found there was not a comprehensive introductory methods text that highlights Canadian health research. The purpose of this book is to provide the reader with substantive and fundamental knowledge of health sciences research methodology while showcasing examples from the Canadian context.

Who is This Book Written For?

This book is targeted at university students who are in the very early stages of their training in research methods. It has been written at an introductory level and does not require any prior knowledge of research methodology. Further, it is intended to be applicable to several health disciplines including nursing, epidemiology, psychology, kinesiology, nutrition, public health, social work, and physiology, among others.

Structure of the Book

As an edited collection with a consistent format, the book has the advantage of drawing on a range of contributions from leading experts in the field. The book is divided into 12 chapters that cover specific research methods topics.

Chapter 2 introduces the paradigms of health research that "frame" research in terms of the knowledge used and methods applied. Paradigms are the sets of beliefs and practices that guide the research process and therefore comprise a fundamental component to the discussion throughout the text. Each paradigm directs the research that is conducted in terms of guiding what questions should be asked, how they should be structured, and what methods are most appropriate for conducting the research. Various paradigms are described, compared, and contrasted in this chapter.

Chapter 3 is designed to guide the reader through the cycle of the research process starting with how to identify a health problem and develop a research question all the way through the various steps in research enquiry to generate new findings and new questions so the process begins again. Subsequent chapters link back to these stages of research. This chapter also highlights the important role of the researcher throughout the research process.

Chapter 4 examines the methods for conducting a literature review—one of the first key steps in the research process. The reader may have to conduct a literature review for a major paper in order to gain a more detailed understanding of the topic. A literature review gives an overview of the research field that is being pursued, describes the questions that are being asked and their findings, and highlights the gaps in knowledge that warrant further exploration. Literature reviews are not only important research tools that provide the researcher with an idea of where their research fits into the "bigger picture" of health research, but they also provide a rationale for pursuit of the research question of interest.

Chapter 5 explores the ways ethical issues impact health research, in particular, the moral conflicts that may arise throughout the research process. This chapter reviews the principles that are involved and how to apply the conceptual principles in practice. One example of this is a detailed discussion of the role and process of applying for ethical approval to a research ethics board. The chapter highlights general guidelines for conducting ethical health research, in particular those that are outlined in the Tri-Council Policy Statement, which is central to any research involving humans in Canada.

Chapter 6 presents the various study designs used in health research. Each design represents a different way of answering a health research question. There can often be more than one design that can be used to answer the same research question so the researcher has to make a decision about which is the most appropriate to use; familiarity with each of the study designs is necessary to make these kinds of decisions. It is also important to understand the different study designs as a consumer of research in order to understand how the research has been done and to critically evaluate the quality of the research. This chapter summarizes the relative advantages and limitations of conventional

study designs including randomized controlled trials, cohort studies, cross-sectional studies, case-control studies, and ecological designs.

Chapter 7 considers measurement—how we assign numbers to phenomena. Measurement allows a researcher to quantify a variable of interest, however, not all variables can be measured in the same way. This chapter outlines the various levels of measurement and how they apply to different types of variables. It explains the step-by-step process of scale development and highlights three key features of scales: reliability, validity, and feasibility.

Chapter 8 covers sampling issues—how to select a sample and the factors to consider when determining which sampling design is appropriate for a specific study. The focus of the chapter is on the application of sampling to survey design, a very common design used in health research. As it is usually impractical for researchers to collect data from every person in the population of interest being studied, sampling is a key method to identify a subset of individuals (i.e., the sample) to collect data from. If the sample is selected carefully, the results will reflect what would have been collected if data were captured from every member of the study population so the researcher can then draw inferences about the study population from this group.

Chapter 9 is concerned with qualitative methods, which include a wide range of various methodologies that aim to more deeply explore and understand health issues. Qualitative health research often seeks to understand how or why a particular phenomenon occurs, and these methods are commonly used on their own for a research study or in conjunction with some of the quantitative methods discussed in the text. This chapter outlines the main approaches used when conducting qualitative research, application of theory to these methods, and core aspects of qualitative research design such as data collection, interpretation, and analysis.

Chapter 10 builds on the discussion of measurement presented in Chapter 7 to illustrate various measures of frequency, effect, and outcome. For health research we are typically interested in these three main categories of measurement and the most fundamental types of these are presented in this chapter. The chapter explains each measure and then provides an explanation of how they can be calculated. This is a particularly useful reference for students, who are often asked to compare and contrast various measures in addition to conducting basic calculations of these measures.

Once you have collected data in a research study, you need to start analyzing that data. Chapter 11 describes the statistical methods commonly used in health research. It provides a discussion of how the types of data collected relate to the appropriate choice of analysis. Important formulas are presented and explained, but the focus of the chapter is on illustrating the underlying concepts and principles for the key statistical approaches.

Chapter 12 is designed to explain the process of writing and reporting the findings of research studies. The approach used varies according to the audience and purpose of the report; this chapter addresses how to develop a research report for these different purposes.

Lastly, Chapter 13 presents knowledge translation (KT)—how to translate the knowledge generated by health research into action so that the findings impact positively on health. The chapter describes the various theoretical foundations of KT, illustrates how KT methods can be applied to research, and how the field of KT can be advanced through these methods.

With this text, we have attempted to present an introduction to health research methods in as clear and concise a manner as possible. Given the spectrum of health research, the breadth of applications that health research can address, as well as the various stakeholders that not only utilize health research methods but utilize health research findings for purposes of improving the health of individuals and the population, we have sought a balanced perspective drawn from a wide range of colleagues across a multitude of complementary backgrounds and experiences. We have chosen as best as possible illustrations of historical and current public health importance, and have tried to achieve a balance between explanations of the methods and their application. Also, we recognize that as an introductory text it is not possible to address all of the nuances and complexities that health research methods entail. With this in mind, each chapter identifies resources for more advanced learning.

References

Babor, T., Caulkins, J., Edwards, G., Fischer, B., et al. (2010) *Drug Policy and the Public Good.* Oxford: Oxford University Press, 2010.

Barreto, L., Van Exan, R., and Rutty, C.J. (2006) Polio vaccine development in Canada: Contributions to global polio eradication. *Biologicals, 34,* 91–101.

Bliss, M. (1982) *The Discovery of Insulin.* Chicago, IL, USA: The University of Chicago Press.

COHRED Working Group on Research to Action and Policy. (2000) *Lessons in Research to Action and Policy—Case Studies from Seven Countries.* Geneva, The Council on Health Research for Development.

Dahlgreen, G. and Whitehead, M. (2006) *European Strategies for Tackling Social Inequities in Health: Levelling Up Part 2.* Copenhagen, Denmark:World Health Organization.

Davis, P. and Howden-Chapman, P. (1996) Translating research findings into health policy. *Social Science and Medicine, 43*(5), 865–72.

Frankish, C.J., et al. (1996) *Health Impact Assessment as a Tool for Population Health Promotion and Public Policy.* Vancouver: Institute of Health Promotion Research, University of British Columbia.

Frankish, J., Veenstra, G., and Moulton, G. (1999) Population health in Canada: Issues and challenges for policy, practice, and research. *Canadian Journal of Public Health, 90*(Suppl 1), S71–S75.

Global Forum for Health Research. (2002) *The 10/90 Report on Health Research 2001–2002.* Geneva: World Health Organization.

Goering, P.N., Streiner, D.L., Adair, C., Aubry, T., Barker, J., Distasio, J., Hwang, S.W., Komaroff, J., Latimer, E., Somers, J., and Zabkiewicz, D.M. (2011) The At Home/Chez Soi trial protocol: A pragmatic, multi-site, randomised controlled trial of a Housing First intervention for homeless individuals with mental illness in five Canadian cities. *British Medical Journal Open, 1*(2), e000323, doi:10.1136/bmjopen-2011-000323.

Hanney, S. R., Gonzalez-Block, M.A., Buxton, M.J., and Kogan, M. (2003) The utilisation of health research in policy-making: Concepts, examples, and methods of assessment. *Health Research Policy and Systems, I*, 2.

Huber, M., Knottnerus, J.A., Green, L., et al. (2011) How should we define health? *British Medical Journal, 343*, d4163.

Kerem, B., Rommens, J.M., Buchanan, J.A., Markiewicz, D., Cox, T.K., Chakravarti, A., Buchwald, M., and Tsui, L.C. (1989) Identification of the cystic fibrosis gene: Genetic analysis. *Science, 245*, 1073–80.

Lavis, J.N., Ross, S.E., Hurley, J. E., Hohenandel, J.M., Stoddart, G.L., Woodard, C.A. and Abelson, J. (2002) Examining the role of health services research in public policy-making. *Milbank Quarterly, 80*, 125–54.

Liu, N., Sprague, A.E., Yasseen, A.S., Fell, D.B., Wen, S.W., Smith, G.N., and Walker, M.C. Vaccination patterns in pregnant women during the 2009 H1N1 influenza pandemic: A population-based study in Ontario, Canada. *Canadian Journal of Public Health, 103*(5), 353–8.

Lohr, K.N. and Steinwachs, D.M. (2002) Health services research: an evolving definition of the field. *Health Services Research, 37*(1), 15–17.

Riordan, J.R., Rommens, J. Kerem, B., Alon, N., Rozmahel, R., Grzelczak, Z., Zielenski, J., Lok, S., Plavsic, N., Chou, J.L., et al. (1989) Identification of the cystic fibrosis gene: Cloning and characterization of complementary DNA. *Science, 245*, 1066–73.

Rommens, J.M., Iannuzzi, M.C., Kerem, B., Drumm, M.L., Melmer, G., Dean, M., Rozmahel, R., Cole, J.L., Kennedy, D., Hidaka, N., et al. (1989) Identification of the cystic fibrosis gene: Chromosome walking and jumping. *Science, 245*, 1059–65.

Rosenfeld, L. (2002) Insulin: Discovery and controversy. *Clinical Chemistry, 48*(12), 2270–88.

Roth, J., Qureshi, S., Whitford, I., Vranic, M., Kahn, C.R., Fantus, I.G., and Dirks, J.H. (2012) Insulin's discovery: New insights on its ninetieth birthday. *Diabetes/Metabolism Research and Reviews. 28*, 293–304.

Steinwachs, D.M. and Hughes, R.G. (2008) Health Services Research: Scope and Significance. Ch. 8. In Hughes, R.G. (Ed.) *Patient Safety and Quality: An Evidence-Based Handbook for Nurses.* Rockville, MD: Agency for Healthcare Research and Quality (US).

World Health Organization (WHO) (1946) Pre-amble to the Constitution of the World Health Organization as adopted by the International Health Conference, New York, 19–22 June 1946, and entered into force on 7 April 1948. Copenhagen, Denmark: World Health Organization.

World Health Organization (WHO) (1984) Health promotion: A discussion document. Copen-hagen, Denmark: World Health Organization.

Zabkiewicz, D., Patterson, M., Frankish, J., Som-ers, J. (2012) The Vancouver At Home Study: Overview and methods of a housing first trial among individuals who are home-less and living with mental illness. *Journal of Clinical Trials, 2*:123. doi:10.4172/2167-0870.1000123.

2 Research Paradigms

Fernando De Maio and Christine Allen

CHAPTER OUTLINE

Introduction

People come to health research from many perspectives. For example, you may be interested in understanding how the health of immigrants changes after settling in Canada. Given that most immigrants experience a better health care system in this country than they did in their country of origin, you might expect that their health improves after settling in the country. Yet empirical research suggests otherwise—and the health of immigrants is thought to deteriorate with time in Canada (Beiser, 2005; De Maio, 2010a). Why does this occur? Are some immigrants more likely than others to experience this worsening of their health? Is this an inequity—an inequality that is avoidable, unnecessary, and unfair? What kinds of public policy are in place or need to be developed to best support the health of immigrants? Researchers working on these questions draw on a variety of research methods, often analyzing large-scale datasets such as the *Canadian Community Health Survey* and the *Longitudinal Study of Immigrants to Canada*, and sometimes carrying out interviews with immigrants and health-care professionals.

Or you may be interested in the very real problems with the health of Aboriginal peoples in Canada. Researchers in this area have engaged with intricate questions of historical trauma, colonialism, cultural assimilation, exploitation, and marginalization—historical and political processes that have led Canada's Aboriginal peoples to experience poor levels of health otherwise unheard of in industrialized countries (Gibson et al., 2005; Samson, 2003). Some of this research involves surveys and statistical analysis—with tools like the *Aboriginal Peoples Survey*. Other researchers have advocated the generation of first-hand knowledge, calling for researchers to spend extended periods of time living with and working with Aboriginal communities. Studies using participant observation may call for prolonged immersion in a culture, often requiring researchers to grapple with the emotions and complex personal ties that challenge the traditional image of a researcher as a detached and "objective" observer.

Or you may be interested in understanding the general pattern of social inequalities in health in this country (Raphael, 2004; Raphael, Bryant, and Rioux, 2006). Why is disease socially patterned, so that the poor are more likely than the middle class (and the middle class more likely than the rich) to have diabetes, suffer from a stroke, and die at premature ages? From this perspective, you may seek to generate theories to explain the social patterning of health and disease, and draw on conceptual tools ranging from patriarchy to racism to structural violence and neoliberalism. Canadian researchers have made important contributions to the study of **intersectionality** (Schulz and Mullings, 2006), the ways in which race, gender, and class combine to influence population patterns of morbidity and mortality.

From a more global perspective, you may be interested in the availability of anti-retroviral medicines for people with HIV/AIDS—comparing, perhaps, the availability of medicines here in Canada with the availability of medicines in countries of the global south. Your work may take on elements of policy analysis, as you interpret data on the pricing of pharmaceuticals, the intricacies of international trade agreements that structure who can manufacture live-saving medicines, and their corresponding legal debates. Or, following Paul Farmer (1999; 2003), you may be interested in understanding how poverty and inequality constrain the choices that people may make in the face of disease—and in this way, seek to understand the structural and personal dimensions of the HIV/AIDS epidemic.

All of these examples conceptualize health as both a *personal trouble* and a *public issue*. As a personal trouble, researchers seek to understand the lived experience of disease—how it affects individuals and their families. What sense can be made of suffering? How do people understand their conditions? How do they make sense of risk? These and other questions enable us to understand important dimensions of health and illness, and can offer important feedback in the evaluation of public health policy. As a public issue, we look beyond the biographies of individuals, and seek to understand the acts of history, culture, economics, and politics that shape our capacities to lead healthy lives. On a local level, this could involve examining local bylaws that enable or restrict the location of fast food restaurants. On a national level, this could involve analyzing laws to restrict tobacco advertising. And on an international level, we can see health as a public issue in that global macroeconomics, climate change, political conflict, and war are inextricably intertwined with the health of populations.

Acknowledging that health is both a personal trouble and a public issue radically expands our way of understanding the causes of disease. Consider the growing burden of chronic diseases—with conditions like obesity rapidly increasing in prevalence not only in Canada (Katzmarzyk, 2002) but also countries of the global south like Brazil (Moura and Claro, 2011) and Argentina (Linetzky et al., 2013). To what extent is obesity caused by individual choices related to unhealthy diet and physical inactivity? To what extent are these choices constrained by an individual's life chances, by the structure in which they live and work? Incorporating questions like these into our thinking about health produces a richer, more nuanced account of lifestyle choices in the context of structural constraints, generating awareness that chronic diseases relate to patterns of inequity. This moves us far beyond traditional epidemiological analysis that focused almost exclusively on individuals and neglected the wider social context in which their choices are made (Davey Smith, 2001).

The great sociologist C. Wright Mills (1959) wrote that the promise of social science involved seeing the connection between personal troubles and public issues. This is arguably just as relevant to **epidemiology** and public health as it is to sociology—for the dual nature of disease as both biological and social demands understanding both troubles at the level of the body and the mind, and public issues focusing on health policy and social determinants of health (De Maio, 2010b).

All of the examples above have something in common. They all frame the research in such a way that health is acknowledged to be biological and social in nature. The examples above also differ in important ways—in the kinds of knowledge they call for, and in the kinds of research methods that they employ. These differences can be understood as reflecting different **research paradigms**.

> ## PRACTICAL TIP
>
> To develop research ideas, take your main area of interest (be it a disease, a population, or a policy) and think of parallel projects on that area of interest that would draw from the different epistemologies, ontologies, and methodologies described in this chapter. You will find that this will help you to be more aware of the assumptions that you have already developed about what kinds of knowledge you value and how that knowledge should be generated.

What is a Research Paradigm?

A research paradigm reflects one's beliefs about what constitutes knowledge and how that knowledge is to be generated. Three distinct dimensions help us to define a research paradigm: epistemology, ontology, and methodology (see Table 2.1).

Epistemology is the branch of philosophy concerned with the nature and definition of knowledge and truth. One's epistemology defines the types of data that would be considered valid and useful. For example, a researcher may privilege data collected from large nationally-representative random samples using validated survey questions. Another may instead focus on personal narratives from a few key informants, perhaps collected in a series of in-depth interviews, focus

Table 2.1	Dimensions of Research Paradigms
Epistemology	The branch of philosophy concerned with the nature and definition of knowledge and truth
Ontology	The branch of philosophy concerned with the nature of reality
Methodology	Approach to data collection and analysis

groups, or oral histories. In the section below, we will contrast three important epistemologies: positivism, interpretivism, and critical realism. Ontology is the branch of philosophy concerned with the nature of reality. **Ontology** orients us to a fundamental question facing researchers: do we study things that can be considered "objective entities," things that have a fixed reality that is independent of our perspectives? Or do we study social constructions, fluid things that change depending on our point of view? Later in this chapter, we will examine two critical ontologies: objectivism and constructionism. Objectivism holds that researchers study phenomena that exist as external objects; their characteristics are independent of our perspective. One's height and weight are objects in this sense. Alternatively, researchers often study socially constructed phenomena: masculinity and femininity, for example, are such socially constructed attributes. They do not exist in the same ontological sense as height and weight. And, lastly, **methodology** describes one's approach to data collection and analysis. A significant methodological divide has pitted quantitative research versus qualitative research—with "mixed methods" an appealing alternative, but whose actual feasibility may in fact be questioned.

Epistemological Foundations

Positivism

Positivism—This branch of epistemology argues that valid knowledge and truth is generated through a scientific process based on observation/measurement and generalization. Positivist science is sometimes labeled "hard science". Indeed, the philosopher most associated with positivism, Auguste Comte (1798–1857) thought that social science should be modelled after physics and the natural sciences. Positivism

emphasizes the rigorous measurement of variables and the analysis of cause and effect relationships. A randomized controlled trial (RCT) falls firmly within this tradition—wherein independent and dependent variables are clearly defined and measurement scales for those variables are tested for validity and reliability. Positivist epistemology is also reflected in other statistical approaches to the generation of knowledge in public health, epidemiology, and social science. Analyses of large-scale datasets like the *Canadian Community Health Survey* typically fall within this tradition as well, with researchers examining a wide range of issues, including health inequalities in mid- and later life (Gee, Kobayashi, and Prus, 2004), correlates of depression and anxiety among young adults (Nguyen et al., 2005), the epidemiology of major depression (Patten et al., 2006), and inequalities based on racialized identities (Veenstra, 2009).

Historically, the positivist approach saw little difference between the natural sciences and the social sciences; both could be based on the scientific process of data collection relying on observation and measurement, on the testing of hypotheses, and ultimately, on the generation of principles and laws (akin to the laws of gravity and motion, for example). These would formalize general principles and patterns identifying the order of relationships in the world. The search for laws of societal evolution has largely been abandoned, yet many important theories in health research retain elements of this tradition. For example, this approach is present in ideas of epidemiologic transition (Mackenbach, 1994; Omran, 1971, 1983), which describe general stages that countries will experience in terms of leading causes of death through the process of economic development (from the "age of pestilence and famine" to the "age of receding pandemics" to the "age of degenerative and man-made diseases"). Similar ideas have shaped thinking around the stages of the global tobacco epidemic (Lopez, Collishaw, and Piha, 1994).

Much of the research on the "healthy immigrant effect" and the "income inequality hypothesis" falls within this epistemological tradition as well (see Health Research in Action boxes 2.1 and 2.2). These studies certainly do share important features of a positivist epistemology. However, they do not seek to generate laws; instead, they look to generate context-specific models describing relationships.

Much of the work in this area uses a type of statistical analysis called **regression**, where the characteristics of individuals are examined as potential predictors of their actions and beliefs. For example, one might study how the diet of an individual immigrant or their family changes over time. This type of research has been criticized for focusing too much on the characteristics of individuals, at the expense of the characteristics of the places in which individuals live and work. An emerging wave of **social epidemiological** studies have attempted to overcome this limitation, and regression analysis now commonly incorporates **contextual factors** (the properties of places), along with **compositional characteristics** (the properties of individuals), as independent variables. This has generated more "realistically complex" positivist accounts of the social patterning of disease, and researchers now routinely incorporate compositional characteristics (e.g., a person's usual diet) with contextual factors (e.g., the presence of "food deserts"—districts with little or no access to affordable fresh food—in their neighbourhood). However, more remains to be done, and a truly global political economy of health inequities has really only started to be mapped out, for example, in the World Health Organization's *Commission on the Social Determinants of Health*. At the same time, many researchers believe that explaining how patterns of disease are generated and experienced call for guidance from other

2.1 Health Research in Action

The Deterioration of Health Status Among Immigrants to Canada

Canadian research on the health of immigrants has engaged with contrasting notions of "sick immigrants" and "healthy immigrants" (Beiser, 2005); the former describing immigrants as carriers of disease and as burdens on health and social welfare systems, and the latter acknowledging that because of a number of factors—including self-selection as well as Canadian immigration policies—immigrants to Canada tend to be healthier than the native-born population at the time of their arrival in the country (Gushulak, 2007; Hyman, 2004).

De Maio and Kemp (2010) analyzed data from Statistics Canada's *Longitudinal Survey of Immigrants to Canada* to examine the role of discrimination as a factor that could explain why the health of immigrants worsens after settling in Canada. Their results indicate that visible minorities and immigrants who experienced discrimination or unfair treatment are most likely to experience a decline in self-reported health status. Their results also suggest an inverse socioeconomic gradient with respect to increasing levels of feelings of sadness, depression, and loneliness. These and other results (see De Maio, 2010a) suggest that discrimination and inequality partly drive the health transitions of immigrants. These factors, which largely operate outside of the formal health care system, need to be understood and addressed if health inequities are to be reduced in Canada.

2.2   Health Research in Action

Inequality as a Social Determinant of Health

Richard Wilkinson's income inequality hypothesis has been one of the most important areas of research in social epidemiology in the past 25 years (Wilkinson, 1996; Wilkinson and Pickett, 2008; 2009b). Broadly speaking, the hypothesis asserts that our health depends not only on our own income but on how income is distributed in the place in which we live. More than 200 statistical studies have examined the relationship between income inequality and population health, and approximately 90 per cent of these have found at least some support for the hypothesized relationship. However, once control variables are taken into account, this figure drops to approximately 40 per cent (Wilkinson and Pickett, 2009a), with little agreement in the literature surrounding what variables should be considered as controls, the geographical level in which the hypothesis should be tested, and the regions in the world where the hypothesis might apply (Lynch et al., 2004; Lynch, Harper, and Davey Smith, 2003; Subramanian and Kawachi, 2003), and which health indicators should be used (De Maio, 2007; 2008). Despite a large and growing body of research, agreement has yet to be reached on the validity of the hypothesis, the mechanisms that underlie it, and the global forces that shape it (Bernburg, 2010; De Vogli, Gimeno, and Mistry, 2009; Deaton, 2002; Starfield and Birn, 2007; Subramanian and Kawachi, 2007).

epistemologies—interpretivism and critical realism, as described below.

Interpretivism

Interpretivism—This branch of epistemology stands in stark contrast to positivism. The term describes a position developed in critique of positivism. In particular, the interpretivist tradition takes issue with the positivist application of the scientific model to the study of social phenomena. Interpretivists argue that there are fundamental distinctions between the social and natural sciences, and that these distinctions lead us to differing ways of knowing. Instead of being based on attempts to *measure*, interpretivist research seeks to generate a *subjective* understanding of social phenomena. Often, this involves understanding what the world looks like through the eyes of those being studied. The goal of this line of research is not to measure the prevalence of a particular condition, but to understand the meaning attached to that condition in the real world. This has been a very important aspect of health research, with interpretivist analyses of tobacco consumption, for example, yielding fascinating insight on why anti-tobacco messaging based on health risk is often ineffective for some groups. Hillary Graham's now classic interpretivist study of women caring for pre-school children in low-income families found that their smoking was a central coping strategy to fight sleep problems, social isolation, and the demands of full-time caring. Anti-smoking campaigns focused on increasing awareness of the pathogenic effects of cigarettes largely missed the meaning of smoking in the lives of these women (Graham, 1987). People in low-income households continue to be more likely to smoke than people in higher income groups.

Within the interpretivist tradition, the purpose of research is to understand how people (social "actors") make sense of their situations. From this perspective, the very nature of reality is subjective and could be seen from multiple perspectives.

Different actors may perceive a situation in different ways—and these different perceptions (or "definitions of the situation") are thought to be real in their consequences. For example, health researchers have grappled with the dynamics of power that are embedded within the medical encounter—the face-to-face meeting of a health care professional and their patient. Researchers have studied the "impression management" that patients with medically unexplained symptoms go through in order to maximize the benefits from their encounter with a health care professional (Werner and Malterud, 2003). Other studies have looked at the medical encounter from the perspective of physicians, in an attempt to understand how they perceive of and work with seemingly non-compliant or uncooperative patients (De Maio, 2010b).

Interpretivist epistemology does not attempt to generate statistical data, nor does it claim to produce generalizable conclusions. Instead, it seeks to generate "thick description" (Geertz, 1973); vivid portraits of the lived experience of individuals and communities. It also seeks to value the insight of research participants—drawing on post-colonial and feminist critiques of traditional research approaches for being inherently authoritative and exploitative (researchers collecting data and giving little back to individuals and communities involved) (Oakley, 1981; Taylor, 1998). An interpretivist epistemology—by seeing the complex and often contradictory perceptions of individuals as the prime source of knowledge—opens the way for the utilization of "empowering methodologies", as described below.

Critical Realism

Critical Realism—Our third epistemological tradition argues that true knowledge and truth is often generated by theorizing, rather than measuring or observing. This position is most closely associated with the philosopher Roy Bashkar (see Benton

and Craib, 2001). The term critical realism is used in different disciplines in different ways, but in health research it has been most productively used by Steven Wainwright and Angus Forbes (2000), along with Graham Scambler (2001), to question the dominance of positivist methods in the study of health inequities. As used by Wainwright, Forbes, and Scambler, critical realism has deep roots in Marxist philosophy. Marx (1818–1883) sought to understand the dynamics of exploitation in capitalist economies primarily through theoretical analysis, using abstract tools like "surplus value" and "alienation". Marx didn't rely on surveys, focus groups, or participant observation—indeed, he believed that "all science would be superfluous if the form of appearance of things and their essence directly coincided" (Tucker, 1978). He called for theories that explained what was going on *underneath the surface* of things—the "motors" of history, and in his case, the contradictions in the capitalist system.

Critical realism offers a unique perspective on what one might define as valid knowledge and truth. It does not privilege that which we can measure, as does positivism, nor does it privilege that which individuals can experience and narrate, as does interpretivism. Instead, it focuses on that which we can theorize—including things which we cannot directly measure or see in our day-to-day lives. For example, consider that "class conflict"—a key Marxist term—is not readily measurable nor can its existence necessarily be verified by the perspectives of individuals.

Critical realism posits that reality exists independently of individuals' perceptions. In that regard, it is quite different from interpretivism, which privileges the perceptions of social actors. From the perspective of critical realism, interpretivism is incapable of going beyond the stated perceptions of social actors—it can be blind to "false consciousness", for example. But unlike positivism, which holds that knowledge about that external reality must be based on observation and measurement, critical realism calls for theoretical analysis of "generative mechanisms" (Scambler, 2001)—deep-rooted structural forces that shape our lived experiences and that influence patterns of morbidity and mortality as well as the very structure of health care systems. Wainwright and Forbes explain:

> To not explore the impact on health inequalities of mechanisms within capitalism such as exploitation and alienation, for example, because they are not seen to exist in either a measurable way or because they are not expressed by those who being researched leads to huge gaps in any subsequent "explanation" and ultimately to partiality and theoretical weakness [sic]. Because the realist position accepts that which is unseen is seen [to] be of equal importance to that which can, this opens up the possibility for researchers to examine and accommodate such forces within their research and subsequent theory. (2000: 271)

Critical realism is therefore an epistemological "third way"—a critique of both positivism and interpretivism, and a position that calls for links between on-the-surface data and deep-rooted theory, which may or may not be amenable to empirical testing.

Ontology

Ontology is the branch of philosophy concerned with the nature of reality. Broadly speaking, we can differentiate two contrasting ontologies found in contemporary health and social research: objectivism and constructionism.

Objectivism as an ontological position holds that researchers study phenomena that exist as external objects—they are beyond the reach or influence of the researcher (Bryman and Teevan, 2005). Physical attributes like height and weight

are such objects. Some would argue that more abstract entities like culture can also be understood in this way; indeed, in many cases we can measure cultural beliefs and practices. In that respect, we can see a logical connection between positivist epistemology and objectivist ontology. Objectivism is also connected to critical realism, but here, while a researcher acknowledges that external reality exists independently of their senses, they do not agree with the positivist position that our knowledge about that reality must be limited to that what we can measure. **Constructionism**, in contrast, holds that researchers study socially-constructed objects; we study beliefs, ideologies, behaviours, and human action. Researchers study identities, and these clearly are socially-constructed objects. A social process underlies our understanding of gender, sexuality, ethnicity and other core aspects of our identities. All of these things take on meaning to the extent that social actors agree on their meaning. In that respect, constructionism has a logical connection to interpretivist epistemology.

Methodology

A key component of a research paradigm revolves around data collection. What kinds of data are to be collected, and how should they be collected? Ultimately, how are they to be used? Will they test pre-existing theories (with *a priori* hypotheses) or will they be used to generate new theories?

The Quantitative Tradition

The quantitative tradition relies on numeric data and statistical analysis. Data are often collected via large-scale social and epidemiological surveys with **fixed response ranges**. This tradition is closely aligned with positivist epistemology and objectivist ontology. It is important to note, however, that quantitative analysis is also used by critical realists (Porpora, 2001). The quantitative tradition is primarily guided by concerns to measure, to test hypotheses, to assess correlation and/or causality, and most importantly, to generalize from *samples* to *populations* (using inferential statistics). Consider Figure 2.1.

The scatterplot displays the hallmarks of the quantitative tradition. In this analysis, two key variables are being measured: the independent variable, displayed on the x-axis of the graph, indicates a city's "median share of income"—the proportion of the total income in that city that is earned by the poorest 50 per cent of people in that city. It is a measure of income inequality—if a city had a perfectly equal income distribution (where all people earned the same amount of income), the median share of income would be 0.50. Of course that is not the case, and even for the most equal North American cities—Barrie and Oshawa Ontario (both primarily working-class cities), the median share is approximately 0.26; the poorest 50 per cent of people in those cities earn about 26 per cent of that city's income. The most unequal cities in North America—shown in the scatterplot to be Bryan and McAllen, Texas and Monroe, Louisiana—have a median share of 0.16 to 0.18.

The dependent variable is shown on the y-axis—it is the mortality rate. In this case, it indicates the number of working-age people (per 100,000) that die every year. There is a remarkable

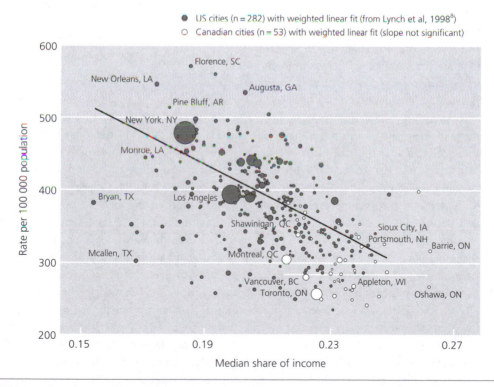

FIGURE 2.1   Mortality in all working age people by proportion of income belonging to the less well-off half of households

Source: Ross, N. A., Wolfson, M. C., Dunn, J. R., Berthelot, J. M., Kaplan, G. A., & Lynch, J. W. (2000). Relation between income inequality and mortality in Canada and in the United States: Cross sectional assessment using census data and vital statistics. *British Medical Journal, 320*(7239), 898–902.

range in the data—from a low of approximately 250 in Canadian cities, to approximately 550 in New Orleans, Louisiana.

The analysis shows a correlation between income inequality and population health; indeed, this is a test of the income inequality hypothesis described in Health Research in Action box 2.2. And statistically, Ross et al. show in their study that a one per cent increase in median share is associated with a decrease of 21 deaths (per 100,000 working age population) every year. In other words, as a city's median share of income improves from 0.20 to 0.21 or from 0.24 to 0.25, we expect a substantial reduction in avoidable mortality. However, the relationship is only statistically significant for cities in the United States—within the Canadian data, an increase in median share was not associated with a decrease in mortality. One interpretation of this pattern is that features of the Canadian welfare system may ameliorate the pathogenic effects of income inequality. Alternatively, researchers have hypothesized that income inequality exerts a significant effect on population health only once a high enough level of inequality has been reached—as a consequence, Canada's income distribution, being more equal than that of the United States, is not unequal enough to manifest in patterns of poor health detectable in macro-level analyses like Ross et al.'s.

Ross et al.'s analysis is firmly rooted in a positivist epistemology, as is most of the literature on the income inequality hypothesis (De Maio, 2012). Most of that literature has focused on statistically verifying the links between income inequality, as an independent variable, and health outcomes. Most studies in this area have utilized some form of regression analysis. Some of the most intense debates in this field have been over measurement issues—the use of morbidity or mortality indicators, the geographical level at which to study the hypothesis, the operational-

ization of income distribution, and the appropriateness of ecological versus multilevel statistical approaches. All of these are indicative of an epistemological approach that is guided by the idea that "to measure is to know".

Critical realist scholars have called for an alternative approach, one that investigates the causes and not just the effects of income inequality. For Canadian sociologist David Coburn, this represents "a broader, more contextualized and more sociologically meaningful causal model" (2004: 43; see also Coburn, 2000; 2001). Coburn argues:

> . . . numerous researchers have explored methods of ameliorating the effects of poor social condi- tions on the health of the underprivileged . . . [but] hardly any have asked about the possible causes of inequality itself. Yet, examining the causes of social inequalities, and not simply their effects, changes our understanding of the causal sequen- ces involved in the income inequality / health status relationship (2001: 50).

From this perspective, the health effects of income inequality are important but should be examined through the wider lens of political economy rather than epidemiology.

Statistical analysis is sometimes criticized for being uncritically supportive of the status quo, of reproducing existing power inequalities (Feagin and Vera, 2008). However, new waves of studies have shown that it is possible to use statistical analysis within the spirit of critical social science—to use a traditional research paradigm to describe *and* challenge social inequalities. Statistical health research has been at the forefront of this—raising critical questions about pathogenic effects of racism and discrimination (De Maio and Kemp, 2010; Krieger, 2011) and the social patterning of disease, both in Canada (Raphael et al., 2006) and across the world (WHO, 2008). Wilkinson's income inequality hypothesis is another clear example of this.

The Qualitative Tradition

This tradition is most closely aligned with interpretivist epistemology and constructionist ontology. Those who choose to approach their research within the qualitative tradition are most likely to ask *open-ended* research questions concerned with meaning. Questions like "*what* is happening in this clinical trial for HIV-drug research?" or "*how* do the patients involved in the trial feel about what they're being asked to do?" for example, would generate descriptive answers and emerge from the people and the *setting* itself, a key aspect of the qualitative tradition. Sometimes this setting is a contained, easily defined space to which the researcher must negotiate access—such as the access Canadian anthropologist Denielle Elliot (2007) negotiated in order to attend the medical clinics in which patients in an HIV trial met with their physicians. Other times, the setting is not as easily defined and may actually be comprised of several places: in this example, then, that may include meetings of the AIDS Foundation, the streets where the homeless patients live, community centres where AIDS activists discuss the trials, and so on. Research like this relies on methods that put the researcher in close contact with people, places and events that become the "research field", which is why qualitative researchers so often refer to what they do as "fieldwork".

Fieldwork methods include immersion in the field, observing and often times participating in the setting in some fashion, and keeping detailed notes of the experience. Other essential qualitative methods include one-on-one in-depth interviews, focus group interviews, collecting oral history, and doing content analysis of written and/or visual material found in or related to the field. Some qualitative researchers describe their work as **ethnography**, the literal meaning of which is "writing culture" and is associated most often with the practice of anthropology (Hesse-Biber and Leavy, 2006) and

participant observation on the part of the researcher. Health research within the *ethnographic* qualitative tradition, then, would be characterized by the underlying belief that the research setting—the doctor's office, say—is not a neutral place, but rather a *cultural* setting imbued with meanings that the researcher can describe in rich detail and analyze through their own written observations, and the words they collect from those in the setting.

Because research in this tradition does rely on close work with people and places, two questions take on a particular urgency: first, what is the role of theory here? While it might make sense to talk of "testing" a theory in the quantitative tradition, it seems somewhat at odds with the open-ended aspect of qualitative methodology. Oftentimes, qualitative research also takes the form of "grounded theory"—an approach to research that values the generation of new abstract concepts and theories *from* empirical data (Corbin and Strauss, 1990; Pidgeon, 1996; Wilson, Hutchinson, and Holzemer, 2002). That is, the qualitative researcher would look for emerging themes in her fieldnotes, interview transcriptions, and materials, and *then* refine research questions which engage these themes, often going back to the field to investigate and analyze these themes further. Grounded theory might also lead a researcher to a body of theory—for instance, if many of the people interviewed defined their own experiences as concerned with "patients' rights", then the researcher might choose to analyze their claims using philosophical and theoretical work on human rights.

The other urgent question within the qualitative tradition is that of ethics, particularly that of *consent*. Doing participant observation, focus groups, and interviews all involve building a research relationship with real people, and responsibilities not to introduce harm and to keep everyone informed of the nature and goals of the qualitative project. Often times, and particularly in health research, this means preparing proposals for ethics review for a board responsible for approving the research. Above all, this means gaining permission from the research subjects or respondents' themselves in order to carry out one's work. It might also involve considering the research design at the outset, and goals about how to exit the field and write about findings when the research has been concluded. Consider, for example, Amy Salmon's (2007) innovative work with women in Vancouver's Downtown Eastside (see Health Research in Action box 2.3).

Salmon's research falls firmly within the qualitative tradition. Salmon argues that the women in her study, by virtue of their experiences, hold unique knowledge. It was her challenge as the researcher to find a methodological approach that would connect her to that knowledge. That meant finding ways of making the research process an empowering experience, a democratic experience.

Deduction and Induction

The examples above hint at two distinct phases of theorization: the testing of pre-existing hypotheses (**deduction**), and the generation of new theories (**induction**).

Deduction refers to the testing of rigidly framed **hypotheses** (a hypothesis is a testable statement about the relationship between variables). In this approach to research, we begin with a pre-existing theory and collect or assemble data to test a hypothesis derived from that theory. Our data may support the theory as is, suggest that a modification in the theory is needed (in the case of mixed findings), and/or suggest that the theory may not actually be correct (in the case of negative findings). Research on the income inequality hypothesis as well as work on the health transitions of immigrants to Canada largely proceeds in a deductive sense.

2.3   Health Research in Action

Research as an Empowering and Democratic Process

Amy Salmon's (2007) research with women in Vancouver's Downtown Eastside who experienced substance use during pregnancy and fetal alcohol syndrome/fetal alcohol effects is a fascinating account of how research can be an empowering and democratic process. Salmon conducted focus group interviews with six young Aboriginal mothers, and worked from an interpretivist epistemology that, above all, valued the perspectives of the women involved in the study. Indeed, Salmon's research is particularly interesting for the degree of respondent validation involved in the data collection and analysis. Salmon did not merely collect data from her "subjects." Instead,

they became partners in the analysis, with Salmon sharing with them rough drafts, and discussing the analysis as a process. Salmon argues that this type of methodology is particularly useful in helping to mitigate the risk of misrepresentation and appropriation of poor Aboriginal women's experiences.

Leslie Robertson and Dara Culhane's *In Plain Sight: Reflections on Life in Downtown Eastside Vancouver* went even further than Salmon in developing an empowering and democratic methodology. Their approach involved stepping away from the researcher's role as author, and instead, they focused on becoming editors of a collection of self-written narratives, with the research participants authoring their own stories.

Induction refers to empirical generalizations that flow from description to abstraction. In this case, findings from a particular study may be used to generate concepts and new hypotheses that are then developed, modified, and tested in other research projects. Graham's (1987) inductive analysis of tobacco consumption by women caring for pre-school children in low-income families is a great example of how research may seek to generate new insight and new ideas, rather than test pre-existing theories.

In practice, deduction and induction form key components of the "wheel of science" (see Figure 2.2).

We derive hypotheses from existing theories. These hypotheses are then tested with empirical observations. Observations, in turn, may be used through the process of induction to generalize ideas and concepts, and it is these ideas and concepts that are the building blocks of theory.

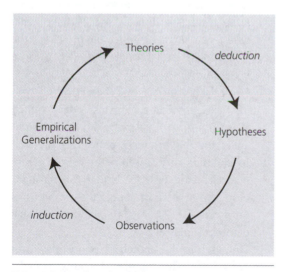

FIGURE 2.2   The wheel of science

Source: Wallace, W. (1971). *The Logic of Science in Sociology*. Chicago: Aldine-Atherton. With permission of Transaction Publishers.

The Quantitative/ Qualitative Divide

There has been a tendency to view quantitative and qualitative research strategies as mutually exclusive (Creswell, 1994). And in fact, research is often divided in this way—with quantitative and qualitative researchers publishing in separate journals, attending different conferences, and in general, proceeding with little engagement with one another. Yet for many years researchers have also called for the use of mixed methods designs—research strategies that could blend the advantages of the two traditions. Interestingly, health research may be the field of research most capable of bridging the quantitative/qualitative divide. It is health research that draws both from quantitative epidemiology and qualitative anthropology. It is health research that examines deep-rooted structural forces as generative mechanisms—for example, in the work of Paul Farmer, who focuses on "structural violence" and the global political economy of tuberculosis and HIV/AIDS while maintaining an ethnographer's close link to the personal narratives and social milieu of research participants.

Canadian researchers have made important contributions on both sides of the quantitative/qualitative divide (Raphael et al., 2006). And new Canadian health research is increasingly showing the value of mixed-methods strategies. Valerie Crooks (2007), for example, has used a mixed-methods approach to understand the life changes experienced by women with fibromyalgia. She used a combination of in-depth interviews (reflecting the interpretivist/qualitative tradition) in combination with a structured standardized test (the Sickness Impact Profile, or SIP, reflecting the positivist/quantitative tradition). She describes this mixture of data collection strategies as "triangulation", noting that "the mixing of qualitative and quantitative approaches within health research is becoming increasingly common" (2007: 578). At the same time, she describes her study as "primarily qualitative in nature" (2007: 578), with the quantitative element added to support the qualitative component. And in this sense, mixed-methods work is indeed more and more common in research—but importantly, the mixture is uneven, with qualitative researchers adding a quantitative element to support the core project, or as with quantitative researchers adding a qualitative dimension to verify their results or perhaps to pilot test a survey question. In these situations, there is still a dominant research paradigm. A mixed-methods design that brings together advanced statistical regression analysis with extended fieldwork/ethnography is certainly a possibility, but such mixture has not been dominant in health research. A mixed-methods approach also raises the possibility of contradictory findings—and these too would call for researchers to privilege one set of data, one research paradigm, over another.

PRACTICAL TIP

To get a sense of how quantitative and qualitative research strategies differ, try this exercise: search www.pubmed.com for quantitative and qualitative studies on a topic that interests you. For example, search for quantitative literature on inequality in asthma by searching for studies on asthma that include the words "survey," "questionnaire," "regression," or "statistics" in the abstract. Repeat the search, but this time look for studies on inequality in asthma that include abstract words such as "focus group," "interview," or "ethnography." What you find may give you ideas for your own research.

Summary

- A research paradigm reflects one's beliefs about what constitutes knowledge and how that knowledge is to be generated. Three distinct dimensions help us to define a research paradigm: epistemology, ontology, and methodology.

- Epistemology is the branch of philosophy concerned with the nature of knowledge and truth. It reflects the type of evidence that one accepts as being valid. Three major epistemologies are found in contemporary health and social research: positivism, interpretivism, and critical realism.

- Positivism is an epistemology that posits that valid knowledge and truth is generated through a scientific process based on observation/measurement and generalization.

- Interpretivist research seeks to generate a *subjective* understanding of social phenomena. Often, this involves understanding what the world looks like through the eyes of those being studied.

- Critical realism calls for theoretical analysis of "generative mechanisms"—deep-rooted structural forces that shape our lived experiences and that influence patterns of morbidity and mortality as well as the very structure of health care systems. Under this epistemology, knowledge of generative mechanisms may call for theoretical analysis, not just empirical analysis.

- Ontology is the branch of philosophy concerned with the nature of reality. Broadly speaking, we can differentiate two contrasting ontologies found in contemporary health and social research: objectivism, and constructionism.

- Objectivism as an ontological position holds that researchers study phenomena that exist as external objects—they are beyond the reach or influence of the researcher. Constructionism, in contrast, holds that researchers study social constructed objects—we study beliefs, ideologies, behaviors, and human action.

- A key component of a research paradigm revolves around data collection. What kind of data are to be collected, and how should they be collected? Ultimately, how are they to be used? Will they test pre-existing theories (with *a priori* hypotheses) or will they be used to generate new theories?

- The quantitative tradition relies on numeric data and statistical analysis. Data are often collected via large-scale social and epidemiological surveys with fixed response ranges. The quantitative tradition is primarily guided by concerns to measure, to test hypotheses, to assess correlation and/or causality, and

most importantly, to generalize from *samples* to *populations*.

- Those who choose to approach their research within the qualitative tradition are most likely to ask *open-ended* research questions concerned with meaning. Research like this relies on methods that put the researcher in close contact with people, places and events that become the "research field", which is why qualitative researchers so often refer to what they do as "fieldwork".

- Deduction and induction form key components of the "wheel of science". We derive hypotheses from existing theories. These hypotheses are then tested through the process of deduction with empirical observations. Observations, in turn, may be used through the process of induction to generalize ideas and concepts, and it is these ideas and concepts that are the building blocks of theory.

- A divide between quantitative and qualitative research has existed for many decades. Health research may be the field of research most capable of bridging the quantitative/qualitative divide.

Review Questions

1. What are the three dimensions of a research paradigm?

2. What do you consider to be the advantages and disadvantages of each of the three epistemologies discussed in this chapter?

3. Epistemology and ontology are rather abstract philosophical terms. Why is it important that researchers grapple with them? What implications do these terms have for our research?

4. Quantitative methods have a long history in health research. What is appealing about this tradition for health researchers?

5. Qualitative research offers unique insight into health issues. What are the advantages and possible disadvantages of this approach?

6. Is "mixed methods" research feasible?

Recommended Readings

Bartley, M. (2004) *Health Inequality: An Introduction to Theories, Concepts and Methods.* Cambridge: Polity.

Provides an excellent overview of the research paradigms that have influenced health inequality research in the past twenty years, with a strong focus on methods.

Benton, T., and Craib, I. (2001) *Philosophy of Social Science: The Philosophical Foundations of Social Thought.* New York: Palgrave.

A book that provides an overview of the dominant epistemological frameworks used in social science. While not explicitly focused on health research, this book is a lucid and valuable resource.

Hughes, C., and Cohen, R. L. (2010) Feminists really do count: The complexity of feminist methodologies. *International Journal of Social Research Methodology*, 13(3), 189–96.

An important article that challenges many mistaken assumptions about the "value" of statistical/positivist research.

Krieger, N. (2011) *Epidemiology and the People's Health: Theory and Context.* New York: Oxford University Press.

An up-to-date and informative account of epidemiological theories and methods. Includes an impressive amount of empirical details which demonstrates the remarkable range of epistemologies, ontologies, and methodologies that are seen in contemporary epidemiological research.

Raphael, D., Bryant, T., and Rioux, M. (Eds.). (2006) *Staying Alive: Critical Perspectives on Health, Illness, and Health Care.* Toronto: Canadian Scholars' Press.

A now-standard Canadian textbook with great discussion of research paradigms in Canadian health research.

Smith, L. T. (1999) *Decolonizing Methodologies: Research and Indigenous Peoples.* London: Zed Books.

An innovative and compelling account of empowering methodological possibilities. Not explicitly focused on health but very useful for researchers concerned with the potential of health research to reproduce existing patterns of oppression and discrimination.

References

Beiser, M. (2005) The health of immigrants and refugees in Canada. *Canadian Journal of Public Health*, 96(Suppl 2), S30–44.

Benton, T., and Craib, I. (2001) *Philosophy of Social Science: The Philosophical Foundations of Social Thought.* New York: Palgrave.

Bernburg, J.G. (2010) Relative deprivation theory does not imply a contextual effect of country-level inequality on poor health. A commentary on Jen, Jones, and Johnston (68:4, 2009). *Social Science & Medicine*, 70(4), 493–95; discussion 498–500.

Bryman, A., and Teevan, J.L. (2005) *Social Research Methods: Canadian Edition.* Don Mills: Oxford University Press.

Coburn, D. (2000) Income inequality, social cohesion and the health status of populations: the role of neo-liberalism. *Social Science & Medicine*, 51(1), 135–46.

Coburn, D. (2001) Health, health care, and neo-liberalism. In Armstrong, P., Armstrong, H. and Coburn, D. (Eds.), *Unhealthy Times: Political Economy Perspectives on Health and Care in Canada* (pp. 45–65). Don Mills: Oxford University Press.

Coburn, D. (2004) Beyond the income inequality hypothesis: Class, neo-liberalism, and health inequalities. *Social Science & Medicine*, 58(1), 41–56.

Corbin, J., and Strauss, A. (1990) Grounded theory research: Procedures, canons, and evaluative criteria. *Qualitative Sociology*, 13(1), 3–21.

Creswell, J.W. (1994) *Research Design: Qualitative and Quantitative Approaches*. London, England: Sage Publications.

Crooks, V.A. (2007) Exploring the altered daily geographies and lifeworlds of women living with fibromyalgia syndrome: a mixed-method approach. *Social Science & Medicine*, 64(3), 577–88.

Davey Smith, G. (2001) Reflections on the limitations to epidemiology. *Journal of Clinical Epidemiology*, 54(4), 325–31.

De Maio, F.G. (2007) Health inequalities in Argentina: patterns, contradictions and implications. *Health Sociology Review*, 16(3-4), 279–91.

De Maio, F.G. (2008) Ecological analysis of the health effects of income inequality in Argentina. *Public Health*, 122(5), 487–96.

De Maio, F.G. (2010a) Immigration as pathogenic: a systematic review of the health of immigrants to Canada. *International Journal for Equity in Health*, 9, 27.

De Maio, F.G. (2010b) *Health and Social Theory*. Basingstoke: Palgrave Macmillan.

De Maio, F.G. (2012) Advancing the income inequality–health hypothesis. *Critical Public Health*, 22(1), 39–46.

De Maio, F.G., and Kemp, E. (2010) The deterioration of health status among immigrants to Canada. *Global Public Health*, 5(5), 462–78.

De Vogli, R., Gimeno, D., and Mistry, R. (2009) The policies-inequality feedback and health: the case of globalisation. *Journal of Epidemiology & Community Health*, 63(9), 688–691.

Deaton, A. (2002) The convoluted story of international studies of inequality and health. *International Journal of Epidemiology*, 31(3), 546–49.

Elliott, D.A. (2007) Pharmaceutical surveillance, medical research, and biovalue among the urban poor. Unpublished doctoral thesis. Burnaby, BC: Simon Fraser University.

Farmer, P. (1999) *Infections and Inequalities: The Modern Plagues*. Berkeley: University of California Press.

Farmer, P. (2003) *Pathologies of Power: Health, Human Rights, and the New War on the Poor*. Berkeley: University of California Press.

Feagin, J.R., and Vera, H. (2008) *Liberation Sociology*. 2nd ed. Boulder: Paradigm.

Gee, E. M., Kobayashi, K.M., and Prus, S. G. (2004) Examining the healthy immigrant effect in mid- to later life: findings from the Canadian Community Health Survey. *Canadian Journal on Aging*, 23(Suppl 1), s61–9.

Geertz, C. (1973) *The Interpretation of Cultures*. New York: Basic Books.

Gibson, N., Cave, A., Doering, D., Ortiz, L., and Harms, P. (2005) Socio-cultural factors influencing prevention and treatment of tuberculosis in immigrant and Aboriginal communities in Canada. *Social Science & Medicine*, 61(5), 931–42.

Graham, H. (1987) Women's smoking and family health. *Social Science & Medicine*, 25(1), 47–56.

Gushulak, B. (2007) Healthier on arrival? Further insight into the "healthy immigrant effect." *Canadian Medical Association Journal*, 176(10), 1439–40.

Hesse-Biber, S.N., and Leavy, P. (2006) *The Practice of Qualitative Research*. Thousand Oaks, California: Sage.

Hyman, I. (2004) Setting the stage: reviewing current knowledge on the health of Canadian immigrants. *Canadian Journal of Public Health*, 95(3), 1–8.

Katzmarzyk, P.T. (2002) The Canadian obesity epidemic, 1985–1998. *Canadian Medical Association Journal*, 166(8), 1039–1040.

Krieger, N. (2011) *Epidemiology and the People's Health: Theory and Context*. New York: Oxford University Press.

Linetzky, B., De Maio, F.G., Ferrante, D., Konfino, J., and Boissonet, C. (2013) Sex-stratified socio-economic gradients in physical inactivity, obesity, and diabetes: Evidence of short-term changes in Argentina. *International Journal of Public Health*, 58(2), 277–84.

Lopez, A.D., Collishaw, N.E., and Piha, T. (1994) A descriptive model of the cigarette epidemic in developed countries. *Tobacco Control*, 3(3), 242–7.

Lynch, J., Davey Smith, G., Harper, S., Hillermeier, M., Ross, N., Kaplan, G.A., et al. (2004) Is income inequality a determinant of population health? Part 1. A systematic review. *The Milbank Quarterly*, 82(1), 5–99.

Lynch, J., Harper, S., and Davey Smith, G. (2003) Plugging leaks and repelling boarders—where to next for the SS income inequality? *International Journal of Epidemiology*, 32(6), 1029–36.

Mackenbach, J.P. (1994) The epidemiologic transition theory. *Journal of Epidemiology and Community Health*, 48(4), 329–31.

Mills, C. W. (1959) *The Sociological Imagination*. New York: Oxford University Press.

Moura, E.C., and Claro, R.M. (2012) Estimates of obesity trends in Brazil, 2006–2009. *International Journal of Public Health*, 57(1), 127–33.

Nguyen, C.T., Fournier, L., Bergeron, L., Roberge, P., and Barrette, G. (2005) Correlates of depressive and anxiety disorders among young Canadians. *Canadian Journal of Psychiatry*, 50(10), 620-8.

Oakley, A. (1981) Interviewing women: a contradiction in terms. In Roberts, H. (Ed.), *Doing Feminist Research* (pp. 30–61). London: Routledge and Kegan Paul.

Omran, A.R. (1971) The epidemiologic transition. A theory of the epidemiology of population change. *Milbank Memorial Fund Quarterly*, 49(4), 509–38.

Omran, A.R. (1983) The epidemiologic transition theory. A preliminary update. *Journal of Tropical Pediatrics*, 29(6), 305–16.

Patten, S.B., Li Wang, J., Williams, J.V. A., Currie, S., Beck, C. A., Maxwell, C. J., et al. (2006) Descriptive epidemiology of major depression in Canada. *Canadian Journal of Psychiatry*, 51(2), 84.

Pidgeon, N. (1996) Grounded theory: theoretical background. In Richardson, J.T. (Ed.), *Handbook of Qualitative Research Methods for Psychology and the Social Sciences* (pp. 75–85). Leicester: British Psychological Society.

Porpora, D.V. (2001) Do realists run regressions? In López, J. and Potter, G. (Eds.), *After Postmodernism: An Introduction to Critical Realism* (pp. 260–6). London: Athlone Press.

Raphael, D. (Ed.) (2004) *Social Determinants of Health: Canadian Perspectives*. Toronto: Canadian Scholars' Press.

Raphael, D., Bryant, T., and Rioux, M. (Eds.) (2006) *Staying Alive: Critical Perspectives on Health, Illness, and Health Care*. Toronto: Canadian Scholars' Press.

Robertson, L., & Culhane, D. (Eds.). (2005). *In Plain Sight: Reflections on Life in Downtown Eastside Vancouver.* Vancouver: Talonbooks.

Ross, N.A., Wolfson, M.C., Dunn, J.R., Berthelot, J.M., Kaplan, G.A., and Lynch, J.W. (2000) Relation between income inequality and mortality in Canada and in the United States: cross sectional assessment using census data and vital statistics. *British Medical Journal,* 320(7239), 898–902.

Salmon, A. (2007) Walking the walk: how participatory interview methods can democratize research. *Qualitative Health Research,* 17(7), 982–93.

Samson, C. (2003) *A Way of Life That Does Not Exist: Canada and the Extinguishment of the Innu.* London: Verso.

Scambler, G. (2001) Critical realism, sociology and health inequalities: social class as a generative mechanism and its media of enactment. *Journal of Critical Realism,* 4, 35–42.

Schulz, A.J., and Mullings, L. (Eds.) (2006) *Gender, Race, Class, and Health: Intersectional Approaches.* San Francisco: Jossey-Bass.

Starfield, B., and Birn, A.E. (2007) Income redistribution is not enough: income inequality, social welfare programs, and achieving equity in health. *Journal of Epidemiology and Community Health,* 61(12), 1038–41.

Subramanian, S.V., and Kawachi, I. (2003) In defence of the income inequality hypothesis. *International Journal of Epidemiology,* 32, 1037–40.

Subramanian, S.V., and Kawachi, I. (2007) Commentary: Chasing the elusive null—the story of income inequality and health. *International Journal of Epidemiology,* 36(3), 596–9.

Taylor, V. (1998) Feminist methodology in social movements research. *Qualitative Sociology* 21(4), 357–79.

Tucker, R.C. (Ed.) (1978) *The Marx-Engels Reader.* New York: W.W. Norton & Company.

Veenstra, G. (2009) Racialized identity and health in Canada: Results from a nationally representative survey. *Social Science & Medicine,* 69(4), 538–42.

Wainwright, S.P., and Forbes, A. (2000) Philosophical problems with social research on health inequalities. *Health Care Analysis,* 8(3), 259–77.

Werner, A., and Malterud, K. (2003) It is hard work behaving as a credible patient: Encounters between women with chronic pain and their doctors. *Social Science & Medicine,* 57(8), 1409–19.

WHO (2008) *Closing the Gap in a Generation: Health Equity Through Action on the Social Determinants of Health.* Geneva: World Health Organization.

Wilkinson, R.G. (1996) *Unhealthy Societies: The Afflictions of Inequality.* New York: Routledge.

Wilkinson, R.G., and Pickett, K.E. (2008) Income inequality and socioeconomic gradients in mortality. *American Journal of Public Health,* 98(4), 699–704.

Wilkinson, R.G., and Pickett, K.E. (2009a) Income inequality and social dysfunction. *Annual Review of Sociology,* 35, 493–511.

Wilkinson, R.G., and Pickett, K.E. (2009b) *The Spirit Level: Why More Equal Societies Almost Always Do Better.* London: Allen Lane.

Wilson, H.S., Hutchinson, S.A., and Holzemer, W.L. (2002) Reconciling incompatibilities: A grounded theory of HIV medication adherence and symptom management. *Qualitative Health Research,* 12(10), 1309–22.

3

The Research Process
Ask the Right Question, Get the Right Answers

Renée S. MacPhee and Jennifer Robertson-Wilson

CHAPTER OUTLINE

Introduction: The Research Process

Health research is diverse and reflects the multidisciplinary and dynamic nature of the health care field. There are many ways to look at the same health-related topic. For example, researchers in the field of epidemiology may conduct research that seeks to determine what factors might increase the likelihood of developing heart disease in individuals who smoke, while someone who conducts research in the field of health informatics might conduct a study that looks to capture data from medical records pertaining to the number and types of in-patient procedures and the length of hospital admissions in order to determine the direct costs related to hospital stays for patients who are smokers with heart disease. Other health professionals, such as paramedics, nurses, and physicians, might be interested in conducting research that examines the use of medications for treating an individual who is suffering a heart attack. Health care professionals who conduct research in the rehabilitation sciences (e.g., physiotherapy, occupational therapy) might be interested in designing an exercise-based research study that will have as its goal the improvement of a reformed smoker's health status after the person has suffered a heart attack.

The phrase *research process* may seem daunting for some, in particular those individuals who have little or no experience in conducting research. What you are about to learn is that when the research process is clearly identified and described it provides the researcher with a step-by-step plan to carry out a research study. The steps in the research process remain relatively the same, regardless of whether the person conducting the study is a novice undergraduate researcher, a full-tenured professor, or an experienced clinician.

Perhaps the most quintessential aspect of health research is that the findings are based on sound evidence. Following its introduction in 1992, this approach was referred to as **evidence-based medicine** (EBM) (Sacket et al., 1996). Use of EBM requires that researchers or health practitioners follow a series of steps in order to arrive at a sound decision. These steps include: analyzing the clinical situation, asking a focused clinical question, accessing the clinical research (i.e.: evidence), appraising the best evidence found, applying the evidence to the problem at hand, and, assessing the effectiveness of care based on this evidence (Buckingham, Fisher, and Saunders, 2007). While EBM found its roots in the field of medicine, with time it began to be used in other health-oriented disciplines such as nursing, psychology, education, and information science, where it has become more commonly referred to as **evidence-based practice** (EBP) (Hjorland, 2011). EPB has further evolved to include **evidence-based behavioural practice** (EBBP), which involves making decisions about how to promote health or provide care by not only using the best available evidence, but also including practitioner expertise and other resources (EBBP, 2013). Readers of this text are encouraged to refer to the web-link located at the end of this chapter that will direct them to the EBBP website, which provides additional information and resources relevant to EBBP.

As you move through this chapter and throughout the textbook, you will learn how to apply most of the steps in EBM and EBP to your research process. In this chapter, we will start our exploration of the research process with a brief discussion of the role of the researcher. We will then present and describe each of the steps in the research process. Practical tips throughout the chapter will help to ensure that you avoid pitfalls and stumbling blocks when conducting your research.

Learning Objectives

When you have finished reading this chapter, you will be able to:

- Explain the concept of evidence-based practice and its role in health-related research.
- Identify the key roles of the researcher when conducting a study.
- List and describe each of the steps in the research process.
- Identify and describe the key components of a well-developed research question.
- Formulate a sound research question using the PICO(T) method.

The Role of the Researcher

Researchers, regardless of their discipline within the field of health, are instrumental in developing a well-designed research question and establishing a logical and manageable research process. But is this all they do? As you read the discussion below, you will soon see that a researcher is responsible for a number of tasks that are essential to the research study. We begin by presenting you with an overview of the *study specific* responsibilities of the researcher, followed by a discussion of responsibilities that pertain to the *administrative* aspects of a study.

Study-specific Responsibilities

In addition to developing the research question, the researcher must *select a study design* that is appropriate for the research question. For example, if the question is attempting to determine cause and effect between two things (e.g., does staying up all night cause someone to fall asleep in class that morning), an experimental design might be selected. However, if the researcher is trying to identify whether or not

there is a relationship between two variables (e.g., is the amount of hours someone studies for an exam related to the score on that exam), a correlational research design would be better suited to answer the question at hand.

Once the appropriate study design has been determined, the researcher must *ensure that the study is ethically sound*. This is determined by a research ethics board (REB) that is responsible for reviewing all research studies before they are conducted. All academic institutions and health care facilities that conduct research have either an REB or an institutional review board (IRB). The primary purpose of any REB or IRB is to ensure the safety and well-being of the individuals participating in the research study. Each and every study that is submitted by a researcher for review will be assessed for the following: risks; risks versus benefits; subject selection; informed consent; and safety and privacy (Neutens and Rubinson, 2002). In some instances the REB or IRB may also review the standards of professional conduct of the researcher conducting the study; the laws and regulations that may have relevance on the study, and previous research done in the area that may have bearing on the study under review. The process, rationale, and the steps involved in submitting an application for a study to be reviewed by an REB or IRB will be described in detail in Chapter 5. It is extremely important to stress that research in academic, health care, or private clinical settings must secure REB or IRB approval prior to starting the study. Students are strongly encouraged to contact the REB or IRB at their school in order to determine what the procedures and requirements are for doing a research study *before* they start their research project.

Having received approval from the REB or IRB to proceed with the study, the researcher can then begin the *data collection phase* of the study. This is where the researcher gathers the information necessary to answer the research question. Once the data have been collected, the next step of *data analysis* begins. During this step, the researcher must be sure to select the types of analyses that will be best suited for the type of data collected. For studies that use a quantitative study design or methodology where the data collected are numeric in nature (e.g., age, height, weight, length of time, etc.), the researcher would conduct the analyses using statistical tests (this is something that you will learn about when you take a course in research statistics). For studies that are qualitative in design methodology wherein the data collected are "words," the researcher would adopt a qualitative analysis paradigm (e.g., grounded theory) that would guide the data analysis process. Additional information about the differences between quantitative and qualitative study designs can be found in Chapters 2 and 6.

Following data analysis, the researcher will *prepare the study findings* in the form of a final report. The REB or IRB may require a copy of this report, including a final budget or financial statement for their records. Further, any agency (e.g., provincial or federal government funding body), organization (e.g., private company), or academic institution (e.g., college, university) that provided any type of funding or in-kind support may also require the same information. Providing the final report and budget and financial statements to the funding bodies will allow them to see that the researcher did what they set out to do, that there were tangible results, and that any funds that were allocated to the study were used accordingly. Based on the findings of the study, the researcher's next step is to *develop a new research question* and begin the research process again.

Administrative Responsibilities

As noted earlier, the researcher has not only study specific responsibilities, but also administrative responsibilities. One of the key administrative responsibilities is that the researcher *establishes a budget*, which must be realistic, feasible, and be based on the funds allocated for the study. The researcher will need to take several factors into consideration during this process including (but not limited to): the cost and number of supplies and pieces of equipment required; salaries (including benefits and taxes) for paid employees (e.g., research assistant, laboratory coordinator); and if necessary and permissible within the REB/IRB guidelines, compensation for the participants (e.g., gift cards, money, gifts, etc.). It is imperative that the researcher follow the budget once it has been set in over to avoid over-spending.

Developing a *timeline* or *schedule* is closely linked to the budgetary process. The researcher should develop a clear timeline that identifies not only the projected start and end dates of the study, but also any milestones that need to be met (e.g., quarterly reporting, due dates for final reports, submission deadlines for conference abstracts, etc). Establishing a well-developed timeline is a skill that requires some experience to master as it requires the researcher to know how much extra time (also referred to as "a cushion") should be built into the schedule. Too much cushion can lead to over-spending, whereas too little cushion may lead to rushing and short-cuts, which can (and usually will) compromise the integrity of the study.

Record-keeping is another administrative responsibility that the researcher undertakes. The researcher must ensure that all records, including items such as financial statements, participant data, and completed data collection forms are kept up-to-date and stored safely and securely, not only during the study but afterwards as well. Each REB/IRB will specify the length of time that records must be kept, along with the manner in which they can be disposed (e.g., confidential shredding service).

In addition, the researcher is also the *supervisor* of all individuals working on the study. This can potentially include undergraduate, graduate, and post-graduate students, as well as animal care technicians, laboratory coordinators, and administrative support staff. As the primary researcher or lead investigator on a study, the researcher may also be responsible for coordinating the research team (e.g., other researchers or co-investigators, research assistants, students, etc.), ensuring that when meetings are set, all members of the team are present (and prepared!) to participate.

Finally, the researcher must ensure that the research team complies with all agency, organizational, and institutional rules, regulations, policies, and procedures (e.g., safety, disposal of biomedical waste, Workplace Hazardous Materials Information System (WHMIS), etc.).

2006; Blaxter, Hughes, and Tight, 2010; DePoy and Gitlin, 2011), there is general agreement that there are key steps or stages that make up the research process. Figure 3.1 outlines the research *road map* that we suggest you follow when conducting a study.

For Blaxter et al. (2010:10) the research process is, ". . .cyclical; can be entered at almost any point; is a never ending process; will cause you to reconsider your practice; and will return you to a different starting place." For instance, some of you may be working with a faculty member in a lab. In this case, the faculty member already has a focused research topic and you are likely working on a specific research question. You may or may not be asked to review the literature on the topic but you are likely collecting data via an established methodology. In other cases, you might be given a research proposal project as part of your research methods course. Here you might be charged with the task of identifying a health-related problem, reading the available literature to get a sense of what we know and do not know on the topic, and then coming up with your own research question and methodology. As you read the literature, your research question and preferred methodology may change and evolve. See the Table of Contents at the start of the textbook which clearly indicates where you can find more detailed information on each of these steps in the research process.

The Research Process: Research Made Easy in 12 Steps

Think of the research process much like travel directions—when followed correctly and in sequence you can arrive at a pretty amazing place. Regardless of which research methods course you are taking or research methods text you are using (e.g., Baumgartner and Hensley,

Step 1: Identify the Research Topic, Idea, or Problem That's Right for You

If you are like most students, you may not have the first idea about how to come up with a research topic let alone a specific question. Durbin (2004: 1195) suggests ensuring you have a ". . . research attitude . . ." or ". . . a desire to question, evaluate, and investigate . . . to answer the questions, 'Why do we do things the way we do them?' and 'Is there a better way?'" Further, a research topic,

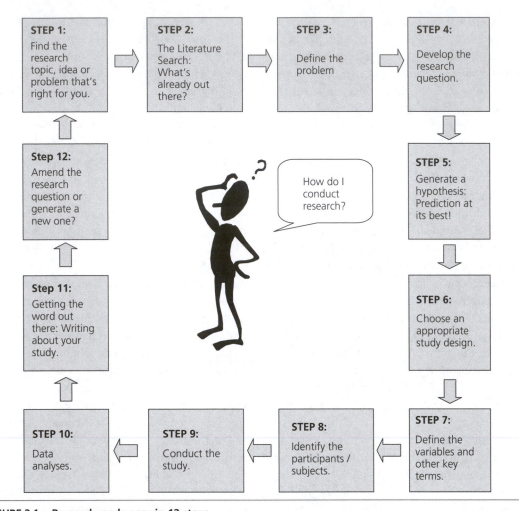

FIGURE 3.1   **Research made easy in 12 steps**
NOTE: Depending on the type of research you wish to conduct (e.g., case-study), you may not need to conduct Step 5 (Generate a hypothesis), and you would simply move from Step 4 directly to Step 6.

idea, or problem may be a ". . . a discrepancy between: (1) the way things are and the way they ought to be, and (2) what is known and what must be known to solve a problem or deal with a situation" (Valiga and Mermel, 1985: 1).

Thabane and colleagues (2009) suggest individuals new to research may differ from more seasoned researchers in their ability to recognize research topics and formulate questions. They then offer a list of ideas for seeking out and

developing a research topic. Following this work, below is a selected sample of questions formulated from the work of DePoy and Gitlin (2011), and Neutens and Rubinson (2010) (see also Thabane et al., 2009; and Valiga and Mermel, 1985 for their reviews of other's suggestions) that may assist you in uncovering a research topic or problem. The first three questions may be more suitable to new researchers, the latter three to the more seasoned researcher.

- *What have been your own experiences and observations (with health, illness, rehabilitation, wellness, fitness, or nutrition, for instance)?* You might develop an interest in a research topic because you came across it during one of your academic courses. For example, if you have ever taken an *Introduction to Health* course, you might have been intrigued by issues around substance use/abuse, sexually transmitted infections, physical activity, or nutrition in different segments of the population. Or, you might want to know more about a health topic because it is affecting one of your family members (e.g., Alzheimer's disease, osteoporosis, type 2 diabetes, cancer, obesity, etc).

- *What does the current research say?* Reviewing the relevant literature (usually through relevant journal articles) is another good place to start.

- *What's making news?* If you watch the evening news, read the newspaper in print or on-line, or subscribe to magazines, current hot or popular research topics may be reported. During the writing of this book chapter, headlines such as "*ER doctors want mandatory CPR training in high school, say it could help save lives*" (Canadian Press, 2011),"*HIV vaccine developed in Canada approved for human studies*" (Ogilvie, 2011), and "*Vaccine-autism tie "an elaborate fraud": journal*" (CBC news, 2011) were all highlighted in the news.

- *What is happening within professional organizations?* Graduate students and faculty are often members of professional societies (e.g., Canadian Medical Association, Canadian Public Health Association, Canadian Nutrition Society, Canadian Association of Gerontology). In addition to holding yearly meetings or conferences (which offer an opportunity to liaise with others and scope the current research), these societies may also provide statements of emerging issues of concern or priority areas for research.

- *What type of research can be funded?* In Canada, the three major sources of funding include the Canadian Institute of Health Research (CIHR), Natural Sciences and Engineering Research Council (NSERC), and the Social Sciences and Humanities Research Council of Canada (SSHRC). The former two are of particular relevance to anyone conducting health-related research. Other organizations (e.g., Heart and Stroke Foundation or the Canadian Diabetes Association) may also fund research specific to a given disease or health issue. It is often useful to know what topics and types of research are being funded by various organizations.

- *How might theory be used and tested?* Theories are ideas or hunches that a researcher has about a particular topic, which in turn serve as potential explanation(s) as to how or why something may or may not occur. In order to be established as viable, theories are developed, refined, tested, and in some cases, developed, refined, and tested again! Ascertaining whether a theory is correct or incorrect requires the collection and analyses of accurate and reliable data.

According to Gravetter and Foranzo (2012) students should be on the look-out for the following in developing their research topic. First, Gravetter and Foranzo believe that students should select a topic they are enthusiastic about. Second, students should explore topic areas that are new to them as long as the topic has a realistic degree of complexity. Third, the topic has to have a specific focus. Fourth, students must be prepared to revise a research topic if needed. Finally, students should ensure that there is sufficient research literature to assist in setting up the topic.

Step 2: The Literature Search: What's Already Out There?

While Chapter 4 of this textbook will go into detail about how to conduct a detailed literature search, here we present you with some of the key terms as well as the rationale for conducting a literature search not only before you start your study, but while your study is ongoing. Once you have identified your topic of interest, it is important that you conduct a literature search to determine what research findings relevant to your problem of interest exist. It will also help you to identify where there are gaps—areas where the research findings may be lacking or missing altogether. Additional reasons for conducting a thorough search of the literature include: the ability of the researcher to demonstrate a familiarity with a body of knowledge; to show the path of prior research and how the current project is linked to it; to integrate and summarize what is known in an area; to learn from others, and hopefully stimulate new ideas (Gravetter and Foranzo, 2012; Thomas, Nelson, and Silverman, 2011).

When conducting your literature search, it is important to be able to distinguish between the different types of materials that are published. When someone refers to a *serial*, they are speaking about publications that are issued on a continuing basis at more or less regular intervals. This would include periodicals, annuals, and newspapers. *Periodicals* are resources that are published "periodically" (e.g., daily, monthly, quarterly.). These resources tend to contain more current information than books because they can be published more frequently and can include publications in the form of magazines (e.g., *Maclean's, Canadian Business Weekly*) and journals.

Journals are periodicals that have a scholarly focus. Researchers should make every effort to have their research findings published in journals when their studies are complete (see Research Process Step 11). Examples of health-related journals include *Canadian Journal of Nursing, Canadian Medical Association Journal*, and *PHYSIO* journal. Many of the health-related journals that are published are classified as peer reviewed (also known as a *refereed journal*). This means that each of the articles in the journal have been evaluated by a panel of experts in the field prior to being published.

There are a series of steps that you should follow when conducting your literature review:

First, you should select and access a database that is relevant to the topic you are researching. Research databases contain thousands of published research articles (both peer reviewed and not peer reviewed). Think of a database like a filing cabinet—one main storage area and within it are thousands of individual files (research articles). The database usually focuses on a particular topic area (e.g., medicine, health, sports, nursing, etc.). Because you will be primarily interested in health-related research, you will want to consider accessing the following databases: PubMed/Medline, CINAHL (Cumulative Index to Nursing and Allied Health Literature), HealthSTAR, PsychINFO. There are many other health databases that exist; consulting a librarian will help you to identify which database is most appropriate for the work you are doing. Second, you will need to search the database for key terms related to your research. Most often searching by "keyword" is the best option as it will search for articles that have the word you have selected anywhere in the document, including the title and reference list. Note

PRACTICAL TIP

Once you have conducted your review of the literature, depending on what information exists, you may have to return to your proposed research question and adjust it accordingly.

that searching by keyword can give you more articles than you may need or that are of relevance to the topic you are studying, and you may need to refine your search in order to produce the best results. Third, you should check the results of your search to determine which articles have been published in peer reviewed journals (these are preferred because they have undergone rigorous scrutiny by subject matter experts prior to publication). Finally, select and retrieve the articles you believe will be helpful for the research that you are conducting.

Besides journal articles, another place to find up-to-date information on a variety of topics is the Internet. Researchers (regardless of level of experience) should be very cautious when accessing health care-related information as some websites are not always what they appear to be. Things to consider include: the author's qualifications, the publisher (i.e., is it a university, scholarly society, government agency, trade, non-profit, or commercial organization?), timelines (i.e., when was the resource published?), accuracy of the information that is posted and, does the source provide a bibliography of related resources? (Wilfrid Laurier University Library, n.d.) For a helpful guide to identifying quality sources on the Internet, please consult the librarians at your college or university.

Step 3: Define the Problem

Once you have come up with a topic or area that you are interested in, it may be too big of a problem area for you to address as an undergraduate, or even as a graduate student. In order to narrow it down to something that is manageable, the next step in the research process is to define what it is you want to study by preparing a problem statement—a concisely written phrase that identifies the *who*, *what*, *when*, and *where* that will be the basis for your study.

The most common reason a problem statement is considered to be poorly defined is because it is either too vague or too wordy. When you are writing about the problem you are interested in studying, it *must* be done in such a way as to be as clear, concise, and specific as possible. You should write in a **parsimonious** manner (in other words, without fluff!).

Narrowing the wording in a problem statement will help the researcher to do several things:

- focus the scope and search parameters with respect to the review of the literature (in some cases, this can mean reducing the number of articles identified by the search engine from 10 000 to 100, the latter being much more manageable, especially for a novice researcher!);
- allow for the selection of an appropriate study design (e.g., experimental, cross-sectional, etc.); and
- provide information that will help the researcher to determine the best method with which to collect the data (e.g., survey, questionnaire, etc.)

PRACTICAL TIP

Librarians are individuals who are trained in the field of library sciences. If you are uncertain of what databases are relevant for your topic area, or if you are unsure about what search terms would be most effective in producing successful searches, make sure you consult the librarian at your college, university, or local public library. Most libraries provide tutorial sessions for students to learn about database searching. Be sure to sign up for one in order to learn all about the in's and out's! You will soon discover that with their assistance, searching for relevant information can be straightforward (and less time-consuming when you do it correctly!).

You should include a description of the specific group or individuals being studied, the location where the study will take place, and the time frame or duration of the study along with the specific "thing" you want to know. The research question should also be practical and feasible—if you will need millions of dollars to study thousands of people, it is highly unlikely that your question or problem statement is appropriate for someone who is an undergraduate student. Be sure to talk the problem statement over with others—ask people with knowledge about the topic (like your professors!) as they may be able to help you narrow down the scope of what it is you wish to study.

Students often ask, "Is my problem statement good enough?" Consider the following example of a poorly written problem statement: *I am going to study drugs and school children.* Before reading on, ask yourself, "why is this a poor statement?," "how could it be improved?" The primary reason it is a poor statement is because the words "drugs" and "school children" are too vague. With respect to "drug"—what is the researcher referring to? Drugs that are bought from a pharmacist with a prescription, or purchased over the counter at a grocery store, or purchased illegally on the street? The phrase "school children" is equally unclear as it could potentially include any individual in school from kindergarten all the way through to grade 12. Perhaps a better way to re-word the problem statement would be the following: *I am going to study the effects of marijuana use on males and females between the ages of 14 and 16 years of age who live in urban city centres.*

The first column in Table 3.1 provides some examples of poorly written problem statements. The second column lists some of the reasons why the question is considered to be poorly developed, while the third column provides you with a problem statement that would be seen as "good." You

are encouraged to cover the second and third columns while you consider what is poor about the example provided (e.g., too vague, too broad, too wordy, etc.). Try to develop your own improved statement and compare it to what is suggested in the table.

Step 4: Develop the Research Question

Students read or hear about research everyday—in the media, in school, when speaking with their professors. When students have a question they would like to investigate and they would like to use research to do so, they are often at a loss as to where to start and what the research process involves. A large part of the research process (the who, the what, the where, the why, and the how of conducting a research study) is driven by the research question. A research question that is vague or unclear will only lead to vague and unclear answers. Researchers (students and professionals) must start with a well-defined research question as this will allow them to meet several important goals. First, it will provide structure and direction for the work that is to be undertaken. Second, it will allow the researcher—whether novice or experienced—to determine if they have the appropriate resources, skills, and time to successfully carry out the study. Third, it will help the researcher to be efficient, particularly when it comes to conducting a search of the literature in order to identify key journal articles and previous work in the field, and in selecting the appropriate measure for data collection and analyses.

Types of questions we can ask

Baumgartner and Hensley (2006, citing Drew, Hardman, and Hart, 1996) discuss three different types of research questions that we can formulate. First, they suggest that *descriptive questions* are those that have as their primary goal identifying

TABLE 3.1	Examples of "Poor" Problem Statements	
"Poor" problem statements	Reasons why it's a poor problem statement	Suggested re-wording for improvement
I am going to study health care among seniors.	"Health care" is too vague. Who is considered to be a "senior"? What type of senior? Where will the study take place and for how long?	I am going to study the number of office visits made to family doctors during one year by males and females between the ages of 65 and 75 who live in rural communities in Manitoba.
I am going to study people with cancer.	The type of cancer is not specified. The demographics of the "people" are unknown. The location and duration of the study are not stated. The "what" about individuals with cancer is not specified.	I am going to study the treatment experiences of males between 50 and 55 years of age who have been diagnosed with prostate cancer and who are undergoing three months of chemotherapy treatment at a cancer centre in Toronto, Ontario.
I am going to study people who live in Canada's Arctic with cancer of the third toe on their right foot that was diagnosed between May 1, 2012 and June 1, 2012.	The type of cancer to be studied is very rare. Limiting both the geographical location and the time of diagnosis to such a narrow field may not yield enough data on which to conduct meaningful statistical analyses. The cost of traveling to the Canada's arctic may be cost prohibitive. Again the "what" about individuals with cancer is not specified.	I am going to study the mobility of males and females between the ages of 30 and 75 living in Manitoba who were diagnosed with a cancer of a lower limb between January 1, 2010 and December 31, 2012.

key features of individuals or groups. For example, if you have a sample of 25 university students, what characteristics could be used to describe the group? You might say that the group consists of males and females, their ages range from 17 to 25 years, they are enrolled in the Faculty of Science, and they are all in the second year of their programs. Study designs that are qualitative in nature (e.g., focus groups) will often utilize descriptive questions to gain an in-depth understanding of a phenomenon. Quantitative studies may also include descriptive questions, but they typically seek to understand a relationship between variables.

The next question type they review are *difference questions*. With these types of questions we are trying to determine how individuals in the same group (e.g., all second-year university students) may be distinct from one another or how groups (e.g., university students in first, second, third, and fourth year) may vary. Baumgartner and Hensley note that researchers will often use difference questions in one of two ways if they are conducting an experiment. First, the researcher may wish to determine what, if any, differences exist between the subjects in the treatment or intervention group compared to the subjects in the control group. Second, this type of question can also be used to determine if there are differences for the same subject. For example, a researcher begins by testing a subject's ability to operate a novel piece of machinery (also referred to as a *pre-test*), followed by an instruction session where the subject is taught how to operate the machinery, and then the researcher tests the subject's ability to operate the machinery after they have received instructions (also known as a *post-test*). The difference in the scores from the pre-test and the post-test will allow the researcher to determine how much the subject learned.

Finally, there are *relationship questions*. When a researcher asks a relationship question, they are trying to determine ". . . the degree to which two or more variables covary or are associated with each other" (Baumgartner and Hensley, 2006: 33). One example of a relationship question could be, "*Does the incidence of asthma increase or decrease in children who live with individuals who smoke in the primary residence?*" Another example might be, "*Does the rate of heart disease decrease when individuals with high blood pressure are prescribed exercise programs?*"

How to develop the best possible question

There are many approaches that can be undertaken when developing a research question. For the purposes of this section, we will address the PICO, PICO(T), and the FINER question strategies.

PICO

According to the Centre for Evidence-Based Medicine at Oxford University (2009, para.1), well-built research questions need to be ". . . relevant to the patients' problems and phrased in ways that direct your search to relevant and precise answers." EBM is often used in clinical settings and as such, this is reflected in the development of the research question and refers to the subjects who will be the focus of the research as "patients."

PICO, a question strategy that is commonly used in EBM research, contains four essential elements (Centre for Evidence-Based Medicine, 2009): **P**, which stands for *Patient* or *Problem*, is how you would describe the patient or problem you are interested in. For example, what is the patient's age, gender, or diagnosis? **I**, which stands for *Intervention*, refers to what main intervention, prognostic factor, or exposure you are considering. For example, in your research study, will you be giving the patient a medication, are you interested in what factors might influence the prognosis of a patient with muscular dystrophy, or are you interested in whether someone was exposed to a certain chemical or toxin? The **C** in PICO stands for *Comparison* and requires you to identify what you will be comparing the main intervention with. For example, are you going to give your patient a medication (treatment) and compare the effects to a placebo group (control group)? Finally, **O** represents the *Outcomes* of interest. What is it that you would like to accomplish, measure, improve, or affect? You have to decide what it is that you are trying to do for the patient (e.g., relieve pain, improve scores on a test, eliminate symptoms, etc.). In essence, PICO tries to frame the context of the research or problem of interest in a question format, specifically with the four questions noted above.

PICO(T)

The PICO method has been expanded and one extension you might find suitable for intervention or clinical studies is PICO(T) (Haynes et al., 2006; Richardson et al., 1995; see Thabane et al., 2009 for review of use). PICO(T) stands for *population*; *intervention*; *comparison*; *outcome*; and *timeframe*. Let's take the example of a researcher interested in the effects of diet and exercise on obesity among middle-aged adults. The researcher might be interested in whether middle-aged adults (*population*) who receive a diet AND exercise program (*intervention*), fare better, worse, or the same as individuals who receive diet only, exercise only, or no intervention (*comparison intervention*) in terms of weight and waist circumference loss (*outcome*), over a six-month trial (*timeframe*). Alternatively, a researcher may be interested in developing a new drug therapy for Alzheimer's. Using PICO(T), the research question could include an older population of adults showing early signs of dementia (*population*) with some being given the new drug-therapy (*intervention*) compared to adults who receive a placebo or no drug-therapy (*comparison intervention*) on memory loss and function (*outcome*) over a five- to ten-year period (*timeframe*).

Not all research is clinical or interventional in nature. Your research may be of a qualitative nature. For example, Sinclair proposed the following study purpose:

> . . . this study explored the impact of death and dying on the lives of key leaders and frontline professionals in palliative and hospice care-individuals who arguably provide society and health care practitioners with the most authoritative discourse on end of life and its effect on life in general. This study was part of a larger ethnographic inquiry on the spirituality of palliative and hospice care professionals in Canada (2011: 180).

While the similarities and differences between qualitative and quantitative research will be explored in greater detail in later chapters of this text, you can appreciate at this stage that Sinclair's question looks quite different from the PICO(T) examples discussed above. For qualitative research questions, Mantzoukas (2008) suggests another set of guidelines (see Table 3.2). The elements of *content*, *coherence*, and *structure* advocated by Mantzoukas are apparent in Sinclair's sample research question. In terms of *content*, Sinclair's question presented a statement focused

on the "impact of death and dying" among a given population. Unlike quantitative studies, there are no *does A cause B* or *does A relate to B* underlying questions. This is what Mantzoukas is referring to as "content". *Coherence* further develops the goal of qualitative research, in Sinclair's case to "explore the impact" which covers the active verb and relevant noun for Mantzoukas. Sinclair's reference to the "larger ethnographic inquiry" provides the methodology of the *coherence* section. Finally, Mantzoukas suggests qualitative research questions require *structure* that follows from identifying the who, what, where, when, why, and/or how. In Sinclair's research question, we see the who ("key leaders and frontline professionals in palliative and hospice care"), what ("the impact of death and dying"), where ("in Canada"), why ("individuals who arguably provide society and health care practitioners with the most authoritative discourse on end of life and its effect on life in general"), and how ("part of a larger ethnographic inquiry").

As you develop your research questions there are three other considerations that you should take into account, including, operationally defining any terms, noting limitations, and delimitations (Thomas et al., 2011). Terms that you may use as part of your research question such as wellness, health, or disease all have varied meanings depending upon the context. If your question centres around health, what does that mean? Are you talking about physical, mental, and/or social health? If it is mental health, which aspect? If your focus is on anxiety disorders, what qualifies in your study as an anxiety disorder? Be sure to define any terms you use.

If you have ever read a journal article, it is likely you have come across study limitations. For example, authors of cross-sectional surveys often note that data generated from this type of design cannot infer causality. Or, authors may note that they did not achieve the desired sample

TABLE 3.2   A Framework for Formulating Qualitative Research Questions

Content	A declarative statement with a period at the end and not an interrogative one with a question mark		
	Should provide focus on the issue that will be studied		
	Should not strictly define relationships between variables		
Coherence	Commence with active verb	Incorporate relevant nouns	Indicate the methodology
	Understanding	Experiences	Interpretative phenomenology
	Exploring	Feelings	Transcendental phenomenology
	Interpreting	Views	Critical ethnography
	Constructing	Perspectives	Classical ethnography
	Explaining, etc.	Knowledge, etc.	Grounded theory
			Action research
			Exploratory study, etc.
Structure	Address five of the following six elements		
	Who will be studied		
	When will they be studied		
	Where will they be studied		
	What will be studied		
	How it will be studied		
	Why it will be studied		

Source: Reprinted from S. Mantzoukas, Facilitating research students in formulating qualitative research questions. *Nurse Education Today*, 28, 3:371–7, © 2008, with permission from Elsevier.

size of participants (e.g., the goal was for 1000 survey respondents to a mental health survey but only 50 completed it). Thomas et al. (2011) note these limitations are typically things outside of the researcher's control while delimitations are ". . . limitation(s) imposed by the researcher in the scope of the study or a choice the researcher makes to define a workable research problem" (p. 60). Typically a researcher may focus on a particular age range of participants, from a particu-

lar location, with or without a certain condition/ disease, or experience, and will selectively decide what will be measured in the study. Researchers cannot typically do it all, so they must narrow the study to fit the FINER approach (explained below) and other criteria.

The Finer approach

There are several things to consider when detailing your research question. For example, Hulley et al.'s (2007) FINER criteria for research questions, suggesting that research questions should be:

- *feasible* (Is your research question doable when you consider things such as resources, skill set, timelines etc.?)
- *interesting* (Are you excited by or passionate about the topic?)
- *novel* (What does your research question add? What gap in knowledge will your research question fill?) Has it been done before?
- *ethical* (Is your research question ethically sound?)
- *relevant* (Why is your research question important theoretically or practically?) (Hulley et al., 2007).

Thabane et al. (2009) then offer strategies for how to attain each criterion.

Step 5: Generate a Hypothesis— Prediction at Its Best!

Once you have a well-developed research question, and if you are going to be using a quantitative research design, the next step is to provide a prediction of what you think the outcome of your study is going to be. In other words, you must generate a hypothesis—a testable statement that offers a predicted relationship between dependent and independent variables (Holosko and Thyer, 2011). In other words, a hypothesis is a statement of what the researcher expects to find. You will need to generate two statements—a null hypothesis and an alternate hypothesis.

The null hypothesis states there is no significant effect of the independent variable on the dependent variable; it is denoted as Ho. An example of a null hypothesis is, "There is no difference in weight between children living in poverty and children who do not live in poverty." On the other hand, the alternate hypothesis says the independent variable has a significant effect on a dependent variable; it is

denoted as Ha. An example of an alternate hypothesis would be, "There is a difference in weight between children living in poverty and children who do not live in poverty." If you want to be very specific, you can specify direction of relationship in the alternate hypothesis. In other words, you can indicate whether the effect you are predicting will result in either an increase or decrease in the levels of the dependent variable. An example for you to try is located at the end of this chapter.

Step 6: Choose an Appropriate Study Design

Types of research studies

Research is often categorized on a continuum from basic to applied (Portney and Watkins, 2009; Thomas et al., 2011). The aim of basic research is to advance theoretical knowledge (disregarding the application of this knowledge in the field or practice setting), typically via lab-based studies (Portney and Watkins, 2009; Thomas et al., 2011). Applied research, on the other hand, is concerned with the direct application of theoretical knowledge in the field with individuals, typically in a practice or therapeutic setting (Portney and Watkins, 2009; Thomas et al., 2011).

As an example, consider the *human papillomavirus* or HPV. At one end of the continuum might be the identification of cellular, chemical, micro-biological or genetic aspects of HPV (e.g., Heller et al., 2011), moving toward the development of the HPV vaccine (see Giles and Garland, 2006 for a review), educational interventions raising awareness about HPV and the vaccine (Reiter et al., 2011), the likelihood of getting vaccinated in no-cost programs (Widgren et al., 2011), the effects of different communication-based interventions on vaccine perceptions and getting vaccinated (e.g., Hopfer, 2012), and discussions on making the vaccine available worldwide (Andrus et al., 2008; Kane, 2010 for overviews).

Before you select the study design that is best suited for your research project, be sure that you have a clear and well-defined research question. By doing so, you will be able to conduct your study in an effective manner, which in turn will allow you to answer your research question well.

Research designs

In addition to the continuum of research, the actual design of research can vary. Chapters 6 and 9 of this book will provide you with specific design information. Here, we will give you a brief overview of types of original study designs with an accompanying Canadian study example.

Portney and Watkins (2009) classify research as *experimental*, *exploratory*, or *descriptive* with various subtypes in each category. As Portney and Watkins note, ". . . randomized controlled trials [are] considered the 'gold standard' of experimental designs" (p. 22). Barr and colleagues (2009) conducted a **randomized controlled trial** (RCT) looking at the impact of different resources on new mothers' responses to their baby's crying (see Health Research in Action box 3.1). One of the main goals of experimental designs is to establish cause-effect and this is accomplished through variable manipulation and control (Portney and Watkins, 2009).

Exploratory research seeks to examine relationships or associations between variables (Portney and Watkins, 2009). Students are often cautioned that a research design might yield a conclusion that one variable *predicts* another variable; but this does not mean that one variable *causes* a particular outcome. One common type of exploratory research design is a **cohort study** (Portney and Watkins, 2009). For example,

---

3.1   Health Research in Action

Can Education Prevent Shaken Baby Syndrome?

In an effort to address shaken baby syndrome, Barr and colleagues (2009) conducted a randomized control trial to see if exposure to information related to crying and shaken baby syndrome (intervention group) versus receiving general/other infant safety information (control group) would impact new mother's responses to their crying baby and their understanding of infant crying and shaking. The authors recruited 1279 mothers from the Vancouver area. Participating women began the study five weeks postpartum. Using random assignment, the mothers in the intervention group received materials from the PURPLE Crying Program developed by the National Centre on Shaken Baby Syndrome. The mothers in the control group were given materials about injury prevention. Mothers in both groups were requested to keep a diary throughout the study. Eight weeks after the start of the study, the researchers asked all mothers to complete a questionnaire about their behavioural responses to their baby's crying, understanding of infant crying and shaking, and whether they had shared the information learned.

One of the key findings from the study was that when their baby was inconsolable, mothers in the intervention group more often reported being able to leave their crying child in a safe place to walk away for a brief break (one key strategy in shaken baby prevention). The authors also found that mothers in the intervention group discussed issues around infant crying and shaking with others more than those mothers who received only general infant safety information.

Emery et al. (2011) detailed a one-year prospective cohort study following mainly male youth hockey players to determine rates of injury, in particular concussions. The authors were specifically interested in the rates of injury/concussion depending upon whether players had played with bodychecking allowed or not.

A second common type of exploratory research, correlational, is concerned with identifying associations between variables and whether one variable may predict another (Portney and Watkins, 2009). For example, Wilson et al. (2010) wanted to know whether depression was linked with adolescents' sexual behaviours. The authors used a survey to assess the predictor variable (risk of depression) and outcomes (sexual activity and engagement in risky sexual activities). In another study (see Health Research in Action box 3.2), researchers wanted to predict the main ways youth who smoke get their contraband cigarettes (Leatherdale, Ahmed, and Vu, 2011).

Finally, research may be *descriptive* in nature with the aim to identify key participant features using quantitative data or perhaps to detail the experiences of individuals on a given topic (Portney and Watkins, 2009). A recent study sought information about how provinces track cardiac arrests experienced prior to an individual reaching the hospital (Vaillancourt et al., 2009). The authors note that Canada has no nationwide tracking program and as such they need to know about the information being collected across different provinces to inform such a program. This provides an example of the former use of descriptive research. An example of the latter use of descriptive research would be qualitative research designs. Qualitative research has been described in the following way:

> . . . since the 1970's more and more researchers have become interested in a "new paradigm" that moves us away from numbers and back to asking people questions and to observing. When we ask questions about human affairs, the responses come in sentences, not numbers. We collect as "data" narratives, or, as I like to call them, stories . . . (Tesch, 1990: 2)

Although the full nuances of qualitative research are described later (see Chapter 9),

---

3.2 Health Research in Action

How Do Contraband Cigarettes Get into the Hands of Youth Smokers?

Adding to our understanding about the culture of youth who smoke is a recent study by Leatherdale, Ahmed, and Vu (2011). Using a representative sample, Leatherdale et al. utilized data previously collected through the Canadian Youth Smoking Survey for their study. The sample utilized included data on 13,300 youth in grades 9 through 12 who smoke contraband cigarettes. The authors grouped smokers according to whether adolescents reported obtaining contraband cigarettes from a store, family member, or friend or others, and then used three categories of variables (sociodemographic, personal, and behavioural) to predict each type of cigarette acquisition.

At least one variable in all three categories of predictors influenced where adolescents obtained their contraband cigarettes. One of the findings the authors labelled as particularly "alarming" (p. 106) was the role that family members (based on parent's smoking status and parents smoking the same contraband type) played in getting contraband cigarettes for youth.

Sinclair's 2011 study where participants (who were professionals working with individuals at the end-of-life) were both observed and interviewed in order to understand how they dealt with death and dying, provides an idea of the differences in methodology from those previously described.

In some cases, you will see a research design using a combination of different methods in the same study. This is called mixed methods. For example, McCay and colleagues (2010) used both surveys and focus groups to gather information on street youth and mental health (see Health Research in Action box 3.3). Whatever design you might choose yourself, always remember that the research design should follow from your research question (Sackett and Wennberg, 1997).

Joining the research question with the study design: A beautiful marriage

Sackett and Wennberg's (1997) point that the research question should precede the study design is an important one, and is echoed by others including Stone (2002). Consider the following: someone conducting an experiment will have a research question that looks different from someone who is conducting a cohort study, even if the broader topic is similar. Stone (2002) provides an example of a cancer-related research question that requires an experimental design and contrasts this with a question requiring a qualitative study design. Expanding upon this idea, researchers have been interested in studying physical activity and mental health. Table 3.3 below provides an example of a research question (adapted from the study's purpose statement) followed by the type of design appropriate for and used in that study.

Step 7: Define the Variables and Other Key Terms

In order to develop your research question, it will be helpful to have knowledge of several key terms that are used in research methodology. Chapter 7 will go into detail about these terms, so for the time being we are only going to provide a brief overview. The terms that are in bold below can be found in the glossary at the end of the book (Holosko and Thyer, 2011).

3.3   Health Research in Action

Citing the propensity of mental health and other risks for homeless young people, and in order to develop intervention programs that are appropriate for this group of individuals, McCay et al. (2010) proposed the need for a mixed methods study to "conduct a comprehensive mental health assessment of homeless youth to increase our understanding of the challenges and strengths pertaining to street-involved youth" (p. 33). To do this, the researcher utilized a convenience sample of youth (ages 16–24) who were drawn from community agencies in Toronto, Ontario. The quantitative arm of the study saw 70 youths complete a survey with questions asking about issues such as the experience of mental illness, abuse (including physical and substance), hopelessness, self-esteem, self-harm, and suicidality. The qualitative arm of the study consisted of two focus groups to further explore youth's mental health and street life experiences. Focus groups housed between 8–10 participants who were different from those who completed the survey. The authors discuss how the findings from both arms of the study mirror one another; in both study arms the difficulties experienced by these youth (e.g., depression, substance abuse) were found along with more positive assets and outlooks (e.g., resiliency).

Variables

The first term that you should be familiar with is *variable*. In a study, the term variable refers to what is being measured, manipulated or controlled. In health research we are most often interested in the effect or influence that one variable will have on another. There are several different types of variables, but it is sufficient for the time being for you to learn about the following key types: independent; dependent, and control or situational (Thomas, Nelson, and Silverman, 2011). Following the discussion of these variables, you will be introduced to *conceptual* and *operational definitions*—two items that are important to include in your study methodology when you describe the independent and dependent variables that you will be using.

Independent and Dependent Variables

For quantitative studies, researchers typically define an independent variable and a dependent variable. If you are using an experimental research design, the primary goal is to assess whether a cause and effect relationship between two items exists and the independent variable is the thought to be the *cause*, while the dependent variable is

presumed to be the *effect* (Portney and Watkins, 2009). For such a design, the **independent variable** is the variable that is manipulated, or altered by the researcher. During the course of the study, this variable is somehow changed in order to see if it will have an influence on another variable, in this case, the dependent variable. The dependent variable represents what the researcher measures or the observed outcome, or disease of interest, in a research study. The **dependent variable** cannot be manipulated. For example, in an experimental study of how *giving different dosages of a medication* are related to the *severity of symptoms of a*

PRACTICAL TIP

- In experimental study designs, remember to ask yourself, "What is being manipulated?" and "What is being measured?"

- When using correlational study designs, variables are not manipulated but rather observed.

- In qualitative studies, researchers are often interested in understanding individuals' experiences, instead of assessing specific variables.

TABLE 3.3   Different Question Formats Based on Study Design

The Research Question	Type of Study Design
What is the ". . . association between physical activity and mental health problems in a cohort of university students"? (Tyson et al., 2010: 493)	Correlational study
What is a ". . . description of the lifestyle physical activity habits of individuals with [severe and enduring mental illness] in an outpatient setting"? (Soundy, Faulkner, and Taylor, 2007: 494)	Qualitative study
What is "the feasibility of delivering a social cognitive theory-based internet physical activity intervention to undergraduate and graduate students receiving mental health services and to examine its effects on physical activity behavior, self-efficacy, anxiety, and depression"? (Mailey et al., 2010: 648)	Experimental study
Is ". . .regular physical activity at baseline . . . prospectively associated with decreased risks of incidence of DSM-IV mental disorders in adolescence and young adulthood as the peak period for first onset of most mental disorders"? (Ströhle et al., 2007: 1658)	Cohort

disease, the administration of the drug in specified doses is the *independent variable* (cause) and the measure of the severity of the symptoms of the disease is a *dependent variable* (effect).

In other study designs, the independent variable is present but is not altered by the researcher. For example, correlational designs (where associations between variables are explored), use the independent variable as a predictor of the outcome or dependent variable (Portney and Watkins, 2009). In epidemiological study designs, the term **exposure** is used (instead of independent variable) to capture whether different individuals have certain risk factors (e.g., smoker or nonsmoker) that may impact a disease outcome (e.g., cancer; Friis and Sellers, 2009; Thomas et al., 2011).

Control variable

A third type of variable is called a **control variable** (also called a **situational variable**). This type of variable is something that the researcher may not be able to manipulate, exclude, or remove. In order to minimize the effect of this type of variable, a researcher would hold it constant throughout the study.

Students often find it difficult to identify these three types of variables in a research question. Tables 3.4 and 3.5 provide you with several research questions for experimental designs—

try to identify the independent variable (what is being manipulated) and the dependent variable (what is being measured) in each of the examples. In the last two examples, try to identify the control variable (what is being held constant).

Conceptual and operational definitions

You have successfully identified the independent variables (that will be *manipulated*) and the dependent variables (that will be *measured*) in Tables 3.3 and 3.4. The next thing that you need to do is develop a conceptual and operational definition for each variable. Don't panic as it is a relatively easy process! For starters, a **conceptual definition** is what you would find in a dictionary (Portney and Watkins, 2009). For example, if you were to look up the word "cat" in the Cat Dictionary, a conceptual definition might read, "a furry, four-footed mammal with whiskers, a tail, and loves to drink milk." Because conceptual definitions tend to be relatively vague, we need to further define the variables.

Portney and Watkins (2009) suggest that ". . . an **operational definition** defines a variable according to its unique meaning within a study . . . Independent variables are operationalized according to how they are manipulated by the investigator . . . Dependent variables are operationally defined by describing the method of measurement . . ." (p. 131, 132).

TABLE 3.4 Independent and Dependent: Can You Spot Them?		
Research question	Independent variable (what is being manipulated?)	Dependent variable (what is being measured?)
Do hot peppers on pizza cause heartburn?	Hot peppers	Heartburn
Does having unprotected sexual intercourse increase the risk of contracting HIV?	Unprotected sexual intercourse	Contracting HIV
Does the number of head injuries sustained during one season of playing hockey cause a person to develop chronic concussion syndrome?	Number of head injuries	Development of chronic concussion syndrome

TABLE 3.5 Independent, Dependent, and Control Variables: Can You Spot Them?

Research Question	Independent Variable (what is being *manipulated*?)	Dependent Variable (what is being *measured*?)	Control Variables (what are being held *constant*?)
An auto manufacturer wants to know how bright brake lights should be in order to minimize the time required for the driver of a following car to realize that the car in front is stopping.	Intensity/brightness of the brake light	Time of onset of brake light until depression of brake pedal by the driver following	Colour of the brake light; shape of the brake light; force needed to apply the brake pedal
A pigeon is trained to peck a key if a green light is illuminated but not if the light is red. Correct pecks get rewarded by access to grain.	Colour of the light (red or green)	Number of pecks	Size of the key; intensity of the light; shade of green and red; number of hours without food

Clearly stated operational definitions allow other researchers to understand exactly what is being measured or altered, and in most cases, how it is being measured.

Consider the following example: The Montréal Canadiens hockey team is interested in finding out whether increasing the type of pre-game music will lead to higher levels of excitement among the fans during the home games.

- What is the independent variable (recall: it is what is being *manipulated* in the study)?

If you said, "pre-game music" you are correct!

- How would you define "pre-game music" (recall: a *conceptual definition* is a general definition that is typically used to describe the independent variable)?

Merriam-Webster defines music as "vocal, instrumental, or mechanical sounds having rhythm, melody, or harmony" (www.merriam-webster.com/dictionary/music)

- How would "pre-game music" be operationally defined? (recall: an *operational definition* will specifically describe what the independent variable entails)

For the purpose of this study, "pre-game music would consist of playing current pop music OR country music on the arena sound system until the puck is dropped on the ice signifying the official start of the game."

- What is the dependent variable (recall: it is what is the outcome being *measured* in the study)?

If you said, "level of excitement" you are correct!

- What is a general definition of "excitement"?

Merriam-Webster defines excitement as "something that…rouses" (www.merriam-webster.com/dictionary/excitement?show=0&t=1369750802)

- How would you measure "excitement" (recall: an *operational definition* will specifically describe how the dependent variable will be measured)?

One example of an operational definition could be, "level of excitement will be measured by the number of decibels being captured on a digital oscilloscope from the time the first note on the organ is played, until the last note is played when the puck is dropped."

You could go into greater detail and indicate that a level of "no" excitement will have a reading of 0 decibels, a level of "medium" excitement will have a reading of 50 decibels, and a level of "high" excitement will have a reading of 100 decibels.

Another example may be, "level of excitement will be measured by the number of fans standing up from their seats from the time the first note of pre-game music is played until the last note of pre-game music is played. No level of excitement will be recorded if no fans are standing; medium levels of excitement will be recorded if 500 fans are standing; high levels of excitement will be recorded if 1000 fans are standing."

If you would like more practice, turn back to Tables 3.3 and 3.4, and try to develop conceptual definitions and operational definitions for the variables. More information on independent and dependent variables can also be found in Chapter 7 on experimental design.

People and Groups

The term *subject* refers to an individual who is participating in an experimental research study. For non-experimental studies, individuals are typically referred to as **participants**.

In an experiment, subjects are assigned to one of two groups. In the **treatment group** subjects receive the item that is being tested or manipulated (e.g., drug, food) whereas subjects in the control group do not receive the item that is being tested.

Subjects can be assigned to either group using what is called **random assignment** (everyone has an equal chance of being placed in either the treatment or control group) or on-purpose assignment where the researcher controls which subjects are placed into which groups.

When assigning subjects to either the treatment or control groups, researchers can also use a blind or double-blind approach. If the researcher uses **blind assignment**, then they know which group the subject is being assigned to (i.e., treatment or control) but the subject does not know. If a **double-blind assignment approach** is used, neither the researcher collecting the data nor the subject knows which group the subject belongs to.

Placebo

The term placebo is one that is commonly found in health-related research, particularly randomized clinical drug trials. A **placebo** is an inactive substance that resembles the medication being tested in all ways except it is inert (it has no medicinal properties). Placebos are generally given for psychological effect or as a control in evaluating a medicine believed to be active. A placebo may be compared with a new drug when no one knows if any drug or treatment will be effective.

Step 8: Identify the Participant/ Subject/Study Population of Interest

Before you develop your research question, you should be clear about *who* or *what* is going to be the focus of your study. In other words, are you going to study people, plants, or animals? Something else? Depending on what you are going to study, you should identify other key descriptors that will help you in the selection of your subjects or participants. At a minimum, you should indicate the age range of individuals who will be eligible to participate (e.g., 18–24 months old; 65–85 years old), and the gender of your subjects or participants (e.g., males only, females only, or both). Depending on what exactly you are studying, there are other descriptors you might want to include such as weight, height, level of education, health status, etc.

The method used to determine exactly how many subjects (*sample size*), participants, or cases are required for a particular study is beyond the scope of this text. It is sufficient for you to know at this time that it is very important for the researcher to determine how many subjects or participants will be needed to provide enough data to adequately answer the research question. Bear in mind that a sample size that is too small will not yield enough information from which to draw accurate conclusions, whereas a sample size that is too large can have a significant impact on the study, particularly as it relates to costs associated with implementing the study, as well as the time that will be required to carry out the study. Finally, thought should be given to whether or not the number and type of subjects or participants that you will require for your study are in fact available. If you are interested in studying a very unique and rare disease, you may need 50 people for your study, but only two live in close enough proximity to you that they could actually participate in the study.

Step 9: Conduct the Study

Congratulations! You have successfully completed all of the previous steps in the research process and you are now ready to conduct your study. But before you do, there are a few more points that you should be aware of that will help you to avoid significant errors/problems during the course of your study. You may want to sit down with your supervisor or an experienced researcher to review each of the following points *PRIOR* to starting your study:

- Do you have signed approval from your REB/IRB to proceed with the study? You must have REB/IRB approval prior to starting your study.
- Have you developed a draft timetable that highlights each of the steps in the research process? Start with the date the findings for your study are due, and work backwards. For

students who have received funding to conduct their study, they should be particularly careful that their timetable will allow them to meet deadlines set out by a funding agency. Failure to do so can result in the agency revoking the funds, or not allowing you to apply for funds in the future.

- Given your study design, the number of subjects or participants to be tested, and the type of analysis that you are going to conduct, have you allocated a sufficient amount of time to do the study? Bear in mind there could be delays because of your subjects or participants (i.e., they could withdraw, get sick, miss testing sessions), your equipment could break down, your research assistants (possibly students themselves) may not be able to test subjects or participants as often as you would like because they have other commitments, and it is not beyond the realm of possibility that you, as the researcher, may also encounter unexpected events (e.g., the dentist appointment you have been waiting six months for is on the same day that you would like to test ten subjects!) Novice student researchers are often keen and enthusiastic but unfortunately they also tend to underestimate the length of time it will take to complete what they have set out to do. Learning how long a study will take from start (developing the research question) to finish (knowledge translation and future recommendations), will come with time and experience. Until then, be sure to have your supervisor, professor, or instructor review your timetable with you and allow them to adjust it accordingly.
- Have you developed a budget that covers all your expenses (and a little bit extra)? Items to consider in your budget include: equipment costs, rental charges for rooms, compensation for your subjects or participants,

PRACTICAL TIP

The motto that researchers should follow when conducting a study is to "expect the unexpected and plan accordingly." Allow the timetable to be adjusted and be generous when setting start and end dates. A good rule of thumb is to build in at least 25 per cent "extra in-case" time!

printing of materials, food for animal subjects, and miscellaneous fees (e.g., parking for your subjects or participants). When developing your budget, if it includes paying research assistants, be sure to contact the human resources department of your school or health care facility to determine what the hourly rate of pay should be, along with the percentage that must be allocated for benefits.

- Given that you probably have relatively little experience with designing and implementing a study, it is important to make sure that you will have support from your supervisor (or their graduate student research assistant, or lab instructor) throughout the course of the study so that they can help troubleshoot if a problem arises.

- When designing your study, make sure that you will have access to the necessary resources (e.g., human, financial, physical) to successfully conduct your study.

Step 10: Data Analyses

Once you have collected all your data, you will want to analyze it in order to determine the results. Determining what statistical tests you need to use in order to do this will depend on the type of study

methodology you used. Chapter 9 (qualitative methods) and Chapter 11 (quantitative methods) will help you sort out what type of analyses you need to conduct.

Step 11: Getting the Word Out there—Writing about Your Study

Your study is completed, you have analyzed the data and you have found some pretty interesting results. The next step in the research process is to write about what you did, how you did it, and what your results are. There are several formats that can be used. First, if you have received funds from an agency (including the university) to conduct your study, you will be required to prepare a written report. The specific information and format of the report will be available from the funding agency. Students are strongly encouraged to follow the parameters set out for them, as well as to submit the completed report in full and on time (failing to do so can affect chances for future funding). Second, with the assistance of your supervisor, you should prepare the written report in the form of a manuscript that can be submitted to a journal for review (and hopefully publication!). By having your work published, you are contributing to the field of literature (much like the one you researched at the beginning of the research process) and you are demonstrating your ability to carry out a study from start to finish. Review the directions for the preparation of the manuscript for the journal that you are interested in submitting to as the instructions for each journal may vary slightly. With respect to authorship, be sure to give credit where credit is due! Individuals who were actively involved in your study should be included on your manuscript (your supervisor can help you with which name goes in what order!), as well as an acknowledgement for others who may have helped along the way.

The process of sharing your written findings with others is known as *knowledge translation* (see Chapter 13 for further details); it is a crucial part of any research study. When preparing your report, be sure to be thorough and accurate in the writing about the information that is being presented.

Step 12: Amend the Research Question or Generate a New One

Just when you think you have finished everything, it's time to start again! Based on what you have learned from your study (and the experiences gained along the way), you now have two choices: (1) amend the research question you developed and adapt your study accordingly; or (2) generate a whole new question and start a new research study. You might want to consider including a section entitled, "Future Directions" when you are preparing your final report. Within this section, you can provide some ideas as to what could/should be changed in future studies based on your experience with this study (e.g., would you recommend that there be more subjects next time? Would you suggest a different way to collect the data?). The "Future Directions" section is often a great launching pad for other researchers to generate new studies.

Remember, the research process is "cyclical; can be entered at almost any point; is a never ending process; will cause you to reconsider your practice; and will return you to a different starting place (Blaxter et al., 2010: 10)."

Summary

Now that you have completed the reading for this chapter, you should be able to complete the learning objectives stated on the first page of the chapter.

Throughout the chapter, you were presented with a lot of information, including the following:

- Chapter Overview
- Learning Objectives
- Evidence Based Medicine: The Foundation of Health Research
- The Role of the Researcher
- The Research Process: Research Made Easy in 12 Steps
- Step 1: Identify the research topic, idea or problem that's right for you
- Step 2: The literature search: What's already out there?
- Step 3: Define the problem
- Step 4: Develop the research question
- Step 5: Generate a hypothesis: Prediction at its best!
- Step 6: Choose an appropriate study design
- Step 7: Define the variables and other key terms
- Step 8: Identify the participants/subjects
- Step 9: Conduct the study
- Step 10: Data analyses
- Step 11: Getting the word out there: Writing about your study
- Step 12: Amend the research question or generate a new one?

Review Questions

1. Identify the 12 steps in the research process outlined in this chapter.

2. List and describe two roles that a researcher has in a research study.

3. What does the acronym PICO stand for?

4. Identify the PICO in the following question:

   For patients with congestive heart failure (CHF), what is the effect of pre-hospital continuous positive air pressure (CPAP) in comparison to hospital application of CPAP on the length of hospital stay for the patients?

5. Identifying the independent and dependent variables:

   Dr Imanut wants to examine whether a new drug increases the maze running performance of older rats. Just like aging humans, older rats show signs of poorer memory for new things. Dr Imanut teaches two groups of older rats to find a piece of tasty rat chow in the maze. One group of rats is given the new drug while they are learning the maze. The second group is not given the drug. One week after the rats learned the maze he retests the rats and records how long it takes them to find the rat chow.

   A.   What is the independent variable?

   Hint: What did the researcher manipulate (allow to vary) in this study?

   a.   *age of the rats*

   b.   *type of maze*

   c.   *length of time it took the rats to run the maze*

   d.   *presence or absence of the new drug*

   B.   What is the dependent variable?

   Hint: What was the measure of the research subjects' responses?

   a.   *age of the rats*

   b.   *type of maze*

   c.   *length of time it took the rats to run the maze*

   d.   *presence or absence of the new drug*

6. Dr Insomniac is interested in determining whether staying up all night before an exam will have an effect on the outcome of the exam.

   State the null hypothesis for the study.

   State the alternate hypothesis, including the direction of his results, for the study.

7. What is one of the main distinguishing factors between experimental and other research designs?

Recommended Readings and Websites

Holosko, M.J. and Thayer, B.A. (2011). *Pocket glossary for commonly used research terms*. Washington, DC: Sage Publications.

Sackett, D.L. Straus, S.E., Richardson, W.S., Rosenberg, W. and Haynes, R.B. (2000). *Evidence-based medicine: How to practice and teach EBM* (2nd edition). Churchill Livingstone: Edinburgh.

US Agency for Healthcare Research and Quality (AHRQ). Retrieved from www.ahrq.gov.

Canadian Institutes of Health Research (CIHR). Retrieved from www.cihr-irsc.gc.ca/e/193.html.

Evidence-Based Behavioral Practice. Retrieved from www.ebbp.org.

Health Canada. Retrieved from www.hc-sc.gc.ca/index-eng.php.

National Council on Research Ethics. Retrieved from www.ncehr-cnerh.org.

Natural Sciences and Engineering Research Council of Canada (NSERC). Retrieved from www.nserc-crsng.gc.ca/index_eng.asp.

Public Health Agency of Canada. Retrieved from www.cihr-irsc.gc.ca/e/193.html.

Social Sciences and Humanities Research Council of Canada (SSHRC). Retrieved from www.sshrc-crsh.gc.ca/Default.aspx.

Statistics Canada. Retrieved from www.statcan.gc.ca/start-debut-eng.html.

The Cochrane Collection. Retrieved from www.ebscohost.com/academic/cochrane-collection-plus.

References

Andrus, J. K., Sherris, J., Fitzsimmons, J.W., Kane, M. A., and Aguado, M. T. (2008) Introduction of human papillomavirus vaccines into developing countries: International strategies for funding and procurement. *Vaccine,* 26(Suppl 10), K87–K92.

Barr, R.G., Barr, M., Fujiwara, T., Conway, J., Catherine, N., and Brant, R. (2009) Do educational materials change knowledge and behavior about crying and shaken baby syndrome? A randomized controlled trial. *Canadian Medical Association Journal,* 180, 727–33.

Baumgartner, T.A., and Hensley, L.D. (2006) *Conducting and Reading Research in Health and Human Performance.* 4th ed. Boston: McGraw-Hill.

Blaxter, L., Hughes, C., and Tight, M. (2010) *How to Research.* 4th ed. Berkshire: Open University Press.

Buckingham, J., Fisher, B. and Saunders, D. (2007). *Evidence-based medicine: mini-manual.* Retrieved from www.library.ualberta.ca/uploads/HealthSciences/200717155.pdf.

Canadian Press. (2011) ER doctors want mandatory CPR training in high school, say it could help save lives. October 13. Retrieved from www.globalnews.ca/Pages/Story.aspx?id=6442500543.

CBC News. (2011) Vaccine-autism tie "an elaborate fraud": journal. January 7. Retrieved from www.cbc.ca/news/health/story/2011/01/05/autism-vaccine.html.

Centre for Evidence-Based Medicine. (2009) Asking focused questions. Retrieved from www.cebm.net/index.aspx?o=1036.

DePoy, E., and Gitlin, L.N. (2011) *Introduction to Research: Understanding and Applying Multiple Strategies.* 4th ed. St. Louis, Missouri: Elsevier.

Durbin, C.G. (2004) How to come up with a good research question: Framing the hypothesis. *Respiratory Care,* 49, 1195–8.

EBBP (2013) *Evidence-Based Behavioral Practice.* Northwestern University. Available from www.ebbp.org.

Emery, C., Kang, J., Shrier, I., Goulet, C., et al. (2011) Risk of injury associated with bodychecking experience among youth hockey players. *Canadian Medical Association Journal*, 183, 1249–56.

Friis, R. H. and Sellers, T.A. (2009) *Epidemiology for Public Health Practice*. 4th ed. Sudbury, MA: Jones and Bartlett.

Giles, M. and Garland, S. (2006) Human papillomavirus infection: An old disease, a new vaccine. *Australian and New Zealand Journal of Obstetrics and Gynaecology*, 46, 180–5.

Gravetter, F.J. and Forzano, L.-A. B. (2012). *Research Methods for the Behavioural Sciences*. 4th ed.Belmont, CA: Wadsworth Cengage Learning.

Haynes, R.B., Sackett, D.L., Guyatt, G.J., and Tugwell, P. S. (2006) *Clinical Epidemiology: How to do Clinical Practice Research*. 3rd ed. Philadelphia, PA: Lippincott Williams and Wilkins.

Heller, C., Weisser, T., Mueller-Schickert, A., Rufer, E., et al. (2011) Identification of key amino acid residues that determine the ability of high risk HPV16-E7 to dysregulate major histocompatibility complex class I expression. *Journal of Biological Chemistry*, 286, 10983–97.

Hjorland, B. Evidence-based practice: an analysis based on the philosophy of science. *Journal of the American Society for Information Science and Technology*, 62(7), 1301–10.

Holosko, B.A. and Thyer, M.J. (2011) *Pocket Glossary for Commonly Used Research Terms*. Washington, DC: Sage.

Hopfer, S. (2012). Effects of a narrative HPV vaccination intervention aimed at reaching college women: A randomized controlled trial. *Prevention Science*, 13(2), 173–82.

Hulley, S.B., Cummings, S.R., Browner, W. S., Grady, D.G., and Newman, T.B. (2007) *Designing Clinical Research*. 3rd ed. Philadelphia: Lippincott Williams and Wilkins.

Kane, M.A., (2010) Global implementation of human papillomavirus (HPV) vaccine: Lessons from hepatitis B vaccine. *Gynecologic Oncology*, 117, S32–S35.

Leatherdale, S.T., Ahmed, R., and Vu, M. (2011) Factors associated with different cigarette access behaviours among underage smoking youth who usually smoke contraband (native) cigarettes. *Canadian Journal of Public Health*, 102, 103–7.

Mantzoukas, S. (2008) Facilitating research students in formulating qualitative research questions. *Nurse Education Today*, 28, 371–7.

Mailey, E.L., Wojcicki, T.R., Motl, R.W., Hu, L. et al. (2010) Internet-delivered physical activity intervention for college students with mental health disorders: A randomized pilot trial. *Psychology, Health, and Medicine*, 15, 646–59.

McCay, E., Langley, J., Beanlands, H., Cooper, L., et al. (2010) Mental health challenges and strengths of street-involved youth: The need for a multi-determined approach. *Canadian Journal of Nursing Research*, 42(3), 30–49.

Neutens, J.J. and Rubinson, L. (2010). *Research Techniques for the Health Sciences*. 4th ed. San Francisco: Benjamin Cummings.

Ogilvie, M. (2011) HIV vaccine developed in Canada approved for human studies. Retrieved from www.thestar.com/news/canada/article/1104653--canadian-developed-hiv-vaccine-approved-for-human-studies.

Portney, L.G. and Watkins, M.P. (2009) *Foundations of Clinical Research: Applications to Practice*. 3rd ed. Upper Saddle River, NJ: Pearson Education.

Reiter, P.L., Stubbs, B., Panozzo, C.A., Whitesell, D., and Brewer, N. T. (2011) HPV and HPV vaccine education intervention: Effects on parents, healthcare staff, and school staff. *Cancer Epidemiology Biomarkers Prevention*, 20, 2354–61.

Richardson, W.S., Wilson, M.C., Nishikawa, J., and Haywood, R.S. (1995) The well-built clinical question: a key to evidence-based decisions. *ACP Journal Club*, 123, A12–A13.

Sackett, D.L., Rosenberg, W.C., Gray, J.A.M., Haynes, R.B., and Richardson, W.S. (1996) Evidence based medicine: What it is and what it isn't. *British Medical Journal*, 312, 71–2.

Sackett, D.L. and Wennberg, J.E. (1997) Choosing the best research design for each question: It's time to stop squabbling over the "best" methods. *British Medical Journal*, 315, 1636.

Sinclair, S. (2011) Impact of death and dying on the personal lives and practices of palliative and hospice care professionals. *Canadian Medical Association Journal*, 183, 180–7. doi: 10.1503/cmaj.100511 p. 180.

Soundy, A., Faulkner, G., and Taylor, A. (2007) Exploring variablility and perceptions of lifestyle physical activity among individuals with severe and enduring mental health problems: A qualitative study. *Journal of Mental Health*, 16, 493–503.

Ströhle, A., Höfler, M., Pfister, H., Müller, A-G. et al. (2007) Physical activity and prevalence and incidence of mental disorders in adolescents and young adults. *Psychological Medicine*, 37, 1657–66.

Tesch, R. (1990) *Qualitative Research: Analysis Types and Software Tools*. New York: RoutledgeFalmer.

Thabane, L., Thomas, T., Ye, C., and Paul, J. (2009) Posing the research question: Not so simple. *Canadian Journal of Anaesthesiology, 56*, 71–9.

Thomas, J.R., Nelson, J.K., and Silverman, S.J. (Eds). (2011) *Research Methods in Physical Activity*. 6th ed. Champaign, IL: Human Kinetics.

Tyson, P., Wilson, K., Crone, D., Brailsford, R., and Laws, K. (2010) Physical activity and mental health in a student population. *Journal of Mental Health*, 19, 492–9.

Vaillancourt, C., Charette, M., Stiell, I.G., Phillips, K.R., and Wells, G.A. (2010) Out-of hospital cardiac arrest surveillance in Canada: A survey of national resources. *Canadian Journal of Emergency Medicine*, 12, 119–27.

Valiga, T.M. and Mermel. V.M. (1985) Formulating the researchable question. *Topics in Clinical Nursing, 7*(2), 1–14.

Widgren, K., Simonsen, J., Valentiner-Branth, P., and Molback, K. (2011) Uptake of the human papillomavirus-vaccination within the free-of-charge childhood vaccination programme in Denmark. *Vaccine*, 29, 9663–7.

Wilfrid Laurier University Library. (n.d.). Finding quality on the internet. Available at https://library.wlu.ca/help/activity/evaluating-sources/finding-quality-internet

Wilson, K., Ashbridge, M., Kisely, S., and Langille, D. (2010) Associations of risk of depression with sexual risk taking among adolescents in Nova Scotia high schools. *Canadian Journal of Psychiatry*, 55, 577–85.

4

You've Been Asked to Conduct a Systematic Review: What You Need to Know

Maureen Dobbins

CHAPTER OUTLINE

Clinical Scenario

You are a third year nursing student in a Bachelor of Nursing program and you have just been informed of your clinical placement for the coming term. You are excited to learn that you have been assigned a placement with the local public health department in the school health program. Upon attending your first day you learn you have been paired with a public health nurse who provides health promotion services to several elementary schools in the city. This public health nurse will be your preceptor during the term, meaning you will work with her at the schools she provides services to during the term. During the course of your first day you participate in a meeting at one of the schools. Those in attendance include your preceptor, the school principal, several teachers, and the school social worker. The purpose of the meeting is to discuss strategies to address school bullying, given it was recently identified as a priority issue amongst students attending the school and their parents. A recent survey indicated that more than 50 per cent of students reported being bullied in the past year, and more than 35 per cent of parents expressed concern over their child being bullied at school. Also, few parents appeared to be aware their child was being bullied, indicating that some children were not informing their parents and potentially trying to deal with the bullying on their own. Several strategies are identified during the meeting to reduce bullying in the school. However, when your preceptor asks for evidence on the effectiveness of these strategies, no one can cite any relevant research evaluating their impact. Your preceptor suggests that no further action be taken until a review of the literature could be done to assess the effectiveness of various school-based anti-bullying interventions. The meeting is adjourned with a plan to reconvene in two months upon which time the results of the literature review would be presented. You are excited to be a part of this initiative until your preceptor indicates this would be an excellent project for you to take on as part of the deliverables for your clinical placement. You have never systematically reviewed the literature before even though you have done research in the past for several papers for your undergraduate courses. Your preceptor suggests you read the Cochrane Handbook to familiarize yourself with how to conduct a systematic review evaluating the effectiveness of interventions. After reading the handbook, you are now ready to get started.

Systematic Reviews

When your preceptor suggested you do a **systematic review** your first question might be, "what is a systematic review?" Your second question might be, "why isn't that single study I heard about recently on anti-bullying sufficient?"

You decide to conduct a Google search of the term "systematic review" and you end up on The Campbell Collaboration website where you find the following definition: "A systematic review is a literature review focused on a research question that tries to identify, appraise, select and synthesize all high quality research evidence relevant to that question" (Campbell Collaboration, 2013). However, while this definition sounds reasonable, you recall discussions in your undergraduate courses about the importance of using high quality sources of information. You realize that Google may not have led you to a high quality source of information and remember that the Cochrane Handbook also provided a definition of a systematic review. You find the following in the **Cochrane Handbook**: "A systematic review attempts to collate all empirical evidence that fits pre-specified eligibility criteria in order to answer a specific research question. It uses explicit, systematic methods that are selected with a view to minimizing **bias**, thus providing more reliable findings from which conclusions can be drawn and decisions made" (Antman et al., 1992; Oxman and Guyatt, 1993). As you consider these definitions it becomes clear to you that your task will have you search for all studies evaluating the effect of school-based anti-bullying interventions, appraise how well those studies were conducted, and finally use the best studies upon which to draw conclusions about the overall effectiveness of the anti-bullying interventions. While intuitively this makes sense, it does not explain why a recently published single study is not sufficient in answering a question about intervention effectiveness.

Purpose of Research

The answer to this latter question causes us to consider what the purpose of research is. Research generally is about testing theories, often generated by previous studies, and applying them to real world situations, to determine definitive and comprehensive answers (Shuttleworth, 2008). For example, if what we want to know is whether a particular anti-bullying intervention is effective in reducing bullying, we conduct a study evaluating one or more anti-bullying interventions. The interventions may be derived from theories that suggest by addressing the underlying reasons for bullying, bullies may be less likely to act in this way. Therefore, we form hypotheses about whether or not interventions are likely to reduce bullying by addressing the factors that underlie that behaviour. The end goal of this inquiry is to apply the knowledge gained from this study to the whole population. However, it is not feasible or ethical to include the entire sample, in this case, school attending children. Therefore, we choose a sample of children to include in our study, with the intent of generalizing what we learn from this sample of children to all children. However, in choosing a **sample** of children we instantly introduce bias into our study: from the way in which we choose the children, and by the

fact that these particular children may not fully represent the whole population of children to whom we want to apply the results of our study. In fact, if we were to rerun the study 100 times, choosing a new sample of children each time, we would end up with 100 unique samples; the mechanics of the sampling process are elaborated in Chapter 8, and analysis in Chapter 9. This is depicted in Figure 4.1.

Furthermore, if we had 100 unique samples of children that represent the overall population to varying degrees, then each of those studies would produce different results. This difference (which could be 100 different results across studies) could vary quite dramatically from showing a large, **statistically significant** positive effect (less bullying), to no effect (no change in bullying), to a large, statistically significant negative effect (more bullying). The "true" result for this population would lie somewhere within this range, and while an oversimplification, one way to determine what the overall result would be across all studies would be to find the average of all these results (this will be discussed in greater

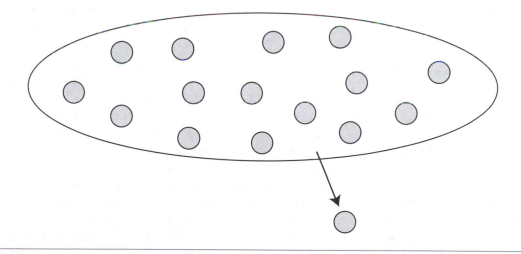

FIGURE 4.1   Samples of single studies drawn from the population as a whole

detail later in this chapter). If one were to rely on the result of just one of these 100 studies to identify the effect of the intervention, that result may be considerably different from the average, and therefore may lead one to draw conclusions about the effectiveness of the intervention that would be different than if the result from another study was used.

This brings us back to the question of why we cannot simply refer to the results of a recently released study on bullying. The results of single studies help health care practitioners stay aware of new emerging knowledge in particular topic areas. However, in instances where decisions concerning the provision of health care services are being made, it is important to base those decisions on all the available studies, so as to ensure that the decision takes into account results that better reflect the effect of an intervention for a whole population, rather than one much smaller sample within that population. Systematic reviews therefore use explicit methods aimed at minimizing bias in order to produce more reliable findings that can be used to inform decision making (The Cochrane Collaboration, 2009).

Steps in Conducting a Systematic Review

Now that you understand what a systematic review is and why a single study is insufficient to base health care decisions upon, you are ready to start working through the steps involved in conducting a systematic review. There are many organizations around the world conducting systematic reviews. The most well-known of those is The Cochrane Collaboration, which is an international, independent, not-for-profit organization dedicated to making up-to-date, accurate information about the effects of health

care readily available worldwide. Cochrane Reviews are intended to help providers, practitioners, and patients make informed decisions about health care, and are the most comprehensive, reliable and relevant source of evidence on which to base these decisions (The Cochrane Collaboration, 2013). To aid in the conduct of systematic reviews of the highest methodological quality, the Cochrane Collaboration developed a handbook that explicitly outlines each step in the process. The handbook is continually updated as new knowledge with respect to systematic review methodology becomes available.

What distinguishes a systematic review from other types of reviews is that the process of conducting the review is clearly articulated, that this process is decided a priori (before the review is started), and that the process does not change throughout the course of conducting the review (The Cochrane Collaboration, 2009). Furthermore, as each step in the process is conducted, more than one person completes each task. For example, when **screening** the results of database searches, two people independently screen the database search results set for potentially relevant studies. The two independent reviewers then meet to discuss and resolve any differences they have. For each step in the process of conducting a systematic review, two **independent raters** complete each task.

There are many steps in conducting a systematic review including: defining the research question; identifying inclusion and exclusion criteria; searching for studies; selecting studies; assessing **methodological quality** of the included studies; extracting relevant data from each included study; analyzing the data; interpreting the results; and drawing conclusions. Each step will now be described in greater detail. However, these steps are more fully described in the Cochrane Handbook, and readers are encouraged to refer to the handbook when conducting a systematic review (The Cochrane Collaboration, 2009).

Defining the Research Question

A well-done systematic review can only be conducted when the research question the review is intended to answer is focused and clearly articulated. A focused and clearly articulated research question addresses the following components as specifically as possible: population of interest; intervention you want to know the effectiveness of; what the intervention is being compared to; and the outcomes you want to learn about. This is referred to as PICO (see Chapter 3 for more details). A clearly articulated research question using PICO as the template is advantageous for at least two reasons: (1) it helps the review authors focus on exactly what their question is; and (2) it helps readers of the review identify very quickly if the review is relevant for their practice question. Let us think about the PICO components that are relevant for the systematic review you are embarking on in the scenario. The population of interest is school attending children. We may want to further refine our question to focus on children attending elementary school; therefore, children aged 5–12. Next we need to identify the intervention(s) we are interested in. For the scenario we could focus our interventions on school-based anti-bullying interventions. Therefore we will limit our search to interventions that occur in the school setting, and are focused on reducing bullying behaviour. We then need to identify what we are comparing these interventions to. For our scenario, we could compare school-based anti-bullying interventions to standard practice; in other words, what schools currently have in place to reduce bullying behaviour. Finally, we need to identify what outcome(s) we want to know about. For our scenario the outcome of greatest interest could be the number of reported bullying episodes during a given school year. The PICO components addressing our scenario are included in Table 4.1. A focused and

TABLE 4.1 PICO Components for Anti-bullying Review

P (population)	children aged 5–12 years
I (intervention)	school-based anti-bullying interventions
C (comparison)	standard practice
O (outcome)	number of reported bullying episodes during school year

clearly articulated research question would read as follows: Among children aged 5–12 years, what is the effectiveness of school-based anti-bullying interventions in comparison to standard practice, on the number of reported bullying episodes during the school year?

It is important to spend time ensuring that the PICO components are fully developed and clearly articulated. Failure to fully develop the research question may result in having to start over again after the review has started, and studies were retrieved and assessed, because it is discovered partway through the process that the research question does not fully address what was needed. For example, if after starting the review you were to determine that any one of the PICO components had to be changed (different population, intervention, comparison, outcome), then the search for all relevant studies would have to be redone. To avoid such events it is well worth spending the time at the outset ensuring the research question and decisions made about the specific PICO components are fully explored a priori.

Inclusion and Exclusion Criteria

The independent reviewers need a set of inclusion and exclusion criteria to follow in order to make consistent decisions about which studies to include or not. Furthermore, all reviewers need to understand how to apply the criteria consistently across studies. **Inclusion criteria** identify what a study needs to address in order to be included in the review (i.e., a particular population, intervention, outcome), and **exclusion criteria** identify situations and circumstances in which a study will not be included (i.e., certain populations, interventions, or outcomes). Inclusion criteria can also delineate the type of research designs that will be included as well as a time frame of when the study was published. In Table 4.2 below, specific inclusion and exclusion criteria relevant for the anti-bullying review are presented.

Inclusion and exclusion criteria are essential to conducting a rigorous systematic review because they reduce bias in the selection of studies. Demonstrating that a study meets certain criteria to be included, or didn't meet certain criteria and is therefore excluded, sets the reader at ease that the studies included in the review are not biased toward finding a particular result by systematically including or excluding particular studies. It is useful to remember that the purpose of conducting a systematic review is to identify all of the studies addressing a particular issue, and to remove those that do not. Therefore, this is a crucial step early in the review process. Once the criteria have been identified and articulated, it is important to determine that all reviewers consistently apply the criteria across all identified studies. This will be described in more detail below under the section "Searching for Studies".

Searching for Studies

In this instance the inclusion criteria stipulate that only **randomized controlled trials** (RCT) will be included in the review, and as such this identifies particular databases in which RCTs are likely to be found. For a refresher on what an RCT is, refer to Chapter 6. It is important to note however that systematic reviews can include research designs other than RCTs. However, for this particular question you expect to find a number of RCTs, and given that they are the most rigorous way to evaluate the effectiveness of an intervention, you decide to limit your search to RCTs. For systematic reviews it is extremely important that a comprehensive search be conducted so that all relevant studies are identified and included. The word all refers to studies that are published or not, and studies published in any language. It is important that the strategy to find studies does not systematically exclude certain types of studies (for example, **unpublished studies**), as this may bias the results in a particular direction. At the completion of the review it is important that readers have confidence that all relevant studies were included in the review.

TABLE 4.2 Inclusion and Exclusion Criteria	
Inclusion Criteria	Exclusion Criteria
• Randomized controlled trials published in the past 10 years	• Interventions implemented outside of school setting
• Includes children aged 5–12 years	• Participants have history of violent behaviour
• Interventions implemented in the school setting	• Interventions focused on anger management
• Interventions focused on reducing bullying behaviour	• Outcome measured as severity of bullying episodes
• Data on bullying events reported	

A comprehensive **search strategy** includes searching relevant electronic databases as well as other approaches, because not all studies will be indexed in electronic databases. In searching electronic databases it is first important to include all databases that address the relevant content. Therefore it is important to understand what content will be found in different databases. For example, Medline includes studies related to biomedical literature, which includes activities and applications of science to clinical medicine (U.S. National Library of Medicine, 2013). The Cumulative Index to Nursing and Allied Health Literature (CINAHL) database includes studies relevant for nursing and allied health (EBSCOhost, 2012), and PsycInfo includes studies relevant for behavioural sciences and mental health (American Psychological Association, 2013). There are a multitude of electronic databases covering various topics worldwide and reviewers must decide which databases are relevant for a particular question. Generally more than one database is necessary to ensure relevant studies are identified. There also exist specialized databases, for example, those that house only certain types of studies such as RCTs. Given RCTs are the only type of research design included in this review, these specialized databases may be particularly helpful in identifying studies. A list of some of the relevant databases to locate trials on anti-bullying are included in Table 4.3.

TABLE 4.3	Relevant Databases for Electronic Search

Databases

General	Specialized
• Medline	Cochrane Central database of trials
• Cinahl	
• PsycInfo	
• Eric	

Once the databases have been identified, keywords with which to conduct the search need to be identified. Each database requires unique keywords resulting in the need to modify search terms across databases. Medline uses **MeSH** which stands for Medical Subject Headings. The creation of a comprehensive set of search terms, and their combination, usually requires the specialized knowledge of a librarian. Particularly for Cochrane reviews, consultation with a librarian with expertise in systematic reviews to develop the string of search terms is strongly encouraged.

Recognizing your lack of skill, you make an appointment with the health department's librarian. Assuming you arrive with your research question formulated using PICO, the librarian gets to work right away generating an appropriate list of MeSH terms and keywords. You leave understanding you will receive electronically the results of the database searches in the next few days.

However, your search for relevant studies is only partially complete, as not all studies are indexed in databases, and despite the creation of a comprehensive and very complicated set of search terms, some studies included in those databases will still be missed. Given this reality it is important to use additional approaches to identify relevant studies. These include: checking the **reference lists** of included studies to identify potentially relevant studies; contacting experts in the content area for additional studies; checking the **conference proceedings**; looking at the table of contents from relevant journals; and searching the websites of organizations that produce evidence on the topic of interest (The Cochrane Collaboration, 2009). The augmentation of the electronic search with these additional strategies increases the likelihood that all relevant studies will be identified.

These additional strategies are particularly useful for identifying unpublished studies, also referred to as grey literature. Research has illustrated that unpublished studies are more likely to report results suggesting an intervention has no effect than a statistically significant effect (Guyatt et al., 2008). As such, if unpublished studies are not included in the review, there is a possibility that the review will be biased toward finding a positive effect when in fact this may not be the case. Therefore it is important to ensure the search strategy is such that unpublished studies will be identified. It is also important to not limit the search strategy to English language only studies. Similar to unpublished studies, studies published in English are more likely to report statistically significant results as compared to studies published in other languages. Therefore, if a review includes English language studies only, the review may be biased toward finding a statistically significant effect, when in fact that may not be the case when all available studies are summarized.

In summary, a comprehensive search strategy consists of multiple strategies for identifying relevant studies, including the searching of multiple electronic databases, reviewing tables of content of relevant journals and reference lists of included studies, key experts, and relevant websites. The employed strategies should also ensure that unpublished and non-English language studies are identified.

Selecting Studies

With the search for studies complete, it is now time to determine which studies will be included in the review. In other words: which studies are relevant to the research question being asked after taking into account the inclusion and exclusion criteria. What is equally important at this stage is documenting why studies were excluded. Therefore it is important to develop a management system that keeps track of these decisions. There are a

number of software packages in existence that not only keep track of the review process, but also allow the work to be completed online, which definitely saves time in the review process.

The use of two or more independent reviewers to screen titles and abstracts for relevance to the research question is strongly encouraged to reduce bias when studies are selected. Generally, the reviewers independently assess each title and abstract, and if necessary the full text of the study, apply the inclusion and exclusion criteria, and make a decision as to whether the study should be included. The reviewers then meet to discuss studies they disagreed on. In many instances it is standard practice that the reviewers discuss their differences until they reach consensus. However, it is also acceptable to have a third reviewer assess the study to break the tie.

Thus, you develop an inclusion/exclusion form. To be included in the review, a study had to receive a YES answer for all inclusion criteria. If a YES answer was received for any of the exclusion criteria, the study was excluded.

Assessing Studies for Methodological Quality

Once relevant studies are identified, attention turns to assessing the methodological quality of those studies. You learn from the Cochrane Handbook that this is known as "risk of bias." The purpose of assessing **risk of bias** is to determine the extent to which studies have assessed intervention effectiveness correctly; in other words, to what extent the results are true (The Cochrane Collaboration, 2009).

In addition to Cochrane's risk of bias, there are a number of well-known, internationally accepted tools available to **critically appraise** randomized controlled trials, one of which is known as the Jadad scale. This scale includes three criteria to assess the methodological quality of trials, namely, **concealment of allocation** (assignment of participants to treatment or control group is not known at time of study recruitment), **blinding** (study participants, intervention providers, and outcome assessors are not aware of who is receiving the intervention or not), and **drop-outs** (number of participants not completing the study). Studies have shown that these three components are most important in distinguishing the methodological quality of randomized controlled trials (Jadad et al., 1996).

However, additional criteria often used to assess methodological quality of intervention studies include: selection bias, study design, confounders, data collection methods, and data analysis (Public Health Resource Unit, 2006). **Selection bias** assesses how likely it is individuals chosen to participate in the study represent the larger population to whom the study results will be generalized to. One way this is determined is by assessing the percentage of selected individuals who agreed to participate. Another is to assess reasons why individuals did not participate, and to determine if non-participants differ systematically from those who did. Study design asks if the most rigorous design was used, giving more weight to RCTs than other designs. In addition it is also important for trials to consider if the randomization process was described and conducted adequately.

Confounders are characteristics that may impact on the outcome as opposed to or in addition to the intervention under investigation. In other words if a change in a health outcome is observed, you need to assess if this change was as a result of being exposed to the intervention, or the result of some other difference between groups that explains the change. For example, in our scenario, participants exposed to an anti-bullying intervention who attend schools previously reporting very low bullying episodes, may respond differently to the intervention than those from schools reporting high levels of bullying behavior. In this instance it would be unclear if a change in bullying behaviour was as a result of the intervention, the baseline level of bullying, or a combination of both. Therefore, it is important to determine at baseline if all characteristics that could impact the outcome were assessed and if significant differences were observed in these variables between the intervention and control group that this be accounted for in data analysis.

The method used for collecting data is also an important criterion. Ultimately, you want to know that the data collection methods produce data that are reliable (the same response is elicited with repeated administration of a questionnaire for example), and **valid** (the data are a true measure of the variable of interest). Authors of studies generally report the level of reliability and validity of the data collection measures or, at a minimum, cite references where these values have been published.

Finally, it is important to assess the percentage of individuals who complete the study compared to those who began the study, and whether there was a difference in withdrawals between the intervention and control groups. Reasons why participants withdraw from either group are also important to assess. Generally, a drop-out rate of 20 per cent or less is considered good; a drop-out rate between 40–19 per cent is moderate; and a drop-out rate of more than 40 per cent seriously draws into questions the validity of the results (Guyatt et al., 2008). Despite the percentage of drop-outs, an **intention to treat analysis** should be conducted, which, put simply, means all participants starting the study are evaluated in the group to which they were assigned regardless of whether they completed the study or not, or ever received the intervention (The Cochrane Collaboration, 2009). Therefore, if someone were to drop out of a study, they would still be accounted for in the data analysis in the group to which they were originally assigned, and they would be assigned a negative outcome. An intention to treat analysis is considered to provide a more conservative and realistic estimate of effect of an intervention, and is considered to be the gold standard for data analysis of intervention studies (The Cochrane Collaboration, 2009).

As was the case for selecting studies, two reviewers independently assess each study for methodological quality using an agreed upon tool a priori and meet to discuss any differences in assessments. Prior to conducting the methodological assessments, all reviewers should discuss the criteria to ensure they are all interpreting the criteria the same way. They should then independently assess one study and meet to discuss their ratings, and then assess additional studies and meet again to discuss their assessments. Once good agreement between raters is achieved, the raters are ready to assess all remaining studies, and then check agreement after all studies have been assessed for methodological quality.

Extracting Relevant Data from Studies

You complete the methodological assessment of all included studies, as well as resolve all disagreements with a second reviewer (your nursing preceptor), relieved to see that there was good agreement between yourself and the second reviewer on most studies and for most criteria. With the methodological assessment complete, it is now time to extract important and relevant data for each study. As was the case for all previous steps in the systematic review process, decisions on which data to extract from each study, how the data will be extracted and by whom must all be made before the review is started. Generally, a data extraction form is developed,

discussed to ensure all reviewers are interpreting the form consistently, and tested on a small number of studies. When good agreement is achieved amongst reviewers, they can then independently extract data on all of the relevant variables from all studies. Once this step is completed they once again meet to discuss any discrepancies in the extracted data. When agreement on all extracted data is reached, the data are entered into a data management package.

Analyzing the Data

With the data entered into a data management package it is time to get down to analyzing the data and interpreting the results. You are eager to determine what impact school-based anti-bullying interventions have on bullying episodes during the school year. While the decision to conduct a meta-analysis rather than narratively combining the results across studies is generally made prior to starting a systematic review, it will be discussed in greater detail now.

Before you start to analyze the findings, you must first decide if you are going to conduct a **meta-analysis** (statistically combine the results across studies) or narratively assess the findings and report results. There are several factors that determine whether it is appropriate to conduct a meta-analysis. First you need to determine if the populations included across the studies are similar enough that it makes sense to analyze them together. For example, it could be that some studies only include children aged 10–12, whereas others include 5–7 year-olds, while still others include children 5–12. In addition, it might also be that the participants vary considerably on other factors from study to study. Some studies might only include participants from very low socioeconomic status, whereas others might include participants from other countries with very different educational systems. The important issue here is that one must assess whether the populations studied, on the whole, are similar enough to warrant combining results across studies. If one were to decide that the populations varied too much across studies, it would then be reasonable to not conduct a meta-analysis, but rather narratively describe the findings across studies. After assessing the population, the student moves on to assess how similar the interventions are across studies. Again the same logic applies here. While all the interventions were implemented in the school setting in order to be included in the review, it might be that the interventions vary so much that it doesn't make sense to statistically combine them into one **effect size**. For example, some interventions might be limited to school assemblies involving skits of bullying behaviour, while other interventions may involve a comprehensive multi-faceted anti-bullying approach. Again, you need to judge if the interventions are similar enough to combine them. The same thinking applies for the outcomes. With respect to outcomes it is important to assess if the outcome measure is the same, as well as if the outcome has been measured in the same way across studies. All of these factors are used to make an overall judgement about whether it is appropriate to conduct a meta-analysis. From the perspective of the populations, interventions, and outcomes included in the studies for our scenario, you might determine that it is appropriate to conduct a meta-analysis.

However, before making the final decision concerning the conduct of a meta-analysis, you must assess if the results from study to study are similar enough to warrant combining them into one overall effect size. You first "eyeball" the results across studies that are presented in a table in descending order of methodological quality, starting with studies of the highest quality. In this first look at the results, you are assessing how much the results from each study vary with respect to

having a statistically significant positive effect, no effect, or a statistically significant negative effect. In this scenario the outcome is the number of bullying episodes during the school year, which is a continuous variable. A **continuous** variable is one in which the variable can be any number along a continuous distribution function (Wikipedia, 2013b). In evaluating the impact of a school-based intervention on the number of bullying episodes, a value of zero would indicate that the intervention had no effect (those in the intervention group experienced no difference in bullying episodes in comparison to the control group— also referred to as the **line of no effect**), while a number below zero would constitute fewer bullying episodes by those in the intervention group in comparison to the control and therefore represent a positive effect, and a number above zero would constitute more bullying episodes experienced by those in the intervention group in comparison to those in the control group and therefore represent a negative effect.

What you can do to quickly assess variation across study results is to plot the result for each study, in relation to the line of no effect. See Figures 4.2a and 4.2b from two different datasets drawn from hypothetical studies evaluating anti-bullying interventions. In Figure 4.2a we can see that all five studies have effect sizes less than zero, indicating that all studies reported fewer bullying episodes among those exposed to the school-based anti-bullying intervention as compared to controls. Said another way: these results illustrate that the intervention had a positive effect by reducing the number of bullying episodes during the school year. Only one of the studies touches the line of no effect, which means that four of the studies reported a statistically significant finding, and only one did not. Based on the data presented in Figure 4.2a, it looks like the results are fairly consistent across studies, and therefore a meta-analysis is likely appropriate.

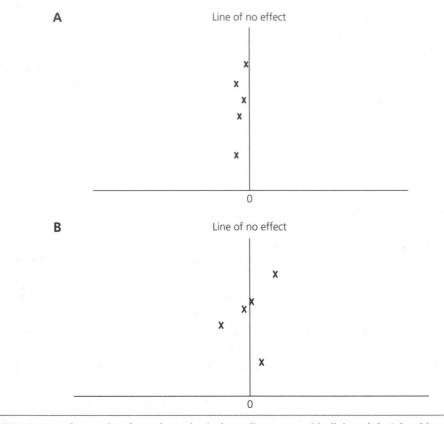

FIGURE 4.2   Sample results from hypothetical studies on anti-bullying (A) School-based antibullying interventions reduce bullying: hypothetical data (B) School-based antibullying interventions yield mixed results: hypothetical data

However, the data presented in Figure 4.2b illustrate a different story. In this instance there is a fair amount of difference across the study results. For example, two of the five studies have effect sizes less than zero, two have effect sizes greater than zero, and one is right on the line of no effect. In other words, two studies showed a positive effect (finding below zero), two showed a negative effect (finding above zero), and one showed no effect (finding touches the line of no effect). It may be that these findings are too different to warrant their statistical combination. Therefore an important first step is to visually look at the findings across studies to ascertain if it is appropriate to statistically combine them. However, as is the case in Figure 4.2b, it may be that visually assessing the findings is insufficient to determine if too much variation exists. Therefore an important component of meta-analysis is to assess the variation in results across studies using statistical tests. Generally, a **test of heterogeneity** is conducted to assess variation across study results. Meta-analysis software will conduct a test of heterogeneity at the time the meta-analysis is being conducted. The test of heterogeneity assesses the extent to which results across studies vary (The Cochrane Collaboration, 2009). There are a number of tests of heterogeneity that can be conducted, although the reasons for choosing one over the other will not be discussed in this chapter. The Cochrane Handbook is a good source for additional reading on choosing a specific test of heterogeneity, and for interpreting the results of those tests. For the purpose of this chapter, it is sufficient to understand that prior to conducting a meta-analysis, it is important to determine if the results are similar enough across studies to warrant combining them and that both visual assessment and statistical methods are needed to adequately assess heterogeneity. In this scenario, you judge the findings across studies to be similar enough to warrant going ahead with the meta-analysis.

The result of the test of heterogeneity is also useful for identifying the statistical procedure that is optimal for combining results across studies. For example, a test of heterogeneity may show that results vary a fair amount across studies however it may still be acceptable to conduct a meta-analysis. However, if this were the case, a different statistical approach would be required than if the test of heterogeneity showed the results were similar from study to study. To understand this concept more fully, it is important to return to the underlying purpose of conducting a meta-analysis. The reason for conducting a meta-analysis is to reduce uncertainty about the effect of an intervention, by combining the results of all studies evaluating a specific intervention. The aggregation of multiple studies provides a more conservative estimate of the overall intervention effect, by taking into account variation between studies. When little variation across study findings exists, then only minor adjustments are required when aggregating the findings. However, if the findings vary a fair amount (meaning the test of heterogeneity is significant), then more adjustments that take into account this greater variation in results across studies is required in order to adequately represent the variation. For these two scenarios different statistical models are needed. It is beyond

the scope of this chapter to go into further detail about the different statistical models that can be used to aggregate data across studies. However, it is important to understand that assessing for heterogeneity must occur and depending on the result of that assessment, a certain statistical model should be used. The Cochrane Handbook should be consulted for further information. In our scenario, the nursing student determines that the test of heterogeneity was not significant.

Interpreting the Results

With the meta-analysis conducted, it is time for you to contemplate what the findings mean. In other words, you must interpret the results. Meta-analysis results are comprised of two parts, both of which are equally important for understanding the impact of interventions on the population we wish to apply the results to. As was illustrated in the previous section every study reports an overall result (if the study is evaluating the effectiveness of an intervention this is referred to as the **effect size**). Those were depicted in Figures 4a and 4b with an X. However, this is only part of the "story" of the effect of the intervention for each study. The whole story requires us to interpret both the effect size and the **95 per cent confidence interval** of the effect size.

The 95 per cent confidence interval is defined as the range of values the true population effect lies within (Wikipedia, 2013a). The following example sheds some light on understanding confidence intervals. When we conduct a study, we take a sample from the whole population and at the end of a study we have an effect size for that particular sample. If we were to conduct the study again, taking another sample from the same population, we might end up with all new participants, or some new participants and some that were in the first study. Nonetheless, this new sample, as a result of being different from the first one, will likely result in a different effect size being reported than in the first study. The effect size may be slightly different from the first study, or quite different. If one were to replicate this study 100 times, understanding that 100 different samples of participants would be drawn for each unique study, then a range of effect sizes will also be observed. The 95 per cent confidence interval therefore, tells us that the true effect size for the whole population, 95 times out of 100 would fall between this range of effect sizes. When we then apply the results of one study back to the whole population, we need to consider not only the effect size of that particular study, but also the 95 per cent confidence interval. It is as likely that the true effect for the population lies at either end of this range as it does in the middle. Let us look at the hypothetical data presented in Figure 4.3. In this figure, we have the same effect sizes reported per study as we saw previously in Figure 4.2a; however, 95 per cent confidence intervals for each study have now been added.

When Figure 4.2a only included effect sizes, we concluded that across the five studies, four depicted a statistically significant positive effect (fewer bullying episodes), and one did not because the X touched the line of no effect. However, a very different story emerges when the 95 per cent confidence intervals are considered. As we can see in Figure 4.3, only two of the five studies have 95 per cent confidence intervals that *do not* touch the line of no effect, and three do. Therefore, our interpretation of the study results changes because for three of the studies, the true effect ranges from fewer bullying episodes to more bullying episodes. Therefore we would say for these three studies that the intervention effect is not statistically significant, even though the actual effect size (the X) is to the left of the line of no effect (meaning fewer bullying episodes). Even for the two remaining studies, whose 95 per cent confidence intervals do not cross the line of no effect, for one study, the confidence interval almost touches the line of no effect. So, in summarizing the evidence presented in Figure 4.3, now that we have a confidence interval included for each study, we are much less optimistic about the effect of school-based anti-bullying interventions.

The final remaining component for the nursing student to interpret in this meta-analysis is the overall effect size, depicted as a diamond. The diamond is found at the bottom of the graph underneath the results of each of the individual studies. The left and right hand points of the diamond represent the 95 per cent confidence interval, while the overall effect size generally is in the

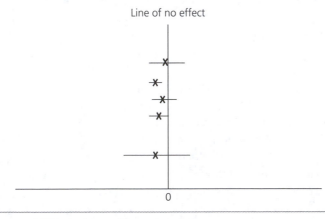

FIGURE 4.3   Effect sizes and 95 per cent confidence intervals

middle of the diamond. The diamond, referred to as the **summary statistic**, takes into account the effect sizes and confidence intervals from each of the individual studies included in the meta-analysis. You will see in Figure 4.4 below, that a (hypothetical) diamond has been added to the plot. What conclusions should you make regarding the effectiveness of school-based anti-bullying interventions as a result of considering the diamond? A quick glance at the diamond tells us that school-based anti-bullying interventions are *not* effective in reducing the number of bullying episodes during the school year in schools exposed to the intervention in comparison to schools not exposed. We know this because the diamond crosses the line of no effect. In addition, given the diamond crosses the line of no effect, we know that the finding is not statistically significant. We can say that there is a trend in the intervention schools toward reduced bullying, but that the effect did not reach statistical significance.

Interpreting the Summary Statistic

Additional analyses could be conducted in the meta-analysis to better understand the reported results: for example, does the result change if only interventions of longer duration are considered, or does the result change if only schools with a low level of bullying at baseline are included; however, that is beyond the scope of this chapter. For additional information on more advanced analyses used in meta-analyses, consult the Cochrane Handbook. Having now completed the meta-analysis, you prepare a presentation for the upcoming meeting with the school representatives. It is important that you clearly articulate the key findings and recommendations for practice with regards to bullying. You write a one-page executive summary that will be distributed at the meeting. The executive summary highlights the following key messages:

the school-based anti-bullying interventions included in the meta-analysis were not effective in reducing bullying episodes in elementary schools; and

as such, you recommend that these school-based anti-bullying interventions not be implemented by the school to reduce bullying episodes at this time.

Your preceptor and you understand that these findings will not be popular at the upcoming meeting, but recognize the importance of ensuring any programs that are implemented in the

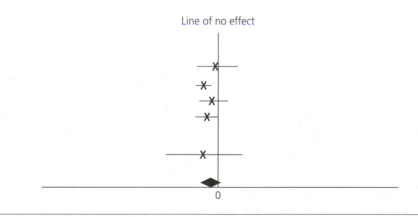

FIGURE 4.4   Interpreting the summary statistic

school have evidence of proven effectiveness. You both prepare a presentation to help the school staff understand why the results of the meta-analysis are more appropriate to guide decision making concerning anti-bullying interventions, rather than the results of a single study. Both of you intend to work with the school staff over the course of the coming months to identify other potential strategies that could be considered to address bullying.

Conclusions

As you reflect on your learning goals and objectives for your clinical placement, you conclude that the opportunity to participate in a meta-analysis, the topic of which was specifically identified by front line decision makers, and thereby held the potential to directly influence practice, was hugely rewarding. Having been involved in all components of the review process, from refining the PICO question, to conducting the search for potentially relevant studies, to identifying inclusion and exclusion criteria, to assessing studies for relevance and methodological quality, extracting relevant data, and then performing the data analysis, interpreting the findings, and presenting the results, allowed you to develop many new skills. As you near the end of your undergraduate program, you feel that you have a good foundation for moving evidence into practice, as you begin working as a new graduate in the nursing profession.

Summary

- Readers learned the steps involved in conducting a systematic review.
- The importance of using a body of evidence to inform decisions was described.
- Readers learned how to turn a practice-based issue into a searchable research question.
- Specific tips on developing an effective and efficient search strategy were identified.

- The importance of assessing methodological quality was described.
- Readers learned how to interpret the results of quantitative findings and how to apply these findings to practice.

Review Questions

1. Why is a systematic review more appropriate for influencing nursing practice than single studies?

2. What components are necessary to develop a focused, answerable research question?

3. What constitutes a comprehensive search strategy?

4. What three criteria are used to assess methodological quality of randomized controlled trials?

5. If the 95 per cent confidence interval is close to, but does not touch the line of no effect, is the result statistically significant?

6. What does the 95 per cent confidence interval represent?

7. What conclusions would you draw based on the hypothetical results reported in Figure 4.3?

References

American Psychological Association (2013) Psych INFO. American Psychological Association. Retrieved from www.apa.org/pubs/databases/psycinfo/index.aspx.

Antman, E.M., Lau, J., Kupelnick, B., Mosteller, F., and Chalmers, T. C. (1992) A comparison of results of meta-analyses of randomized control trials and recommendations of clinical experts: Treatments for myocardial infarction. *The Journal of the American Medical Association*, 268, 240–8.

Campbell Collaboration (2013) What is a systematic review? Retrieved from www.campbell-collaboration.org/what_is_a_systematic_review/.

EBSCOhost (2012) Cumulative Index to Nursing and Allied Health Literature: CINAHL available via EBSCOhost. Ebsoco industries Inc. Retrieved from www.ebscohost.com/biomedical-libraries/the-cinahl-database.

Guyatt, G.H., Drummond, R., Maureen, M., and Cook, D. (2008) *Users' guides to the medical literature: A manual for evidence-based clinical practice.* (2nd ed.) New York, NY: McGraw-Hill Professional.

Jadad, A.R., Moore, R.A., Carroll, D., Jenkinson, C., Reynolds, D.J., Gavaghan, D.J. et al. (1996) Assessing the quality of reports of randomized clinical trials: Is blinding necessary? *Controlled Clinical Trials*, 17, 1–12.

Oxman, A.D. and Guyatt, G.H. (1993) The science of reviewing research. *Annals of the N.Y. Academy of Sciences*, 703, 125–33.

Public Health Resource Unit (2006) The Critical Appraisal Skills Tool: Making sense of evidence about clinical effectiveness. Public Health Resource Unit. Retrieved from www.casp-uk.net/wp-content/uploads/2011/11/CASP_Cohort_Appraisal_Checklist_14oct10.pdf.

Shuttleworth, M. (2008) Purpose of Research. Explorable. Retrieved from http://explorable.com/purpose-of-research.

The Cochrane Collaboration (2009) Cochrane Handbook for Systematic Reviews of Interventions. Retrieved from www.cochrane-handbook.org.

The Cochrane Collaboration (2013) About Us. The Cochrane Collaboration. Retrieved from www.cochrane.org/about-us.

U.S. National Library of Medicine (2013) MEDLINE/PubMed Resource Guide. U.S.National Library of Medicine: National Institute of Health. Retrieved from www.nlm.nih.gov/bsd/pmresources.html.

Wikipedia (2013a) Confidence Interval. Wikipedia, The Free Encyclopedia. Retrieved from en.wikipedia.org/wiki/Confidence_interval.

Wikipedia (2013b) Variable (mathematics). Wikipedia, The Free Encyclopedia. Retrieved from http://en.wikipedia.org/wiki/Continuous_variables.

5 Applied Ethics in Health Sciences Research

Dario Kuzmanović and Solomon R. Benatar

CHAPTER OUTLINE

Ethics and Health Research

The terms ethics and morals are often used interchangeably but they are distinguishable. **Ethics** (or moral philosophy) is the branch of philosophy that is concerned with systematic examination of, and argumentation for, right and wrong conduct through theories and principles that can be applied universally. **Morals** may be defined as the observed ways in which individuals or groups behave. Morals vary across geographic groups and eras and are thus considered to be relative to cultures, time, and place.

In constructing frameworks and guidelines for ethics in research, the focus is on developing a universal approach that applies to all research everywhere, rather than allowing different ethical standards in different places and times. This is important if some of the unethical research that has taken place in the past (most typically in Nazi Germany, but also subsequently and elsewhere) is to be avoided. As contexts vary this is more difficult to achieve than may be imagined. The challenge is to develop an ethics of research that can be applied with consideration of morally relevant contextual factors without reverting to moral relativism. Ethics differs from the law, guidance, and regulation, although law, guidelines, and regulation of conduct should ideally be based on ethical considerations. As history is replete with laws and guidelines that were incompatible with what could be considered right and good, the challenge for ethics is to formulate justifiable arguments for human conduct generally, and of relevance in this chapter for research specifically.

The two major theories of ethics are **consequentialism** which, simply stated, judges actions on the basis of whether they produce good or bad consequences (utilitarianism is one example within this category), and **deontology**, which judges actions based on whether they are inherently right or wrong actions, without emphasis on their consequences (Beauchamp and Childress, 2001). **Utilitarianism** strives to reach a balance between benefits and risks to people in order to maximize the best outcome for the greatest number of people. In other words, it focuses on means to ends. The deontological approach posits that acts themselves are inherently right or wrong, good or bad in a universal sense, and requires that every person should be treated as having intrinsic moral value, and thus treated as an end in itself and never as the means of achieving good for others. Deontology lies at the heart of the idea of universal human rights and has greatly influenced ethical deliberation in research. Neither deontology nor utilitarianism can provide all embracing and water-tight guidance on every ethical dilemma. Several prima facie ethical principles have been derived for use

in practice and these can be justified from both dominant theories.

Determining what is ethical often starts with consideration of these broad guiding principles. However, these are not ranked hierarchically; they may conflict with each other and there can be ambivalence about how they should be applied. While knowledge of the guidelines and regulations for research are necessary, it is understood that this may not be sufficient. Researchers also need to develop both sensitivity and moral reasoning skills to resolve ethical dilemmas. As there is often no obvious single or "correct" answer to an ethical dilemma it is important to support whatever position is taken with sound arguments based on a clear knowledge of the facts of the case and on how universal ethical principles can be justifiably applied.

Research on humans has a long and checkered history. Awareness of the extent to which experimental subjects could be abused first received a high profile internationally with the revelation of atrocious experiments carried out by the Nazis during the Second World War. The **Nuremberg Code** (see Figure 5.1), promulgated in 1949 after the Nuremburg Trials, was the first international endeavour to instill respect for research subjects and to guide human research. The 1948 Universal Declaration of Human Rights provides additional potential protection and extends respect for human dignity beyond the realm of medical research. Prominence given in the 1960s to ongoing unethical research on humans in prestigious medical schools in the US and the UK, and the public outcry in 1972 on exposure of the 40-year-long US Public Health Service Tuskegee study of the natural history of untreated syphilis in a cohort of African-American men, further boosted interest in regulating human research.

The World Medical Association's Declaration of Helsinki in 1964 (modified several times since then) and many other national and international guidelines have since facilitated universal

Nuremberg Code (1947) was the first guideline stating that consent is necessary for research. It was a landmark document since it established principles for medical practice and influenced many research ethics documents that followed, including the Canadian TCPS (Tri-Council Policy Statement).

1. The voluntary consent of the human subject is absolutely essential.
2. The experiment should be such as to yield fruitful results for the good of society.
3. The experiment should be so designed and based on the results of animal experimentation and knowledge of the natural history of the disease.
4. The experiment should be so conducted as to avoid all unnecessary physical and mental suffering and injury.
5. No experiment should be conducted where there is an a priori reason to believe that death or disabling injury will occur.
6. The degree of risk to be taken should never exceed that determined by the humanitarian importance of the problem to be solved by the experiment.
7. Proper preparations should be made and adequate facilities provided to protect the experimental subject against even remote possibilities of injury, disability, or death.
8. The experiment should be conducted only by scientifically qualified persons.
9. During the course of the experiment the human subject should be at liberty to bring the experiment to an end.
10. During the course of the experiment the scientist in charge must be prepared to terminate the experiment at any stage, if he has probable cause to believe, in the exercise of the good faith, superior skill and careful judgment required of him that a continuation of the experiment is likely to result in injury, disability, or death to the experimental subject

FIGURE 5.1   The Nuremberg Code

Source: Nuremburg Military Tribunal. "The Nuremburg Code," from *The Trials of War Criminals Before the Nuremberg Military Tribunals* (Government Printing Office: Washington, DC, 1948).

approaches to the regulation of human research through research ethics committees in universities and other organizations conducting research. New dilemmas arising from biotechnological progress, for example in neuroscience, and genetic research, continue to stimulate scholars of ethics. This applies with added complexity in regions inhabited by people of more than one set of cultural values, and of course when researchers from one culture move across the world to do research on people from other cultures. The challenge here, as indicated above, is to apply universal concepts with morally justifiable contextual balance.

In Canada, research is defined as "an undertaking that is intended to extend knowledge through a disciplined inquiry or systematic investigation" (TCPS, 2010). Obligations to ensure that study findings are valid may sometimes come into conflict with patients' and research participants'

best interests. The goals of research ethics are to systematically analyze ethical issues that may arise during research, to ensure that study participants are protected, and that research is conducted in a way that serves the needs of participants and society at large while avoiding exploitation of vulnerable persons. It is now widely acknowledged that ethical issues permeate research and must inform every aspect of research, ranging from study design and genesis of research questions to the dissemination of results.

Requirements for Ethical Research

First, the scientific design of the study and the methodology used should provide the means of answering the research question, and the researchershould be sufficiently familiar with the design of a research project and the methods to be used. Sample size, inclusion and exclusion criteria, measurable end points, consideration of potential adverse effects and of benefits, and informed consent obtained through an appropriate process—all need to be considered. Secondly, there is a need to sensitize researchers to the range of ethical issues that may arise in the course of research on humans. These include the complexities of obtaining informed consent in some contexts, maintaining confidentiality, appropriately balancing harms and benefits of research, and avoiding exploitation and conflicts of interest. Guidelines for authorship also need to be established to ensure fair treatment of all who contributed to the generation of new knowledge (including junior staff) and to preserve the freedom and integrity of scholarly work. Thirdly, in order for high scientific standards in research to be supplemented by high ethical standards, it is necessary for researchers to receive some education about research ethics. This can enable them to strive for ethical standards as high as the scientific standards to which scientists aspire, and thus avoid the idea that the ethics review process is merely one of policing. Studying the substantive body of knowledge on research ethics and internalization of a desire for ethical excellence by researchers is the route to non-exploitative and ethical research practices. Several procedural requirements also need to be met to ensure appropriate accountability.

There should be little doubt that health research has dramatically improved and enriched our lives. Reduction in infant mortality, vaccinations, and treatments for HIV and diabetes are only a few examples of the benefits of these inquiries. One category of research, known as clinical trials, has been particularly beneficial in the development of new drugs and treatments, with the main objective being to provide the most

reliable data on the effects and safety of a drug, device, or other intervention.

Clinical trials are categorized into four phases: I, II, III, and IV. Phase I clinical trials are sometimes known as "first-in-human" trials and raise the most safety concerns because of little or no previous experience with the intervention in humans. These studies are usually conducted on a small number of healthy humans to determine the rate at which the drug is absorbed, excreted, and whether it has toxic effects. Phase I trials are meant to provide early information about the safety of the potential use of the drug or intervention. After a successful completion of this phase, the intervention is tested for safety and efficacy on a larger number of individuals with the disease or condition for whom the new treatment is intended. These trials, known as Phase II trials, aim to explore therapeutic efficacy in target patients and to estimate proper dosage for future studies. After a drug is shown to be reasonably effective it enters a Phase III trial. Here participants are randomly assigned to either an experimental or a control group, with the experimental group receiving the new drug or intervention, while the control group receives either a placebo or the currently standard treatment. Double-blinding, whereby neither the participant nor the research personnel know who is receiving the experimental agent, is aimed at minimizing bias, so that any observed differences in results in the two groups can be confidently attributed to the intervention. The primary objective of Phase III trials is to demonstrate or to confirm a statistically significant therapeutic benefit of new drugs and thus provide the scientifically justifiable basis for marketing approval. Once an intervention is approved for distribution or marketing, Phase IV trials (post-marketing) may begin. These trials assess long-term safety and effectiveness since earlier trials are of limited duration, and pre-market clinical trials (Phase I to Phase III) normally detect only half of all serious adverse reactions that eventually come to be associated with the drug or intervention (Oberle and Allen, 2006).

One problematic issue in clinical trials is the fundamental misunderstanding that research participants may have about the purpose of clinical trials. It is now well recognized that despite detailed processes of providing accurate information about the purpose of the study and obtaining consent before they are enrolled into trials, participants often have difficulty fully understanding the goals of research and recognizing how this differs from clinical care. Specifically, they may misunderstand that research is meant to create generalizable knowledge and not to provide medical treatment according to individualized clinical needs. Participants also frequently fail to understand terms such as randomization, blinding, and placebo, and that the use of these techniques is to ensure study results are statistically valid and not specifically for the participants' best clinical interests. This difficulty in differentiating between clinical research and clinical treatment is a phenomenon known as the **therapeutic misconception** (Lindz et al, 2004; de Melo-Martin and Ho, 2008).

Regulations Guiding Research in Humans in Canada

The foundations of research ethics have been influenced by many fields of study and through professional codes and practices. In Canada, the guiding document for all research involving humans is the *Tri-Council Policy Statement: Ethical conduct for research involving humans, 2nd edition* or "TCPS" for short (Canadian Institutes of Health Research, Natural Sciences and Engineering Research Council of Canada, and Social Sciences and Humanities Research Council of Canada, 2010). The three major funders of research in Canada created the original document in 1998 and have

revised it significantly since that time with a view to making it as comprehensible and accessible as possible (see Review Question 1).

The document lays out the framework for ethical research and covers many topics broken down into different sections. The first part of the document lays out the ethical framework and the core principles. According to the document the core principles for conduct of research are:

- respect for persons;
- concern for welfare; and
- justice.

These three principles are broad enough to be applied to a variety of contexts. The underlying value articulated within the TCPS, as in most other research ethics documents, is respect for persons. Respect for persons means that all research participants carry an inherent value which must be validated by seeking their voluntary, informed, and ongoing consent. All research is, on some level, an intrusion into people's lives. Therefore, the mechanism through which researchers show deference to the humanity of others is by seeking permission to include them in the processes required to advance medical knowledge. Participation in research is always a matter of choice and people must be free to exercise both the choices of being included in trials, or exiting from these at any time. Informed consent should always be based on a full understanding of the reasonable risks and possible benefits, what the research study entails for participants, as well as any other salient features that may influence participation.

Seeking free and informed consent may not always be possible. There are certain factors that may diminish a person's ability to adequately decide whether or not to participate in research. Individuals with diminished capacity, such as children or those with mental health issues, may lack the ability to make their own decision. Researchers will need to seek consent from a third party who is authorized to make decisions on their behalf. A two-stage consent is required when doing research on those with diminished ability to decide. For example, individuals with schizophrenic disorders may have legal guardians who can decide if they should enrol in research, but the individuals with the disorder also need to provide consent. This second component of seeking consent is usually referred to as **assent** and demonstrates that even in situations where lack of competence prevents obtaining free and informed consent, researchers should involve those individuals in the decision making process. Dissent from a prospective participant, regardless of consent provided by their caregiver, must be respected and the individual should not be included in the research against their will.

Obtaining consent and assent is one way of showing researchers' concern for the welfare of their potential participants. Concern for welfare also means respecting the quality of the participants' lives in all possible dimensions—family, community, employment, health status, and social participation. Researchers strive to protect participants from harm and increase their overall wellbeing and safety. Research should never intentionally injure or cause harm to participants, regardless of what possible benefit may flow from the research in the future. A key aspect of concern for welfare extends beyond individuals and can be applied to whole communities. While health research may have many benefits, research findings can also promote stigmatization and further marginalization of whole groups of individuals. Researchers therefore need to engage relevant community members in order to maximize benefits and minimize possible harms.

Justice in research means treating people fairly and equitably. This principle arises out of the strong recognition that in many instances in the past, the burdens of research have fallen to groups that are marginalized, while the benefits of medical innovations have traditionally been enjoyed by those much better off, or who have a vested interest in the research. One concrete way researchers can ensure that they are treating people justly is by making sure that their inclusion and exclusion criteria are justified. Historically, some groups were excluded from research arbitrarily (e.g., women) while other groups were used because of how easy they were to access (e.g., prisoners). Injustice occurs when groups are included or excluded for logistical or arbitrary reasons.

Research Ethics Boards

As all research that involves humans has the potential for ethical concerns, any Canadian institution, for example a university or hospital that receives federal funding for research, must establish a **Research Ethics Board** (REB). REBs are independent, multidisciplinary teams of individuals who review the ethical acceptability of research proposals, as defined by TCPS and other regulatory requirements and standards.

The function and composition of the REB as outlined in the TCPS requires that there are at least five members on the board. Meeting the minimum quorum for a meeting requires that at least two of those members have expertise in the area or discipline of research reviewed. For example, REBs that review nursing and health services studies should have members on the board who are familiar with research methods in nursing and health services. There must be at least one member who is knowledgeable in the relevant laws, and who is typically (but not necessarily) a lawyer or a privacy expert. There must also be one member who is knowledgeable in ethics. The role of this person is to guide the REB in assessing and addressing ethical issues within defined ethical frameworks. The final requirement for

REB quorum is a community member who is not affiliated with the institution. The role of the community member is to reflect the perspective, concerns, and interests of potential research participants.

Due to high workloads and diversity in the disciplines and methods employed by their researchers, most REBs in Canada require more than five members and typically have from 10–15 members. The TCPS encourages the inclusion of community members in a ratio of 1:5, which means that an REB typically has two or three community representatives. Having larger boards facilitates retaining a quorum at any given meeting. Institutions are required to provide sufficient administrative and financial support for ethics reviews. REB responsibilities are administered through a research ethics office, with staff to coordinate meetings, manage membership, and provide training, orientation, and other support. Financial resources are important to provide recognition of service, as REB members are mostly volunteers. Most individuals who serve on these boards are doing so in addition to all their other duties, such as regular jobs, or if they are faculty members, in addition to teaching, supervising, and their own research. Providing honoraria to chairs, sending members to continuing education meetings and even serving food, at what are usually long meetings, are ways of facilitating recruitment and retention of REB members.

All researchers, including students, conducting research involving human participants in institutions who receive federal funds must follow the requirements for ethical research set out in the TCPS. This means that all those who wish to do research must receive approval from their REB before they begin recruiting participants or analyzing data. Fundamental to REB review, as discussed in TCPS, is the concept of **proportional review**. This means that the level of scrutiny should be dependent on the level of foreseeable risk to participants. REBs review research through two streams: delegated review is reserved for **minimal risk** protocols, and full board review is required for all research that poses more than minimal risk. Full board review is the default process, and this is achieved through face-to-face meetings of the REB, where quora are required and protocols are reviewed for their ethical acceptability, according to TCPS and other requirements. The delegated review process does not involve a meeting, and instead can be conducted by one, two, or a few REB members. Based on specific criteria (discussed below), REBs are mandated to approve, reject, or propose modifications to any proposed or ongoing research. Most of the time, REBs neither reject nor immediately approve the research, but rather request further information, clarification, or explanation of specific issues. The process of research ethics review is meant to be iterative and educational for both researchers and board members.

REB Review

While REBs review studies for ethical issues in general, there are some fundamental concepts that they must examine. These include minimizing potential risks to participants, ensuring that consent is free and informed, that the scientific merit of the research is sound, and that any conflicts of interest have been properly managed. We will now discuss these concepts in more detail.

Risks of harm to participants are always possible since most research seeks to find answers about something that is unknown. Given the uncertainty of finding answers and possibility of harm that may result, researchers are required to take all reasonable steps to minimize risks of harm to participants. Harms can vary from minor inconvenience to severely adverse physical, emotional, social, or legal effects. Risks to participants can also occur at the individual level or community level. While historically, REBs have concentrated primarily on risks of harm to participants as individuals, the revised TCPS reminds REBs that potential harms of research extend beyond individuals to also include participants' families and communities. All these must be taken into account when reviewing the ethical acceptability of research.

As discussed above, free and informed consent is a cornerstone of ethical research. Participants must understand the purpose of research, all the potential risks and benefits, precisely what they are being asked to do to meet study requirements, and how information about them will be used. Consent to participate in research should not be understood as merely a signature on a document, but rather as a documented, continuous dialogical *process* between the participant and the researcher. Because it has such significance in research, consent is often scrutinized by REBs to ensure that it is voluntary, informed, and acquired through discussions in group-appropriate language. Since REB review is done prospectively and the consent process is rarely monitored, board members spend a significant part of their review focusing on the consent documents and making sure they cover all the information participants need to make an informed decision. Researchers often want to know exactly which information and how much of it they should provide to participants in informed consent documents. While the answer to this question is case-dependent, a useful piece of practical advice would be to consider what and how much information would be sufficient for a layperson. The researcher may consider their significant other or a family member enrolling in the study and how much detail they would provide in order to ensure that the participant understands what the study entails, the risks and benefits of participation, and any other relevant considera-

tions, so that agreeing to participate would be voluntary and informed.

Another condition of ethical research is the scientific merit of the proposed research. While REBs are not normally scientific review committees, they are often compelled to comment on the design of the study and the methods of the proposed projects, especially if they are concerned that these may not be sound. Additional scientific expertise may have to be obtained to reach a decision. If a study design cannot answer a scientifically significant question or generate useful or generalizable knowledge, then there is no justification for exposing people to risk. Research that lacks scientific rigour is unethical and may waste participants' time or even put them in harm's way.

Given the variety of health research and study designs, REBs can focus on any aspect of the project that gives rise to ethical concerns. Some projects raise concerns that deal with compensation for participation in the study, while others are problematic because they lack meaningful sharing of research results. The ethical review process is meant to flag some of these concerns for the researchers but it is only one step in a very long process toward ensuring ethical conduct of research. Ideally REB review is meant to make researchers more introspective and honest about their study while also sensitizing them to the range of possible ethical dilemmas in research.

Privacy and Confidentiality

Privacy and confidentiality are key considerations for the conduct of research. **Privacy** usually refers to the individual's right to control personal data and information about themselves. **Confidentiality** is related to privacy but refers to the researchers' obligation to safeguard and protect information that participants provide during research. Privacy is a right that participants have, while confidentiality is a duty that researchers must respect. There are many types of data that researchers collect, use, and analyze, and the potential for harm increases substantially when the data is directly identifying and of a sensitive nature. Although there are some discrepancies in how data identifiability is defined, in general, there are five categories of identifiability:

- Directly identifying information—the information identifies a specific individual through direct identifiers (e.g., name, social insurance number, personal health number).
- Indirectly identifying information—the information can reasonably be expected to identify an individual through a combination of indirect identifiers (e.g., date of birth, place of residence, unique personal characteristics).
- Coded information—direct identifiers are removed from the information and replaced with a code. Depending on access to the code, it may be possible to re-identify specific participants (e.g., the principal investigator retains a list that links the participants' code names with their actual name so data can be re-linked if necessary).

- Anonymized information—the information is irrevocably stripped of direct identifiers, a code is not kept to allow future re-linkage, and risk of re-identification of individuals from remaining indirect identifiers is low or very low.
- Anonymous information—the information never had identifiers associated with it (e.g., anonymous surveys) and risk of identification of individuals is low or very low (Chapter 5, Section A, TCPS).

In research, data are described as **anonymous** when no one, not even the researcher, can attribute responses to individual participants, and there is no possibility of re-identification. In some instances, researchers may choose to not collect any data that can render individuals identifiable since that may put the research or the participants at risk. A typical example of sensitive data that researchers may not wish to collect would be names of individuals involved in illicit activities that might be of interest to legal authorities which, if divulged, could put the researcher and participants in harm's way (see Health Research in Action box 5.1).

5.1 Health Research in Action

One of the more well-known examples where the collection of sensitive data resulted in legal conflict occurred during Russel Ogden's graduate research at Simon Fraser University (SFU) in 1994. Ogden conducted interviews with people who were present during assisted suicide or euthanasia of individuals with AIDS. During the consent process, he assured participants that he would provide them with "absolute confidentiality." However, when his research was published in the media, the Vancouver Coroner's office submitted a subpoena to find out the identity of one of the participants. Ogden refused to reveal the identity of any of his participants because he promised he would not do so (Palys and Lowman, 2000). He was taken to court and successfully protected his research and the confidentiality of his participant. The legal fight was not an easy one and SFU did not provide any support, except for a small monetary amount to apply to his legal bill. The institution shortly thereafter created a policy prohibiting researchers from guaranteeing confidentiality of research participants. This case is important in highlighting the issues that can arise when ethical obligations to participants conflict with legal obligations of duty to report. Researchers can be put in uncomfortable situations of balancing competing interests and priorities.

Misconduct in Health Research

Much like other professional activities, health research is open to interpretation, imperfections, and misuse of power. Over the years, research misconduct of a few scientists has threatened the safety and wellbeing of patients and participants, and has eroded public trust in the scientific enterprise. While likely under-reported, there have been a few high-profile cases of scientific misconduct in Canada that have caused a stir globally and nationally.

Research misconduct is a serious problem that needs both prevention and strong action. Addressing it is complicated by the fact that we do not know how frequently it happens. Estimates of misconduct range from as low as 0.001 per cent up to one per cent of all research (Kondro, 2007). Even at lower estimates of incidence, research misconduct has the potential to harm the entire research enterprise and erode public trust. As scientific inquiry and exploration are based on prior discoveries and theories, misconduct may hamper scientific progress—with knowledge, financial, scholarly, and reputational consequences.

It is important to clearly define types of research misconduct, as there are several varieties of offences under the umbrella of misconduct. These may occur together or in isolation. The *Tri-Agency Framework for Responsible Conduct in Research* (2011) describes the following types of breaches that qualify for misconduct.

Fabrication is the making up of data, methodologies, or findings. **Falsification**, which is slightly different, refers to the manipulation or omission of data, methodologies, or findings, without appropriate acknowledgment resulting in inaccurate findings. **Plagiarism** refers to the appropriation of someone else's work without appropriately referencing, or in some cases, without obtaining permission.

Other offenses, as defined under the *Tri-Agency Framework* include destruction of research records (to avoid detection of wrongdoing), redundant publication (also known as self-plagiarism or "salami publications"), invalid authorship, whereby an individual who has not provided intellectual contribution is given authorship (this includes both guest and ghost authorship), inadequate acknowledgement, whereby an individual who has provided intellectual contribution is not properly acknowledged as doing so, and mismanagement of conflict of interest. All of these are problematic in their own way, to varying degrees of severity. It is not uncommon for there to be more than one type of breach within the same misconduct case (see Health Research in Action box 5.2).

The case of Dr. R.K. Chandra, a nutrition researcher from Memorial University in Newfoundland, caused a big ethical controversy. His research specialty was infant allergies and the role of nutrition in cognition. He submitted a paper for publication that claimed that minerals and vitamins greatly improved cognition in seniors. The paper was originally submitted for publication in the *British Medical Journal* (BMJ) in 2000 but the journal editors had serious concerns about the data presented and noted that the paper "had all the hallmarks of having been entirely invented" (Smith, 2006). They contacted Memorial University and asked them to investigate the matter. The first response the BMJ editors received was from Chandra's lawyer asking them to identify the scientific reviewers. They declined. The University hastily investigated the matter and said they found no problems (Smith, 2006). Chandra resigned from the university and left Canada. He stated that he had lost all the raw research data. Shortly thereafter, the BMJ editors discovered that the same paper they rejected

5.2   Health Research in Action

One of the more notorious cases of scientific misconduct was discovered in the early 1990s in Montreal's St. Luc Hospital. Dr. Roger Poisson was the one of the investigators on a large study known as National Surgical Adjuvant Breast and Bowel Project (NSABP) that changed the way doctors treat breast cancer. Before the study reached its conclusions in 1985, breast cancer patients frequently had a mastectomy, which is a removal of the entire breast. However, this study showed that a less invasive procedure known as lumpectomy, whereby only the tissue surrounding the tumour is removed, was an equally effective treatment option in early stages of the disease. The study manager noticed some discrepancies in the data submitted by Dr. Poisson and reported him to the auditors. After a thorough investigation by the US Office of Research Integrity, Dr. Poisson was found to have fabricated and falsified data related on tests and dates of procedures in 115 separate instances. This matter was profoundly unsettling as the falsified data provided the basis for treatment options. Luckily, NSABP was a multi-centre trial and Dr. Poisson was only one of hundreds of researchers. The study conclusions held up even after his results were removed from the analysis. A follow-up study done a few years later confirmed earlier findings about lumpectomies (Angell and Kassirer, 1994). While the science held, the circumstances still left some people feeling uneasy and suspicious about health research.

was published in another journal in the field—*Nutrition*. They notified the journal and the study was retracted. However, over his career, Chandra had dozens of clinical trials published and only one of those has been retracted. Even today, a search on PubMed or Google Scholar displays many of his studies with no caveats whatsoever. The Canadian Broadcasting Corporation did an exposé on the story and found that Chandra had a long history of misconduct and that Memorial University had found serious research violations in the past.

Another case of scientific misconduct involved a physiologist, Dr. Eric T. Poehlman, a researcher at the University of Vermont, studying energy expenditure after menopause. One of his graduate students discovered altered data and reported him to the university, which investigated and laid criminal charges against him. Poehlman pleaded guilty to the biggest case of research misconduct in US history, admitting to falsifying grant applications and fabricating data in several articles (Sox and Rennie, 2006). While the investigation against him was under review, he departed to Université de Montréal, where he was awarded a CAD $1 million Canada Research Chair in nutrition and metabolism. His Canadian employer knew nothing of the ongoing investigation until Poehlman retracted an article he published earlier and there was a public outcry.

Given these and some other cases, 2005 was named by *Nature* as the year of "Scientists behaving badly" and Canadian research institutions were forced to consider the impact and magnitude of research misconduct nationally. The Canadian Research Integrity Committee was formed in 2006 and held their first meeting the following year. As a result of the meeting, a comprehensive report on research integrity in Canada was contracted to a private consulting firm, Hickling Arthurs Low Corporation (2009). This report included recommendations on how to strengthen Canada's research integrity system.

One option is the formation of an independent, national research integrity agency. This agency would be similar to the integrity agencies that are already operative in the US, as well as some European countries. Currently, charges of misconduct are investigated by local universities and this may put a lot of stress on smaller institutions that lack the requisite resources to investigate. Canadian researchers remain hesitant to form another regulatory body and the movement to create one seems to have stalled (Kondro, 2007). A recent report by a panel of experts on research integrity, has advocated creation of such a body that would enhance transparency and accountability in research (CCA, 2010). This federal body for research integrity could have significant impact on health research since it would assist in setting standards the scientific community should follow, provide information gathering on a case-by-case basis, and aid in dissemination and reporting of misconduct information. This integrity agency would not be involved in sanctioning or enforcement, but provide advice and guidance to the research community.

In 2011, the three federal granting agencies created the Panel on Responsible Conduct of Research, and changed the name and mandate of the Secretariat on Research Ethics to Secretariat of Responsible Conduct of Research. These changes were to reflect the emphasis the agencies were placing on research integrity, and dealing head-on with allegations of misconduct. The *Tri-Agency Framework: Responsible Conduct of Research* (2011) was adopted in the same year binding research institutions that received federal funds to educate their researchers on the importance of responsible conduct, and to handle allegations with transparency and accountability. While the reach of this policy is only within the context of institutions receiving federal monies (as is the case with TCPS), it is a good

first step toward a comprehensive research integrity policy in Canada. Each allegation of research misconduct is potentially harmful and merits a thorough investigation of the facts. Researchers who are found to be delinquent often claim that competing pressures of their jobs (a so-called culture of "publish or perish") contributed to their misconduct. Not all cases of misconduct are the same but they do all have some negative outcomes. Care should be taken not to be overzealous in accusing researchers of misconduct, and it should be possible early on to identify errors and honest mistakes that could give the appearance of falsification or plagiarism at first glance. All human endeavours, including research are open to error as well as to misconduct.

Interests and Conflicts of Interest in Health Research

Another issue that may arise in the conduct of research is a **conflict of interest** (CoI), which is also defined as a type of research misconduct. Ethical issues concerning conflict of interest have received increasing attention in recent decades because of growing financial influences on the research endeavor. A widely used definition states that a CoI occurs in situations where "a professional judgment concerning a primary interest tends to be unduly influenced by a secondary interest" (Lo and Field, 2009). The definition reflects the fact that people have many interests and that not all of them give rise to ethical concerns.

Primary interests vary depending on the position or the role we play. For example, the primary interest of a researcher working to advance knowledge for public health is different from the primary interest of a clinician who treats individuals, where the aim is to benefit the patient. When the clinician who is caring for patients recruits patients into their research study, this can pose a conflict of interest. Secondary interests also include financial gain, academic advancement, or the desire to benefit family members. Secondary interests are not always inappropriate in and of themselves but they may conflict with primary duties in a way that exerts negative influence. Researchers, just like everyone else, live in a tangled web of obligations to their employer, themselves, their profession, participants, funders, and others. COIs are not measurable units because human behaviour and motivations are often difficult to ascertain. A further complication in determining undue conflicts of interests is that a COI is distinct from conflicts of obligation. A conflict of obligation is a situation where an individual or an institution has duties that require different actions but only one action can

be taken given the circumstance. For example, a research participant who has a non-notifiable infectious disease may potentially be of harm to others but the researcher has an obligation to maintain confidentiality. While most of the literature on the topic of conflict of interests focuses on individuals, institutions can also have conflicts of interest. These types of conflict arise when an institution or its senior officials impose risks or undue influence on decisions involving the institution's primary interests (Lo and Field, 2009). A famous case of institutional COI occurred in Canada and is often referred to as the Olivieri affair (see Health Research in Action box 5.3).

Whether at the individual or institutional levels, there are ways to deal with conflict of interest situations. In health research, the wellbeing of individual research participants must take

5.3   Health Research in Action

Dr Nancy Olivieri was a researcher at the Hospital for Sick Children located in Toronto. She was doing a study on a blood disorder known as thalassemia. The study was funded by the pharmaceutical company Apotex. During the course of her research, Dr Olivieri found that the drug she was studying might cause some harm to her patients. She felt she had a duty to report those risks to her patients. However, Apotex disagreed with her interpretation and threated to take legal action against her if she were to disclose. Apotex claimed that the contract Dr Olivieri signed with them contained a non-disclosure clause, which prevented the researcher from disclosing any confidential information about the drug. In other words her legal obligation to the sponsor conflicted with her moral and clinical obligation to patients (Schafer, 2004).

Dr Olivieri was the subject of many reports and internal as well as external investigations. In the end, with next to no support from her

hospital or the University of Toronto, she received full exoneration by her professional college and several independent reports. One of the more interesting discoveries during this time was that her employer, University of Toronto, was negotiating a CAD 20 million donation from the same drug company that was suing Dr Olivieri (Schafer, 2004). The University's president at that time had gone as far as to lobby the Canadian government on behalf of Apotex. It has been argued that when private pharmaceutical companies sponsor studies, they usually do so because they wish to see results that are favourable to their products and that biomedical researchers and universities should not be in a situation of financial conflicts of interest (Schafer, 2004). Such activities placed the university in a situation of institutional conflict of interest that prevented it from being a fair broker (Kondro, 2007).

precedence over all other interests. Institutions need to foster an environment of openness and accountability. A key component of fostering this culture is to declare and then appropriately manage organizational and research COIs. The task of identifying and managing COIs is both complex and time-consuming. Disclosure of COI allows all those involved to adjust their expectation of one another but this is not necessarily a remedy for all conflicts (Tonelli, 2007). Disclosure is only effective when it is done in concert with management techniques. These can be tailored to specific circumstances and can range from full prohibition of certain interests to avoidance of others.

Research with Special Populations

Marginalized communities are frequently the focus of health research. Research with these communities often invites considerations of vulnerability. Research involving vulnerable persons is quite broad but may include children, persons with disabilities, those who are institutionalized, minorities, or those involved with illicit activities. Vulnerability may be considered as a joint product of participant characteristics and research design; and it should be acknowledged that all of us are potentially vulnerable at certain points in our lives. Research with especially vulnerable populations raises unique ethical issues. The notion of vulnerability is associated with limited capacity or limited access to rights, opportunities, and power. Groups whose circumstances or historical injustices have caused them to be marginalized may need to be afforded special protections in order to ensure they are treated justly in research. This does not mean that vulnerable groups should be inappropriately excluded from participating in research; however, the ethical obligation of the researchers is to ensure that the participants'

interests are properly safeguarded. Researchers need to engage communities in research and ensure that prominent cases of research controversy do not jeopardize the participants' trust.

Research with First Nations, Inuit, and Métis (Aboriginal) people of Canada has been particularly marred by unethical cases of conduct by researchers that have caused concern. People from those communities have often felt they have been researched extensively with very little or no real benefit to their communities. The majority of these research studies were conducted by university or government researchers who had approached their communities with completed research designs that did not address the communities' most pressing health issues. Several of these researchers have benefited greatly from this research but have failed to create any capacity in Aboriginal communities. One of the main ethical issues has focused on the inability to obtain free and informed consent from study participants (see Health Research in Action box 5.4). Individuals from these communities report being persuaded to take part in studies without understanding risks to health and safety, or misapplication of research outcomes (Schnarch, 2004). These are just some of the recurring grievances about the research process, which they perceive to be very colonial in its approach.

In response to these and other related grievances, Canadian Aboriginal communities have mobilized to create a research-based political response that aims to create an ethical framework for knowledge production within their communities. The **ownership, control, access, and possession** (OCAP) principles aim to enhance community's self-determination in the research process. Ownership means that a community or a group owns information collectively. Control means that those communities or groups control all aspects of data management that may impact them—from formulating the research question

5.4 Health Research in Action

The Nuu-chah-nulth people are a group of First Nations tribes that live along the northwestern coast of Canada. They have high rates of rheumatoid arthritis, and in 1986 they agreed to take part in a research study done by a University of British Columbia (UBC) genetic researcher, Ryk Ward. The study was funded by the government of Canada and approximately 900 individuals donated their blood. The results of the study were inconclusive but Dr Ward soon left UBC and took the tissue samples with him without consent from the research participants. He continued to do research on the samples and produced many research papers that covered everything from studies on HIV/AIDS to migration (Kovach, 2009; Wiwchar, 2004). The tribe never gave their consent to these additional studies. In 2000, these studies came to the attention of tribal members and many felt misled and betrayed. As a direct response to this case, the tribe created its own research ethics board that would review all research taking place in their communities.

- Identify and analyze the ethical issues from the perspective of participants.

- Identify and analyze the ethical issues from the perspective of the researcher.

- What would you do in this situation as a student conducting research on your supervisor's protocol?

to dissemination of results. Access gives the communities rights to manage and make decisions regarding use of their data. The final principle, possession, refers to the mechanism by which ownership can be asserted (Schnarch, 2004). All of the principles are meant to be ethical guides to researchers in order to assist them in their decision making processes.

Applied Ethics in Health Sciences Research

Despite concerted efforts to ensure ethics in research and a vast literature on the topic, some unethical research continues. For example, in recent years federal agents temporarily shut down the entire research programs at two US research universities following the death of research subjects, in order to scrutinize their ethics review processes. In the case of the gene therapy death at Penn State University the subject had not been adequately informed of the potential dangers of the study. At Johns Hopkins University, an avoidable death resulted from failure to perform an adequate literature review that would have revealed previously documented fatalities from use of the experimental drug. The Olivieri case in Canada and growth of conflicts of interest associated with commercialization of research, remind us of vulnerability within Canada to participation in unethical research.

Increasingly, it is being acknowledged that the ethics of medical research on humans is also applicable to research in the social sciences and other disciplines where research may be associated with considerable psychological harm and the exploitation of vulnerable people. The HIV/AIDS pandemic has greatly increased sensitivity to the range of psychological and physical harms that may follow unethical medical and social science research. These concerns have been buttressed by (1) the growth of research as an international collaborative endeavour—often driven by the interests of powerful nations—with the potential to exploit vulnerable participants from alternative cultures in developing countries; and (2) sensitivity to the need to reduce such exploitation. This led the US National Institutes of Health to fund through its Fogarty International Centre 18 centres around the world (budget of USD $4 million per year) to promote capacity building education in research ethics in developing countries.

The focus on this chapter has mostly been on research ethics issues in the Canadian context. However, it is notable that in a globalizing world 90 per cent of annual global health research expenditure is on diseases that cause 10 per cent of the global burden of disease, and Canadian researchers are frequently involved in international projects at several sites. Before researchers embark on any international projects they should have a thorough understanding of the social, economic, and political environment of these countries (Benatar, 2002), and some understanding of evolving new ethical requirements in international collaborative research (Benatar and Singer, 2010). These proactive actions could promote understanding of community needs and better guide researchers in addressing some of the large disparities in global health. Research should be a tool for promoting positive change in the lives of those who need it the most. By incorporating community needs in the design of international studies, researchers can build hope for a better future.

Conclusion

The planning and execution of research requires researchers to have an ethical framework for decision making. Health researchers must understand the ethical dimension to their work and apply sound judgements. Ethical dilemmas can arise at the level of personal behaviour of the research team and in all stages of research: design, recruitment, analysis, and dissemination of study results. The ethical obligation does not begin and end at the REB level but is instead a continuous process involving researchers, research participants, and society at large. Over the past 60 years, research ethics frameworks have evolved from dominance of paternalism through more detailed regulations, to considerations of research subjects' participation in the choice and design of studies, and more recently to considerations of community engagement in order to link research to capacity building, human development, and application of research in practice. A major challenge for junior health researchers will be to move from an intellectual understanding of abstract ethical principles to applying them in their daily practice.

Summary

- Ethics is a branch of moral philosophy that aims to systematically address concepts of what is right and wrong, or what is good and bad. Morals are related but focus on observed behaviours of individuals or groups based on their traditional beliefs and values.
- Two major approaches to ethics are consequentialism and deontology.

- Awareness of the extent to which research participants could be abused first came to prominence following experiments done in the Second World War.
- There are many requirements for ethical research. In addition, researchers should be sensitive to ethical issues and receive some education on research ethics.

- The pre-eminent guidance document for all research in Canada is the *Tri-Council Policy Statement* or TCPS. According to the TCPS, the core principles are respect for persons, concern for welfare, and justice.
- Seeking free and informed consent from participants is an ethical and legal cornerstone of good research and a way that researchers show respect for participants.
- Research ethics boards (REBs) may approve, reject, or propose modifications to a study under review. REBs review research to ensure that risks are minimized, consent is free and informed, the study is scientifically sound, burdens are equitably distributed, and that any conflicts of interest are properly managed.
- Clinical trials are important in health research since they are central to registration of new drugs and treatments.
- Much like other human endeavours, health research is open to interpretation, imperfection, and misuse of power. Notable examples of research misconduct in Canada include the cases of Poisson, Chandra, and Poehlman.
- With a view to reducing misconduct, federal granting agencies have created several initiatives to address research integrity and misconduct.
- Research with First Nations, Inuit, and Métis has been marred by several cases of questionable conduct. As a response, Canadian Aboriginal communities have mobilized to create the ownership, control, access, and possession (OCAP) framework for research ethics.
- The researchers' ethical obligations do not begin and end at the REB but form part of a continuous interactive process with research participants and society.

Review Questions

1. In order to ethically carry out their research, it is essential that all stakeholders involved in human research understand the guidelines and best practices that facilitate research. Canadians interested in research can complete an online research ethics tutorial. This self-paced tutorial features multi-media and interactive exercises, and can be found on the following website: http://tcps2core.ca/welcome#.

2. Try to create a draft informed consent document for the following hypothetical study. You are a nursing student who wishes to do a qualitative study using one-on-one interviews with approximately 10 HIV-positive individuals to find out how they view their health and sexual well-being. You plan to recruit participants by posting flyers in a local hospital clinic and conduct the interviews over the phone. The semi-structured interviews will be audio recorded. You will take notes during the call and anticipate that each interview will be no longer than one hour. You have no funding so you will not provide any financial compensation. Write an informed consent document for this study that explains all the key points of your research and is no longer than 1500 words.

Recommended Readings

Annas, G.J. (1992) *The Nuremberg Code: Human Rights in Human Experimentation*. New York: Oxford University Press.

Detailed book on the crimes committed by Nazi physicians and researchers that promoted the creation of one of the most important research ethics documents of all time—the Nuremberg Code.

Beauchamp, T.L. and Childress, J.F. (2008) *Principles of Biomedical Ethics*. 6th ed. USA: Oxford University Press.

One of the most insightful texts on ethics in the health professions. Includes the use of the four well-known principles (respect for autonomy, non-maleficence, beneficence, and justice) to guide moral reasoning.

Emanuel, E.J., Crouch, R.A., Arras, J.D., Moreno, J.D., and Grady, C. (Eds.) (2003) *Ethical and Regulatory Aspects of Clinical Research: Readings and Commentary*. 1st ed. Baltimore, Maryland: The Johns Hopkins University Press.

A collection of readings and commentaries geared toward undergraduate students interested in learning more about different aspects of research ethics and public health.

Jones, J.H. (1993) *Bad Blood: The Tuskegee Syphilis Experiment*. Revised Edition. New York: Free Press.

A thorough account of the US government-funded study in Macon County, Alabama that studied the effect of untreated syphilis in African-American males.

Kovach, M.E. (2010) *Indigenous Methodologies: Characteristics, Conversations, and Contexts*. Reprint. Toronto: University of Toronto Press, Scholarly Publishing Division.

A brief book on indigenous research methodologies, which offers guidance for students and all those wishing to work with traditional communities.

Lavery, J.V., Grady, C., Wahl, E.R., and Emanuel, E.J. (Eds.) (2007) *Ethical Issues in International Biomedical Research: A Casebook*. 1st ed. USA: Oxford University Press.

A comprehensive book that examines 21 cases of controversial issues in research ethics in developing countries.

Lo, B. and Fields, M.J. (Eds.) (2009) *Conflict of Interest in Medical Research, Education, and Practice*. 1st ed. Washington, DC: National Academies Press.

This Institute of Medicine report examines conflict of interest by examining the available evidence on the extent of the industry relationship with researchers and how different institutions have decided to manage or limit conflicts.

Skloot, R. (2011) *The Immortal Life of Henrietta Lacks*. Reprint. New York: Broadway.

A personal look at the life of a woman whose cells became one of the most valuable tools in medical research. Henrietta Lacks's cells (known as HeLa cells) were used for developing many important advances, yet were taken from her without her consent.

Note

1. While the use of animals for research or testing carries ethical imperatives and has strong emotional overtones for some people, such considerations are beyond the scope of this chapter.

References

Angell, M. and Kassirer, J.P. (1994) Setting the record straight in the breast-cancer trials. *New England Journal of Medicine,* 330(20), 1448–50.

Benatar, S.R. (2002) Reflections and recommendations on research ethics in developing countries. *Social Science and Medicine,* 54, 1131–41.

Benatar, S.R., and Singer, P.A. (2010) Responsibilities in international research: a new look revisited. *Journal of Medical Ethics,* 36(4), 194–7.

Beauchamp, T.L., and Childress, J.F. (2009) *Principles of Biomedical Ethics.* 6th ed. New York: Oxford University Press.

Canadian Institutes of Health Research, Natural Sciences and Engineering Research Council of Canada, and Social Sciences and Humanities Research Council of Canada. (2011) *Tri-Agency Framework: Responsible Conduct of Research.* Ottawa, Ontario: Government of Canada.

Canadian Institutes of Health Research, Natural Sciences and Engineering Research Council of Canada, and Social Sciences and Humanities Research Council of Canada. (2010) *Tri-Council Policy Statement: Ethical Conduct for Research Involving Humans.* Ottawa, Ontario: Government of Canada.

Council of Canadian Academies. (2010) Honesty, accountability and trust: Fostering research integrity in Canada: The Expert Panel on Research Integrity. Retrieved from: www.scienceadvice.ca/uploads/eng/assessments%20and%20publications%20and%20news%20releases/research%20integrity/ri_report.pdf.

De Melo-Martin, I. and Ho, A. (2008). Beyond informed consent: the therapeutic misconception and trust. *Journal of Medical Ethics,* 34, 202–5.

Hickling Arthurs Low. (2009) The state of research integrity and misconduct policies in Canada. Canadian Research Integrity Committee, www.hal.ca/index.php?option=com_content&view=article&id=65:hal-publishes-research-integrity-report&catid=39:news%Itemid=43.

Kondro, W. (2005) Université de Montréal in the dark about fraud. *Canadian Medical Association Journal,* 172(10), 1278.

Kondro, W. (2007) Call for arm's-length national research integrity agency. *Canadian Medical Association Journal,* 176(6), 749–50.

Kovach, M. (2009) *Indigenous Methodologies: Characteristics, Conversations, and Contexts.* Toronto, Canada: University of Toronto Press.

Lidz, C.W., Appelbaum, P.S., Grisso, T., and Renaud, M. (2004) Therapeutic misconception and the appreciation of risks in clinical trials. *Social Science and Medicine,* 58, 1689–97.

Lo, B. and Field, M. (2009) *Conflict of Interest: In Medical Research, Education, and Practice.* Washington, DC: Institute of Medicine of the National Academies.

Oberle, K. and Allen, M. (2006) Ethical considerations for nurses in clinical trials. *Nursing Ethics,* 13(2), 180–6.

Palys, T., and Lowman, J. (2000). Ethical and legal strategies for protecting confidential research information. *Canadian Journal of Law and Society*, 15(1), 39–80.

Schafer, A. (2004) Biomedical conflicts of interest: A defense of the sequestration thesis-learning from the cases of Nancy Olivieri and David Healy. *Journal of Medical Ethics*, 30, 8–24.

Schnarch, B. (2004) Ownership, control, access, and possession (OCAP) or self-determination applied to research: A critical analysis of contemporary First Nations research and some options for First Nations communities. *Journal of Aboriginal Health*, 1, 80–95.

Smith, R. (2006) Research misconduct: the poisoning of the well. *Journal of the Royal Society of Medicine*, 99, 232–7.

Sox, H.C. and Rennie, D. (2006) Research misconduct, retraction, and cleansing the medical literature: lessons from the Poehlman case. *Annals of Internal Medicine*, E7–E11.

Tonelli, M. (2007) Conflict of interest in clinical practice. *American College of Chest Physicians*, 132(2), 664–70.

Wiwchar, D. (2004,). Nuu-chach-nulth blood returns to west coast. *Ha-Shilth-Sa*, pp. 1–4.

6 Overview of Study Designs in Health

Martin Tammemägi

CHAPTER OUTLINE

Introduction

A fundamental purpose of research is to obtain knowledge. This may be to obtain descriptive information or identify new associations, in particular causal associations, to validate suspected associations, and to predict future events or new relationships. In the health sciences, such knowledge helps us to control, manipulate, prevent, detect and treat medical conditions. All research requires a study design, that is, a plan or strategy. The study design identifies who the study participants will be, how they will be sampled and how many will be sampled, which in turn determines what and how measurements are taken, and the most appropriate analysis for answering the study question. When the details of a study design are incorporated into a formal document, it is often referred to as the *study protocol*. In this chapter we introduce (1) qualitative research methods, such as focus groups, and (2) quantitative methods, which include **experimental study** designs, such as randomized clinical trials, and observational study designs, including the cohort, cross-sectional, case-control, and ecological study designs.

It is through scientific study that medical advances have occurred at a rapid rate in the last 100 years and have made possible great leaps in the general health of the public. Consider that global life expectancy at birth in 1800 was just 28.5 years (Ferguson, 2011) and in Canada in 2009 it was 80.7 years (World Development Indicators, 2011). This remarkable increase in life expectancy can be attributed in large part to scientific study and advances in health studies. Almost all of the research study designs described in this chapter have come into existence in the last two hundred years, and most have come into common research practice in the last 70 years.

Many factors go into making an excellent health researcher. Curiosity, ethics, objectivity, and a deep understanding of subject knowledge come to mind. However, one of the most important is the understanding of scientific methodology, including the many aspects of study design.

Background Concepts

Much of health research concerns developing an understanding between some "exposure" and "disease" or other health-related "outcome." Exposure can have a wide range of meanings. For example, exposure could be an environmental toxin such as lead, a health-related behaviour such as smoking, a personality type, a genetic mutation, a dietary pattern, a prevention program such as a smoking cessation program, a cancer screening program, or a treatment for a disease.

Similarly, disease or outcome in health studies can represent a multitude of different things, for example, getting a specific disease, having a disease recurrence after successful treatment, time to relapse, or death due to disease. We may start with disease-free individuals and investigate which exposures increase their likelihood of getting the disease, or start with diseased people and study what factors influence their recovery. What may be the endpoint (outcome) in one study may be a starting point (exposure) in another study. For example, one study may investigate whether smoking decreases quality of life, and another study may investigate whether quality of life impacts the survival of cancer patients.

Study designs are determined by how one chooses or samples and measures the exposures and disease or outcome states. Studies that have hypothesis and comparison groups which allow statistical testing to find out if a difference exists between groups or if an association exists between the exposure and disease or outcome are *quantitative* studies. Studies that are descriptive in which hypotheses are not tested are *qualitative* studies. Qualitative studies are used to discover new knowledge and answer questions which cannot be answered using quantitative study methods. Qualitative study methods are described in the second half of this chapter.

To understand how to relate exposure and disease/outcome in different study designs, it is important to develop some knowledge regarding measures of health. Some common health measures include incidence, prevalence, and mortality rates. To evaluate causal relationships we usually attempt to evaluate the risk or probability of disease/outcome in the exposed group and see if it is different from the risk or probability in the unexposed group. In health studies, the optimum measure of risk or probability is obtained from incidence rates. *Incidence rate* is the number of new cases of disease in a defined population at risk per unit time. In the absence of such data, alternative health data are sometimes used. For example, if most of the people with the disease die of that specific disease after a relatively short period, then *prevalence proportion* or *mortality rates* may be used, *prevalence proportion* being the number of existing cases in a defined population at risk during one point in time (*point prevalence*) or during a period of time (*period prevalence*). In diseases that have a long duration, such as multiple sclerosis or arthritis, the prevalence proportion may be quite different from the incidence rates. *Mortality rate* is the number of deaths per population per unit of time. Mortality rates would not be a good surrogate for incidence data, if accurate cause-specific mortality data were not available or the disease was usually non-fatal. Different study designs provide different measures of health events, and thus provide different strengths of evidence for causal relationships. To control health-related events, we usually try to understand causal relationships, not mere correlations that might not be causal.

In some study settings, the researcher has control over which study participants receive or do not receive the "exposure" under study. These are *experimental* study designs and usually involve exposures thought to be safe. It would be unethical to administer a harmful exposure in a research study setting, for example, cigarette smoke to a non-smoker. Researchers investigating the effects of potentially harmful exposures must rely on observational studies. These are studies in which some of the study participants received the exposure under study due to self-selection or accident.

PRACTICAL TIP

Sometimes students and even some scientists think that to study the relationship between exposure and disease, the "unexposed" group must have zero exposure. Indeed, one scientist came onto the radio denouncing the INTERPHONE study investigating cell phone use and brain cancer (Interphone Group, 2010), because she said that no one in the control group was free of exposure. This thinking is not correct. It is valid to study the rate of disease over a range or gradient of exposures. For example, it is well-known that blood pressure or body mass index (BMI, weight in kilograms/height in metres squared) are determinants of health outcomes; yet no living human has a blood pressure or BMI of zero.

Study Designs

For a new study, the optimal study design is driven by the study question, the available population for study, resources, and the current state of research. Different study designs vary in cost, time required to conduct them, complexity, vulnerability to bias, and the evidence they contribute to establishing causal relationships. Although some study designs are more optimal than others, it is often not possible, feasible or even necessary to start off testing the study question/hypothesis with the most elaborate study design. Most study designs can contribute valuable information, if well-conducted and interpreted in light of their weaknesses. Scientific knowledge and causal relationships in health are rarely, if ever, advanced by one study in isolation. The scientific process is iterative and depends on replication of findings in different populations by different researchers in different settings using different approaches. Some examples of study questions which are suitably answered by the different study designs are presented in Table 6.1.

TABLE 6.1   Example Study Questions That can Appropriately be Answered by the Specific Study Designs

Study Design	Study Question
Randomized controlled trial	Does vitamin E and beta carotene supplementation protect smokers against developing lung cancer?
Cohort	Does smoking cause lung cancer?
Case-control	Is childhood leukaemia associated with parental occupation during conception?
Cross-sectional/prevalence	What is the prevalence of cigarette smoking in Canadian high school students?
Ecological	Does the national intake of fat calories correlate with national breast cancer mortality rates in various countries around the world?

Randomized Controlled Trial (RCT)

The **randomized controlled trial** (RCT) is a study design often used to evaluate the therapeutic effects of treatments in diseased individuals, or the beneficial effects of a protective agent or screening procedure. This study design is *experimental* in that the researcher controls who receives the treatment or intervention, that is the "exposure", and who gets the alternative. Those receiving the alternative are called the *controls*, and the alternative may consist of a placebo, no intervention, or the currently accepted treatment. A *placebo* is a simulated agent or sham procedure that has no specific intended therapeutic effect but is intended to make the recipient thinking that they might be receive treatment.

The RCT is a **prospective** study in that the study participants receive the intervention or become controls, and are then followed over time to determine the rates of the study outcome in both groups. A key element of the RCT is that study participants are randomly assigned into the intervention or control arms of the study. The components and flow of the RCT are illustrated in Figure 6.1. It is important to appreciate that the researcher does not get to pick and choose who gets the intervention and who does not. Such a practice could lead to selection bias, for example, this could occur when a researcher, who believes in the new treatment under study, assigns

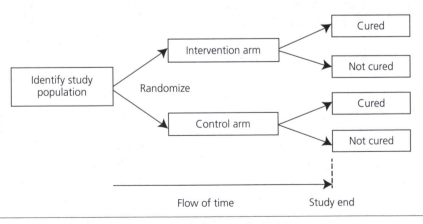

FIGURE 6.1   Components and flow of the randomized controlled trial

healthier patients to the treatment group and the sicker ones to the **control group**. In the properly randomized trial, the researcher has no control over who ends up in the intervention and control arms. In addition, when it is feasible, the evaluation of study outcome is done blinded to which study arm an individual belongs to. If randomization was successful and the study is sufficiently large, other factors which influence the study outcome, for example age and severity of disease on survival, are usually distributed roughly equally in both study arms and balance out in analysis. This is an example of *confounding* being controlled for in RCTs.

The "randomized controlled trial" (RCT) is sometimes referred to as a "randomized clinical trial". The former name is preferred, because the RCT is often used to evaluate prevention programs to reduce subsequent disease in a healthy population. In this situation, the word "clinical" is not appropriate, because "clinical" usually refers to diagnosis and treatment of patients in medical practice.

Sometimes, some interventions are evaluated best at the community level. For example, the beneficial effect of fluoridation of drinking water on reducing dental disease (caries) was first convincingly demonstrated in randomized community trials. The impact of public health policies or teaching practices would be best evaluated when randomized to districts or classrooms, respectively. When the unit of randomization is a group of individuals sharing one or more defining characteristics, then the study is referred to as a *randomized community trial*.

6.1   Health Research in Action

A Cautionary Story

The randomized controlled trial is thought to be the ideal study because it reflects a true experiment, and true randomization can minimize confounding and selection bias. So how can one explain the following story?

Prostate specific-antigen testing (PSA) was adopted for screening men for prostate cancer in general medical practice in many western countries in the 1980s. This adoption took place without strong scientific evidence to support it. Recently, two large RCTs, the *European Randomized Study of Screening for Prostate Cancer* in Europe (Schroder et al., 2009) and the *Prostate, Lung, Colorectal and Ovarian Cancer Screening Trial* (PLCO) in the United States (Andriole et al., 2009), evaluated whether annual screening with PSA reduced prostate mortality. The European study found that PSA screening significantly reduced prostate cancer mortality, and the US PLCO found no reduction in mortality. These findings, with opposite conclusions, come from what is considered to be the highest type of study design. This is perplexing! What happened? The studies looked at the same question using similar study designs and came to opposite conclusions. It turns out that the populations under study were different. In Europe, PSA testing was not commonly carried out in routine practice. In the US, PSA testing is often routinely carried out in older men in annual checkups. In the PLCO control group a high proportion of men were getting PSA testing outside the trial. This lead the two groups to be similar with regard to the "exposure" under study and no difference in mortality could be found. Such studies are complex and interpretation is not always straightforward. Considerable thought needs to be given to all aspects of the study, from its design, conduct, analysis, and interpretation.

Cohort Study Design

In the *cohort study*, individuals without the disease of interest are sampled and they are classified according to whether they have the exposure of interest or not. They are then followed over time to see who develops disease and who does not (Figure 6.2). Cohort studies are sometimes referred to as prospective studies. The health measurements of primary interest are incidence rates, and these rates are compared between the exposed and unexposed groups. Sampling of study participants generally can take two approaches. *Population-based sampling* attempts to select participants so that they reflect the general population of interest or some component of it. This is useful for relatively common exposures. When an exposure is uncommon or rare, then sampling is often *exposure-based* to ensure adequate numbers of exposed individuals in the study. For example, to study the impact of inhaling high temperature combustion particles on respiratory cancers in firemen, one would not sample the general population, but rather would sample firemen and a comparison group similar to firemen except for the exposure under study, for example, policemen. Sometimes studies are carried out using data that have been collected in the past. But even in these *historical cohort* studies, exposure measurements were made in disease-free individuals who were subsequently followed to determine if disease occurred at some later point in time.

Because cohort studies have exposures measured before disease has occurred, inferring causal associations between exposure and disease is more convincing than with other study designs in which the order of events is unclear. Cohort studies measure disease or outcome rates over time, and thus make possible estimation of rates of disease in the exposed and unexposed groups. This makes possible the direct calculation of risks related to exposures under study. In prospective cohort studies, more accurate and detailed measurements of exposures are possible than in retrospective studies.

However, the distribution of other factors that affect the outcome may differ between exposed and unexposed groups and may distort or *confound* the association under study. In cohort studies such potential confounders must be dealt with to obtain valid results. Some diseases have long incubation periods between exposure and disease, and a cohort study of

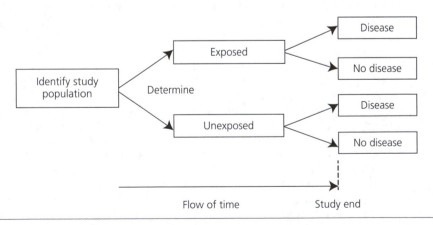

FIGURE 6.2   Components and flow of the cohort study

their relationship would require a long time. For example, it is estimated that the time between asbestos exposure and mesothelioma, a cancer of the lining of the thoracic cavity, is between 30 to 40 years. A cohort study of the association between asbestos exposure and mesothelioma may well span more than one researcher's career. Some diseases are uncommon or rare. A cohort study of such diseases would have to be very large to draw meaningful conclusions. Follow-up of cohort members must be done systematically and rigorously. Loss of follow-up can lead to biased study findings and must be minimized. However, this can be time-consuming and challenging because participants often move or lose interest in the study over time and drop out. For example, consider a study of the association between cigarette smoking and lung cancer survivorship. What will be the impact on the study conclusions if smoking in truth does lead to shorter survival, but smokers are more likely to quit the study before their follow-up is complete?

Case-control Study

In the **case-control study** cases from a specified population are sampled. Controls (non-

cases) who are free of the disease under study are also sampled. Ideally, the controls should come from the same referent population that gave rise to the cases. In other words, if controls had been diagnosed with the disease of interest, they should have a similar likelihood of being enrolled in the study as the cases in the study. Sometimes the controls are selected to be similar to cases with regard to some characteristics such as age, sex, race/ethnicity, socioeconomic status, or smoking status. This is called *matching*. Following enrollment in the study, the past exposures of cases and controls are measured (Figure 6.3). In the case-control study there is no carefully measured follow-up time, so it is not possible to directly calculate incidence rates and relative rates between exposed and unexposed groups. Instead in the case-control study, the measure of association is the exposure odds ratio, that is, the probability of exposure divided by the probability of no exposure in the cases versus in the controls.

Case-control studies are good for studying rare or uncommon diseases. Also, multiple exposures can be evaluated in one study. Generally, case-control studies are cheaper and faster to complete than their cohort counterparts.

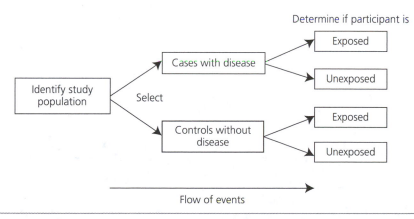

FIGURE 6.3   Components and sequence of events in a case-control study design

PRACTICAL TIP

When designing your own study, be careful to sample participants appropriately, based on the study design selected. If conducting a cohort or case-control study, be sure to sample your study participants consistently, either based on exposure for a cohort study or disease status for a case-control study, not a mixture of both. For example, a student wanted to study if having diabetes increases the risk of developing colorectal cancer using cohort data. Selected for study were colorectal cancer patients who had diabetes (exposure) and individuals who had not developed colorectal cancer (disease/outcome) during follow-up, who had or did not have diabetes. In this case, correct calculation of odds ratios or relative risks is not possible.

However, case-control studies are more vulnerable to biases than cohort and RCTs. Choosing unrepresentative case or control groups can lead to *selection bias*. This is especially likely when using hospital or medical system controls compared to using population-based samples drawn from the community at large because individuals who are sick and under medical care may well have had exposures different from the general population. *Recall bias* occurs when cases, because of their illness, reflect more about their past exposures than healthy controls, and report past exposures in a manner that is systematically different than controls. For example, a mother of a baby born with a congenital abnormality may be more likely to report having been exposed to toxic substances than a healthy control.

Variations on Cohort and Case-control Study Designs

There are several variants of cohort and case control studies. For the cohort design, they include the nested case-control study, the case-cohort study, and the case-crossover study. These designs are advanced methods, which are not detailed further in this text. Further details can be found in standard epidemiologic textbooks, such as by Gordis (2009).

Cross-sectional or Prevalence Study

When a population is sampled and the exposure status and disease status are measured at the same time, the study design is called a **cross-sectional** or **prevalence study** (see Figure 6.4).

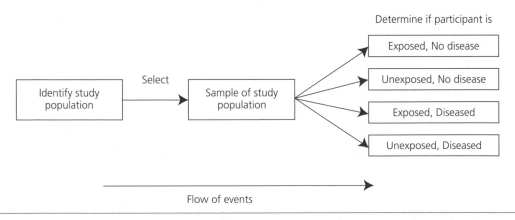

FIGURE 6.4   Contingency table stratifying exposure versus disease status for a cross-sectional study

This study design has a number of limitations. Because the element of time is not measured incidence rates cannot be calculate. As with the case-control study, associations are measured by the odds ratio. And, because temporal sequence is often unclear, that is, we don't know whether the exposure was followed by disease, or vice versa, arguing a causal relationship between exposure and disease is weak. When studying fatal diseases, cross-sectional studies are over represented by survivors, which may be unrepresentative of the disease in general, especially when studying disease etiology (cause). Many cross-sectional studies rely on self-reported disease status, which may not be as accurate as doctor-diagnosed disease status. Further, for rare or uncommon disease a large sample size is required.

Regardless of these limitations, the cross-sectional study design is much used and makes important contributions. It is good for estimating the burden of exposures and diseases in populations, and because multiple exposures and diseases or outcomes can be investigated in one study, it is useful for exploring and discovering new associations. Some chronic diseases have an insidious onset, making accurate incidence of disease hard to measure. With these types of diseases, such as multiple sclerosis or dementia, cross-sectional studies provide an alternative to cohort studies. Generally, cross-sectional studies are relatively cheap and fast to conduct.

Cross-sectional studies also provide valuable information used to design cohort and case-control studies. For example, to calculate the sample size needed in a case-control study of genetic variations and disease, the prevalence of the genetic variants (polymorphisms) in the population is required. Such information often comes from cross-sectional studies.

Large national cross-sectional studies repeated over time play an important role in monitoring unhealthy exposures, behaviours and diseases, and trends in them over time, and can provide a sense of whether current health promotion programs are working or are needed. An example of a cross-sectional study is the Canadian Health Measures Survey, which began collecting data in 2007 in two-year cycles. The survey collects direct physical measures, including blood and urine samples for laboratory testing, as well as data on environmental exposures to contaminants and infectious diseases, lifestyle characteristics, and the extent of chronic diseases. For each two-year collection period about 5500 participants across Canada between the ages of three and 79 are surveyed. The intended end users of this information are policy makers, health professionals, and researchers.

Ecological Studies

The studies described in this chapter so far, collect exposure and disease status data at the individual level. In **ecological studies**, we do not have individual level data, but data summarizing the exposure and/or disease in samples or populations. If we collect these summary data for a large number of samples or populations (usually ≥ 10) then we can statistically test if there is a correlation between exposure and disease. For example, one published ecologic study found that the density of fast food outlets in Ontario correlated significantly with cardiovascular mortality rates in the community (Alter and Eny, 2005).

PRACTICAL TIP

Some students mistakenly thinking that ecological studies have something to do with ecology, the study of the relationships between living organisms with each other and the environment. In the context of health studies, the ecological study design means something completely different.

Ecological studies are vulnerable to many weaknesses. For example, using ecological data it would be easy to demonstrate that the average number of cars per capita correlates with national average breast cancer incidence rates. However, common sense tells us that cars do not directly cause breast cancer. One important weakness of the ecological study design is the *ecological fallacy*; that is, results that apply at the group level may not apply at the individual level. Applied to the previous example, the study did not demonstrate that those individuals who had the cardiovascular deaths ate at fast-food outlets.

Sometimes the results of ecological studies are clearly wrong. For instance, the *Seven Countries Study of Hypertension and Stroke* found that hypertension was protective against stroke at the ecological level, whereas the individual level data confirmed the accepted association between hypertension and increase risk of stroke (Menotti et al., 1996).

Ecological studies can fail to control confounding variables and often present weak evidence supporting a causal relationship. For instance, in the previous example of fast-food restaurant-cardiovascular mortality, it may well be that some other aspects of life in the communities where there is a high density of fast-food restaurants are the direct causal links to heart attacks. In other words, if one forcibly closed fast-food restaurants, cardiovascular death rates may be unaffected.

Although ecological analysis can lead to spurious conclusions, they often do lead to important correct conclusions. In some situations, inter-country variations in an exposure are considerably larger than intra-country variations, and associations with disease are easier to identify. In addition, some exposures, such as health policies, food availability or smoking regulations, are administered at the group level and can only be studied with ecological designs. Because ecological studies are cheap and can be run quickly, they are a good early step in studying

hypothesized relationships or discovering new relationships.

Validity Pyramid of Quantitative Study Designs

Of the quantitative study designs, not all studies have equal potential for drawing valid conclusions. Some studies are more vulnerable to bias while some more closely reflect a true experiment and thus are considered to have a higher likelihood of producing valid or truthful findings.

Figure 6.5 attempts to represent an ordering of health study designs, working up from least to most potential validity. If the RCT is optimal, why not use the RCT design in all studies? Because it is unethical to expose individuals to harmful exposures. That is why almost all studies of potentially harmful exposures are observational. Non-serious exceptions sometimes occur, for example, in the study of the adverse effects of sleep deprivation in healthy volunteers. In addition, some exposures are more suitably administered to groups and the community trial design can be more appropriate than an RCT. Also, usually as one climbs up the Validity Pyramid, the studies become more complex, time-consuming, and expensive, so it makes sense to work one's way up from lower to higher study validity.

Some researchers do not like the idea of a "Validity Pyramid" because it might stigmatize studies lower in the pyramid. It is important to recognize that studies lower down the pyramid can produce valuable, valid information and lead to correct conclusions, but it is also important to be aware of their limitations. In medical science, no one study alone can irrefutably demonstrate a causal association. In the scientific process, validation of a new association by different researchers, in different settings, in different populations, and using different study designs, is much more

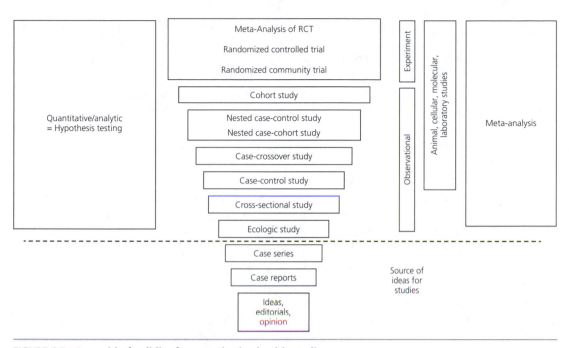

FIGURE 6.5   Pyramid of validity for quantitative health studies

convincing than an isolated finding, regardless of what study design was used.

Some have incorrectly argued that only the RCT can demonstrate a causal relationship because it is the only truly experimental study design for health studies of human populations. However, there is no doubt in the scientific community that smoking causes lung cancer, and yet no RCT was ever conducted to test this hypothesis. The first strong evidence for a link between smoking and lung cancer came from case-control studies followed by cohort studies in the 1940s and 1950s, which occurred before we had an understanding of the biological effects of smoking carcinogens on tumor suppressor genes and oncogenes.

Pilot or Feasibility Studies

Sometimes, to support a larger, more expensive, time-consuming, and complex study, prelimin-

ary studies are conducted to get information prior to carrying out the larger more definitive study. They may test the logistics of running the larger study so as to improve its quality and efficiency. **Pilot** or **feasibility studies** are not large enough to have enough statistical power to answer the specific proposed study question. Pilot studies may identify optimal methods for conducting the study, and sometimes evaluate whether a larger study is even feasible or affordable. Pilot studies may obtain data to more accurately calculate the sample size and study recruitment period for the larger study. This may entail measuring the **frequency** of the exposure of interest in the study population and the ability to recruit participants into the study, or to recruit cases in a case-control study. A pilot study may pre-test research tools, such as measurement instruments. Simply put, a pilot study may be said to "work out the bugs" before launching the larger study.

Qualitative Research

There is no one simple definition that describes all the features of qualitative research and different authors describe qualitative research in different ways. The following paragraphs provide a sense of what qualitative research is and does.

Qualitative research attempts to find out what is going on, what is happening, and the nature of "something" from the perspective of those involved in the situation under study (Bouma, Wilkinson, and Ling, 2009). In contrast to the ideal RCT setting, qualitative research is used to study what happens in the everyday world.

Qualitative research can involve feelings and impressions, which by their nature are not readily described numerically. This is in contrast to **quantitative research**, which involves measurements and numeric (statistical) descriptions of distributions or relationships between factors. Answers to questions such as how much, how often, what proportion, and what rate, involve counting and numbers, and by their nature entail quantitative research. The study question determines whether quantitative or qualitative methods are more appropriate.

Qualitative research can focus on beliefs and perceptions of truth that individuals have. Such things are difficult to quantify and measure at the population level. Consider studying the concerns and issues that people who are terminally ill have. Attempting to evaluate such issues with a structured close-ended quantitative questionnaire would not be effective as it would fail to capture many important concerns, many of which cannot be easily expressed in such a format.

Subjective "meaning" influences how individuals make decisions regarding health-related matters. Qualitative research attempts to interpret such subjective meanings and understand how they explain health-related behaviours (Green and Britten, 1998). For example, some individuals,

though already underweight, perceive themselves to have issues with their body, and diet when it is detrimental to their health. Qualitative methods can be used to investigate such perceptions and their link to eating disorders. Similarly, inappropriate use of some medications are attributed to patient perceptions, which can best be studied by qualitative methods (Green and Britten, 1998).

Qualitative researchers are also interested in the *process*, that is, how "meanings" change over time, and *interaction*, for example, between patient and physician. In addition, "reality" can look different from different perspectives, for example, from the physician's and patient's views. Qualitative health researchers are interested in studying such *relativism* (Green and Britten, 1998).

Often quantitative and qualitative research go hand-in-hand to develop true understanding and successful application of knowledge. For example, an RCT (quantitative research) suggests that annual screening for colorectal cancer using flexible sigmoidoscopy examination of the bowel significantly reduces deaths due to colorectal cancer (Weissfeld et al., 2012). Flexible sigmoidoscopy involves inserting a flexible endoscope through the rectum and visually inspecting the large bowel for abnormalities. Attempts to implement flexible sigmoidoscopy screening into public health practice may have disappointingly low participation rates and thus fail to provide the benefits projected from the RCT results. This is where *qualitative research* is invaluable. It can listen to individuals in the target population to find out the reasons why they are not participating in a flexible sigmoidoscopy screening program. Lack of participation may be due to a fear of discomfort, embarrassment, poor transportation availability, unaffordable costs. The researchers would not have been able to explain the failure of the program and how to modify it effectively, if they had not asked the right questions and listened to responses. In this case, researchers could use in-depth interviews or focus groups to identify the reasons for low participation.

Quantitative health studies usually have the outcome as the primary study focus (e.g cure vs. no cure in response to treatment), whereas qualitative studies evaluate the process or natural history of how one gets to the outcome (why was diagnosis not sought earlier when the disease was more curable).

Qualitative data has the *natural setting* as the direct source of data (Neutens and Rubinson, 2010). The researcher wants to study the situation in context so they often go to the location under study because situations can be best understood when they are directly observed (Neutens and Rubinson, 2010).

Phenomenologism is the idea that individuals have a voice, that understanding their story is essential to understanding social issues (Bouma, Wilkinson, and Ling, 2009). Qualitative researchers who are trying to understand a phenomenon do not only want to understand the individual's feelings, thoughts, and perspective, but also that of those in the participant's life. For example, in developing a complete understanding of the end-of-life experience of a terminal patient, the patient's spouse, family and friends, would also be interviewed. By talking to all stakeholders, new issues, concerns or understandings may arise. Most qualitative researchers use the *phenomenological perspective* (Neutens and Rubinson, 2010).

Methods Used in Qualitative Research

Qualitative research uses many methodological approaches, a few of which are outlined below. In many qualitative studies, multiple approaches are used.

1. A fundamental method for data collection is the **in-depth interview**, in which the researcher talks with the study participant about the study themes. Usually the interviewer does not use close-ended questions, but rather engages the interviewee in an open-ended conversation to extract ideas and interpretations.

2. Often individuals are interviewed in groups called **focus groups**. This can be particularly useful when individuals are reluctant to offer opinions or when it is inappropriate to ask questions on an individual level, for example, when asking about poor health services. Usually a moderator acts as a group leader directing discussion to make sure all planned topics are covered. Group size is often around five to 12 individuals.

3. What people actually do is often different from what they say they do. For this reason observing them can be an important source of data. **Observation** is a discovery-oriented approach in which data are collected in the natural setting, minimally influenced by the researcher. In some situations, observation is the optimal choice of study, for example, in the study of infants or dementia patients. The observation method can be unstructured or structured. In the **unstructured** method a digital camera, recorder, or an alternative method may be used to recorded events. Unstructured observations are best used to generate hypotheses.

   In contrast, **structured observation** studies are set up more formally. The researcher can pre-select activities to focus on and methods of data documentation (Neutens and Rubinson, 2010). Recording of activities, events, and behaviours can be continuous, or focus on the duration of a particular event, or the count or frequency of a specific behaviour, or what is happening at specific intervals. For example, the length of time physicians spend listening to a patient's problems during an office visit could be measured by structured observation, and time can be measured by stopwatch. Whether physicians consistently ask patients if they smoke and recommend smoking cessation programs to smokers could be evaluated by using frequency count recording. Structured observational studies may employ pre-prepared data entry forms, which anticipate important responses and simplify data collection.

Consistency and high quality observer data collection requires development of a detailed observation manual, observer orientation and training, all of which have to be adequately completed prior to onset of the study.

In order to develop a thorough understanding of a program, a qualitative researcher might obtain a detailed description of the program setting, that is the physical environment it occurs in, program activities and participant behaviours, informal interactions and unplanned activities, nonverbal communications, and unobtrusive measures (Neutens and Rubinson, 2010). In a study of smoking cessation, searching garbage for evidence of cigarette butts is an example of an unobtrusive measure.

Participant observer. Sometimes the qualitative researcher does not stay a detached observer, but rather participates to a varying degree in the group or program under study. Such methods have advantages and may allow greater access to information, often more accurate information, and provides deeper insights into what is going on, frequently stimulating new ideas. Participant observation has disadvantages. It may also alter behaviours so that the researcher is no longer observing what would have taken place if they had not participated. Ethical issues may arise if participant observation is carried out in a way that deceives study participants. Observer acceptance into a group depends on establishing social relationships, which may lead to emotional involvement and loss of objectivity. In addition, because observations cannot be documented as events unfold, data recording occurs at some later time, relying on memory, and can be incomplete and inaccurate. An example of participant observation is the following: To study the issues and problems facing patients in long-term care homes, a participant observer could pose as a staff member.

4. Some qualitative research involves **document study**, in which institutional, public, or personal documents are systematically reviewed. For example, Rosella and colleagues (2013) incorporated document analysis into their study of developing Canadian public health policies for the H1N1 pandemics of 2009. When novel infectious disease outbreaks occur, public health policies are made rapidly, with uncertainty, and can have unexpected consequence. This study examined four highly debated issues, including use of adjuvanted vaccine in pregnant women, vaccination of priority groups, school closures and personal protective equipment. Across Canada, 40 public health officials and scientific experts were interviewed, and 76 pandemic policy documents were reviewed. Among other things, the study concluded that clarification of roles and responsibilities and improved transparency would lead to reduced duplication and improved public credibility.

5. **Ethnography** is the method of identifying and describing social and cultural groups and subgroups (Liamputtong, 2013). Ethnography initially was most used in social anthropology to study non-Western populations, and more recently it has been adopted by sociology to describe subgroups in modern contemporary societies. Ethnographic

methodologies are now applied by qualitative researchers in medical and health research.

Techniques for collecting qualitative data include field notes, participants' written words, photography, videos, and official statistics (Neutens and Rubinson, 2010). Field notes are the mainstay of qualitative research and are used to capture all information thought to be of any value. Field notes start with descriptive details of when and where an event took place, who was there, and what happened, including interactions between people. Quotations of what people said are documented. Observer insights and reflections are also recorded.

Qualitative versus Quantitative

Is quantitative research superior to qualitative research? This is not a sensible question. It cannot be said that one is better than the other, because they seek to answer different questions and get at different knowledge claims, both of which are important. Qualitative research is used to study how family, community, cultural, and other factors influence the attitudes, beliefs, motivations, and preferences of medical care providers and patients, and can provide an understanding of how evidence from quantitative studies can be turned into practice (Green and Britten, 1998). Whereas quantitative research is used to identify measureable numeric relationships and pat-

terns, which may range from simple to complex, between "exposures" and health outcomes, and can quantify the burden of disease.

In addition, in health research the two approaches often work together. Preliminary qualitative studies can provide important information, which can improve the design of subsequent quantitative study. Often a study that starts out as a qualitative study can transition into a quantitative study. Consider the earlier example of low uptake of flexible sigmoidoscopy screening for colorectal cancer. Once the qualitative study finds the reasons for poor uptake of screening, a quantitative study is used to estimate the proportions of each reason, and look at the relationship between different reasons and the impact of combined reasons, and identify which sociodemographic groups are at highest risk to have these reasons for lack of screening.

Regarding quantitative versus qualitative, although one is not more important than the other, they do use different study approaches and require different skill sets to conduct. It should be noted that although some lines of medical research are triggered by anecdote, a case report, or a case series report, these should not be thought of as representing typical qualitative research. Green describes qualitative research as a rigorous process that entails "explicit sampling strategies, systematic analysis of data, and commitment to examining counter explanations" (Green and Britten, 1998).

Summary

- Study design refers to the study plan or strategy.
- The study question/hypothesis should drive the study design.
- Many different study designs exist, and they fundamentally differ in how they sample

the population under study and collect the exposure and disease/outcome data.
- Qualitative studies do not have a comparison group and do not test hypotheses, but are useful for idea development and hypothesis generation.

- In contrast, most quantitative studies with comparison groups are hypothesis testing.
- In experimental study designs, such as RCTs and community trials, the researcher has control over which study participants receive the exposure under study.
- The impact of adverse or harmful exposures on populations is studied using observational study designs, of which cohort and case-control studies represent two of the most commonly used study designs.
- Different study designs vary in their vulnerability to biases.
- Qualitative research can answer questions and find out answers that quantitative studies cannot, and can help make implementation of evidence-based knowledge from quantitative studies more successful.

Review Questions

1. A graduate student in her MSC thesis defence was asked: "To answer your thesis question, what is the most appropriate study design?" The student thought about it and replied: "It depends on your point of view and who is doing the study." Do you agree or disagree with the student's answer? Why?

2. If the RCT is the optimal study design and comes closest of epidemiological studies to the experimental design, why not use it all the time?

Recommended Readings and Websites

Standard texts on research methods

Jacobsen, K.H. (2012) *Introduction to Health Research Methods: A Practical Guide.* Sudbury, Massachusetts: Jones & Bartlett Learning.

Neutens, J.J., and Rubinson, L. (2010) *Research Techniques for the Health Sciences.* 4th ed. San Francisco: Benjamin Cummings.

Free Books on the Internet

They contain useful information. However, some of them do contain mistakes, as almost all books do, so read critically.

Bonita, R., Beaglehole, R., and Kjellström, T. (2006) *World Health Organization. Basic Epidemiology.* 2nd ed. Geneva: World Health Organization.

Coggon, D., Rose, G.A., and Barker, D.J.P. (2003) *Epidemiology for the Uninitiated.* 5th ed. London: BMJ Books.

(This book was initially published as a series of articles in the journal Lancet. *The articles are still available online as separate postings.)*

Pearce, N. (2005) *A Short Introduction to Epidemiology*. 2nd ed. Wellington, New Zealand: Centre for Public Health Research.

World Health Organization. Regional Office for the Western Pacific (2001) *Health Research* *Methodology: A Guide for Training in Research Methods*. 2nd ed. Manila: World Health Organization, Regional Office for the Western Pacific.

References

Alter D.A. Eny K. (2005) The relationship between the supply of fast-food chains and cardiovascular outcomes. *Canadian Journal of Public Health*. 96(3):173–7.

Anderson, C.M., Yip, R., Henschke, C.I., Yankelevitz, D.F., Ostroff, J.S., and Burns, D.M. (2009) Smoking cessation and relapse during a lung cancer screening program. *Cancer Epidemiology, Biomarkers & Prevention*, 18(12), 3476–83.

Andriole, G.L., Crawford, E.D., Grubb, R.L. 3rd, et al. (2009) Mortality results from a randomized prostate-cancer screening trial. *The New England Journal of Medicine*. 360(13), 1310–9.

Bouma, G.D., Wilkinson, L., and Ling, R. (2009) *The Research Process*. Canadian ed. Oxford: Oxford University Press.

Ferguson, N. (2011) *Civilization: the West and the Rest*. New York: Penguin Press.

Gordis L. (2009) *Epidemiology*. 4th ed. Philadelphia, PA: Saunders/Elsevier.

Green, J., and Britten, N. (1998) Qualitative research and evidence based medicine. *British Medical Journal*, 316(7139), 1230–2.

Interphone Group (2010) Brain tumour risk in relation to mobile telephone use: Results of the INTERPHONE international case-control study. *International Journal of Epidemiology*, 39(3):675–94.

Liamputtong, P. (2013) *Qualitative Research Methods*. 4th ed. New York: Oxford University Press.

Menotti, A., Jacobs, D.R. Jr., Blackburn, H., et al. (1996) Twenty-five-year prediction of stroke deaths in the seven countries study: The role of blood pressure and its changes. *Stroke*, 27(3), 381–7.

Neutens, J.J. and Rubinson, L. (2010) *Research Techniques for the Health Sciences*. 4th ed. San Francisco: Benjamin Cummings.

Rosella L.C., Wilson K., Crowcroft N.S., Chu A., Upshur R., Willison D., et al. (2013) Pandemic H1N1 in Canada and the use of evidence in developing public health policies—a policy analysis. *Social Science & Medicine*. 83: 1–9.

Schroder, F.H., Hugosson, J., Roobol, M.J., et al. (2009) Screening and prostate-cancer mortality in a randomized European study. *The New England Journal of Medicine*, 360(13), 1320–8.

The World Bank. (2011) *World Development Indicators 2011*. Washington, D.C.: International Bank for Reconstruction and Development.

Weissfeld, J.L., Schoen, R.E., Pinsky, P.F., et al. (2012) Flexible sigmoidoscopy in the randomized prostate, lung, colorectal, and ovarian (PLCO) cancer screening trial: Added yield from a second screening examination. *Journal of the National Cancer Institute*, 104(4), 280–9.

7 Measurement

David L. Streiner

CHAPTER OUTLINE

Introduction

Measuring phenomena plays a central role in health sciences research. The primary discipline in which this is true was originally psychology. Indeed, one could probably trace the history of psychology by looking at what psychologists were measuring at the time: subjective experiences of internal states in the latter part of the nineteenth century; intellectual capacity among Army recruits during the First World War; psychodynamic functioning in the middle of the century; personality traits in the latter half of the century; and more recently an emphasis on models of personality. Not surprisingly, psychologists have been responsible for developing a large number of measurement tools. The most recent edition of *Tests in Print* (Murphy, Impara, and Plake, 1999) lists over 4000 commercially available scales; and this is only one-quarter the number of instruments that have not been published commercially (Goldman and Mitchell, 2008). Given this level of interest in measurement, it is equally unsurprising that psychologists have been in the forefront in the development of theories and techniques that underpin scale construction. This chapter will discuss what we mean by the term "measurement"; briefly review the steps in constructing scales, including establishing their reliability and validity; and discuss factors that influence how people respond to scales. Entire books have been written about these topics (e.g., Anastasi and Urbina, 1997; Nunnally and Bernstein, 1994; Streiner and Norman, 2008), so this will be at best (or at worst) a brief overview.

The Process of Measurement

At its simplest level, measurement consists of giving a numerical value to some phenomenon. This seems fairly easy and straightforward; after all, we have all used a ruler to measure the length of some object, and people who are concerned (or obsessed) about their weight have the daily experience of stepping on a scale to determine if their diet is working or if they ate too much over the holidays. Life becomes a bit more difficult, though, when we try to measure phenomena we encounter in health research; ones such as pain, quality of life, continuity of care, or patient satisfaction with care. The problem with these and other such attributes is that they are not directly observable; they are what Cronbach and Meehl (1955) called **hypothetical constructs**. Hypothetical constructs consist of behaviours, attitudes, processes, and the like, that tend to occur together. For example, we don't directly see intelligence (some have argued because it's in such short supply). Rather, we observe that an impressive vocabulary, wide knowledge about the world, good problem-solving ability, and other such skills tend to be correlated, and we attribute this to an underlying, unseen construct

that we call intelligence. Similarly, we directly see that a person may be pessimistic about the future, be slow in their movements, cry often, have disturbed sleep patterns, and express thoughts about suicide; and we would say that the person is depressed. Note that we do not observe the depression itself; we see only the outward manifestations, and say they are correlated because they all reflect this unseen phenomenon that we label depression.

Much of measurement in the health field consists of trying to assign a number to these hypothetical constructs. Problems arise, though, because people may disagree about which observable phenomena should be included in the construct. Should a scale that measures pain, for instance, include items that tap interference with **activities of daily living** (ADL) such as bathing, work, or grooming? The answer to this (and, as we'll see, to many other questions in this field) is, "It all depends." If your definition of pain is purely physiological, then the answer is "No"; and the scale should be limited to questions about its location, intensity, duration, and what it feels like. However, if you take a more comprehensive view of pain, then its effects on people, including ADL, would be included in your definition and therefore in your measure of it.

One reason that many scales exist to measure the same construct (in addition to the unworthy ones of the author wanting his or her name on it or the royalties from it) is that different people have varying conceptualizations of the phenomenon. This means that users of scales must be clear about their own definition of a construct—how they conceptualize it, what they believe should and should not be included, and how the construct should best be operationalized—and select an instrument that is congruent with their definition. Using a scale simply because others have or it is readily available may result in not assessing what you really want to know.

Variables

Types of Variables

Simply saying that measurement consists of assigning numbers to a phenomenon skims over the fact that what we are trying to measure differs from one attribute to another, and the numbers assigned to them have different interpretations. Consider the differences among determining if a person is disabled by pain; the number of ADLs affected by the pain; and the intensity of the pain. The first, whether or not a person is disabled by pain, divides the population into *categories*; in this case, only two—the person is or is not disabled. Categorical variables must satisfy two conditions. The first is that the categories are *mutually exclusive*; that is, a person cannot be placed into two or more categories. The second condition is that the categories must be *collectively exhaustive*— all possible options must be covered. Classifying hair colour as black/brown/blond/thinning violates both of these conditions: it doesn't include red heads (the scheme is not exhaustive), and those of us with brown but thinning hair can be put into two categories. Some diagnostic schemes satisfy both conditions. Using the second version of the Diagnostic and Statistical Manual (DSM-II; American Psychiatric Association, 1968), psychiatric patients could fall into only one of several mutually exclusive categories: organic, psychotic, neurotic, personality disorder, and so forth. Medical diagnoses, on the other hand, are not mutually exclusive (you can have both ulcers and migraine headaches); and are collectively exhaustive only by having terms like "cryptogenic" or "idiopathic," which is medical-speak for "We don't know what the heck is going on here," and are equivalent to an "other" category for everything that can't be put into one of the named categories.

Counting the number of ADLs affected by pain is a *discrete* variable, in that the answer is constrained to be a whole number, and cannot take on any value between the whole numbers. Pain can interfere with 0 or 5 ADLs, but not 2.38 of them. Similarly, scores on a test and answers to a Likert scale (e.g., Strongly Agree / Agree / Neutral / Disagree / Strongly Disagree) are limited to discrete values. On the other hand, variables such as height, weight, blood pressure, and the like are continuous, in that they can assume any (reasonable) value. To say someone's height is 170 cm is an approximation. If we want, we could use a ruler with more divisions and measure to the nearest millimeter, but that again is just rounding to the nearest unit. Obsessives could use more and more sensitive instruments, and record the height as 170.2 or 170.21 cm because the underlying variable is continuous. Measuring pain intensity is similar; we may constrain the person's answer to a 7-point scale, or a mark on a 10 cm line, or whatever, but the gradations of pain itself that the person feels are continuous and do not increase in a step-wise fashion.

Levels of Variables

Another way of describing variables was first proposed by S. Smith Stevens (1946). He divided them into four levels—**nominal, ordinal, interval, and ratio**—which are differentiated by three attributes: (1) the rules for assigning numbers to different values of the variable; (2) the mathematical properties of the resulting scales; and (3) the types of statistics that can be used with them.

Nominal variables are equivalent to categorical ones we just discussed, and consist of named categories: diagnosis, religion, political affiliation (which, to some people, is another form of religion), hair colour, sex, and the like. As with categorical variables, the assigned values must be mutually exclusive and collectively exhaustive. We can assign numbers to the categories to keep computer programs happy (e.g., Male = 1, Female = 2), but they are simply labels. That is, we can change the numerical assignment, and have Females = 1 and Males = 2, without gaining or losing any information. From a statistical point of view, nominal scales are quite limited: all we can do is determine which category has the most members (the **mode**; if you need help with measures of central tendency and dispersion, see the Practical Tip box below). Even this is of little use, because in some cases, two categories can be just about equal (**bimodal distributions**), and, especially if the sample size is small, the modal value can change a few times as new people are added to the sample.

Let's take the assumptions of a nominal scale (that the categories are mutually exclusive and collectively exhaustive) and add another assumption—that the categories have to be in rank order. What we now have is an **ordinal** scale (yes, the names actually do make sense, which isn't always the case in measurement theory). Simply naming the political parties would be a nominal scale, as we've seen, but if we ordered them along a left-wing to right-wing continuum (NDP/Liberal/Progressive-Conservative), it would form an ordinal scale. They key point is that the distances between successive values are not constant: the change in the amount of "liberalness/conservatism" from NDP to Liberal is not the same as that between Liberal and Progressive-Conservative. The same is true for points along a Likert scale: the difference in a person's attitude between answers of Strongly Agree and Agree is not necessarily the same as the distance between Agree and Neutral, or between Disagree and Strongly Disagree. The total scores for most scales used in health research are, in fact, ordinal in nature. Although the Beck Depression Inventory (Beck, Steer, and Brown, 1996) yields a number between 0 and 63, there's no guarantee that the change in depression from a score of 5 to one of 10 is the same as the change between 30 and 35, although both represent five points on the scale.

PRACTICAL TIP

Descriptive statistics are ways of summarizing data with just a few numbers. The two numbers that are of most concern to us are measures of central tendency and dispersion. Measures of central tendency indicate where the bulk of the data lie. For nominal variables, that measure is the *mode*, which is the most frequently used category. For ordinal data, the measure is the *median*—the data are put in rank order from lowest to highest, and the median is the value for which half of the numbers lie below it and half above it; it divides the data into two equal halves. With interval and ratio variables, the measure is the *arithmetic mean*, usually called simply the mean or the average. The numbers are summed and divided by the number of numbers.

Measures of dispersion indicate how widely or narrowly the data are spread out. For nominal data, it is simply the number of categories that have been used. There are two indices for ordinal data. The easier, and less useful, one is the *range*, which is the difference between the highest and the lowest value. A better measure, because it is less affected by one or two extreme scores, is the *interquartile range* (IQR). We begin with the median, and then find the median of the lower half of the distribution and the same with the upper half; the IQR is the difference between the two. With interval and ratio data, the measure of dispersion is the *standard deviation* (SD). It is a reflection of how much each data point deviates from the mean.

Statistical tests for data that follow a normal distribution require knowledge of the two parameters that define the distribution—the mean and SD. Hence, they are called *parametric statistics*. Some tests do not assume a normal distribution, and are therefore called *non-parametric*.

Strictly speaking, we must use the **median** to describe the **central tendency** of an ordinal scale, and the **range** or the **interquartile range** for its **dispersion**; and the statistics we can use are limited to **non**-**parametric** ones (again, see the Practical Tip box if you need help with this term) based on ranks (e.g., Spearman's rho or Kendall's tau for correlation; the Mann-Whitney U for differences between groups). However (and there's always a "however"), not all ordinal scales are created equal. When the scale has many points—"many" being a deliberately vague term that's sometimes interpreted as meaning seven or more—and if the data are not highly skewed, then some authors state that you can get away with using the mean, standard deviation, and **parametric statistics** (e.g., Norman and Streiner, 2008).

Because they are both analyzed with parametric statistics, let's discuss interval and ratio scales together. If we add to the two restrictions of an ordinal scale one more condition—that the values have to be equally spaced—we have an **interval scale**. When we add yet another condition—that there be a meaningful zero—we have a **ratio scale**. True interval and ratio scales are relatively rare in the health sciences; even Stevens (1946) didn't give any examples in his seminal article. The difference between the two is usually illustrated with the various scales we use to measure temperature. The Celsius and Fahrenheit scales are examples of interval scales; the fact that they use different temperatures to define zero degrees (the freezing point of water in the case of the Celsius scale, and the lowest temperature that could be achieved in a lab at the time the Fahrenheit scale was developed) is an excellent clue that it's an arbitrary value and not a meaningful one. The Kelvin scale begins at absolute zero—the lowest possible temperature—so it is an example of a ratio scale.

The difference between interval and ratio scales lies in the mathematical operations we can do with each. For both of them, *differences* are meaningful: a five-point change is a five-point change anywhere along the continuum. That is, because the intervals are equal, we can add and subtract values and the answers are meaningful. On the other hand, ratios between values are meaningful only for ratio scales (yet again, the name really does connote something). We can say that 10° Kelvin (or 10 Kelvins, to be pedantic about it) is twice as hot as 5° because it is a ratio scale. But, despite what many TV weather announcers say, if it's 10° Celsius today, it is *not* twice as hot as yesterday's temperature of 5° Celsius, because Celsius is an interval scale and the zero is arbitrary. To see this more clearly, we can simply transform the values to the Fahrenheit scale: 10°C = 50°F and 5°C = 41°F, and 50 is not twice as big as 41.

Although, as we've said, there are very few true interval scales in our field, we often treat ordinal scales as if they were interval scales. From a statistical point of view, we can usually get away with it; the tests are robust (that is, they can tolerate deviations from their underlying assumptions of the statistics), and we get an answer that's usually meaningful. But, they are most assuredly not ratio scales: a score of 20 on a depression scale is not twice as high as a score of 10; and someone with an IQ of 130 is *not* twice as bright as a person with an IQ of 65.

For both interval and ratio scales, the measure of central tendency is the **mean**, and the measure of dispersion is the **standard deviation**. Unless the data are highly skewed, parametric tests (Pearson's correlation and Analysis of Variance types of tests) are the ones of choice.

Constructing Scales

A Touch of Psychometric Theory

For the past 100 years or so, scale development has been guided by what is now called **classical test theory** (CTT), which assumes that the score that's obtained on a scale actually consists of two parts—the (unobserved) true score plus some error. The reason that CTT is so prevalent is that the assumptions underlying it are considered to be "weak"; that is, they apply in most situations. But in order to understand the assumptions, we have to begin with the basic premise of scale construction. As we've said, that premise is that the score we observe (X_O) is made up of two parts: the **true score** (X_T) and some **error** (ε), or:

$$X_O = X_T + ε$$

This means that we never see the true score, because there is always some error associated with it. It is also assumed that the error has a mean of zero. That is, sometimes it adds to the true score and sometimes it makes it smaller, but if we added up the errors for a large number of items, the average value would be zero. The true score is the score the person would obtain if the scale had an infinite number of items or if the respondent completed it an infinite number of times (which is decidedly time-consuming), so that the error terms for each of individual items or of each of the individual administrations can cancel each other out (Allen and Yen, 1979). Actually, "true" is a poor choice of terms, because it implies that the number is accurate and cannot change. But if the person lies about his or her actual state (and we will discuss such biases later in this chapter) and does so consistently, every one of the infinite times the scale is completed, we will get a true, but not an honest, value. Also, if the person's condition changes, as might happen following therapy, then the true score should change. "True," then, simply means that the score is free from random error (Streiner, 2003).

With that as background, we can return to the two assumptions of CTT. The first is that the error is unrelated to the true score. That is, the amount of error is the same throughout the entire range of the scale's possible scores. The second assumption is that the expected value of the error for each item is zero, and that the errors will cancel each other out as we add the items up to arrive at the total score, as we said previously. The implication, then, is that longer scales are freer from random error than shorter scales, because there is greater opportunity for the errors to cancel.

Now we are in a position to discuss what scale designers and scale users should know. We'll go through the steps in the same order that scales are constructed: devising the items, checking the items to determine their usability, combining them into scales, and finally checking the resulting scale for reliability and validity.

Devising the Items

Most of the phenomena that we measure in the health field are hypothetical constructs, and this has direct implications for what items do and do not appear on a scale. For example, there are (at least) three conceptualizations of what is meant by "social support" (Barrerra, 1986). For some, it refers to *perceived* social support (i.e., a subjective assessment that there are others who will help in times of need); while a second theory holds that is a function of *enacted* support (the amount of support actually received); and a third camp defines it in terms *of social integration* (the size of one's social network). These theories determine what items do or do not appear on a given social support scale. Not surprisingly, there is little correlation among scales that measure social support from these different perspectives (Barrerra, 1986; Uchino, 2009).

In this case, what the scale should encompass arises from one's theory or conceptualization of the construct. Other times, the domains may come from previous research or clinical knowledge about the area. For example, we know from both clinical experience and research that anxiety affects people in various ways: what they experience physiologically (e.g., rapid heart rate, sweatiness); how they feel emotionally (feelings of apprehension and dread); how they think (difficulties with concentration); and how they behave (avoidance of some situations). Consequently, anxiety scales should include items that tap each of these four domains.

In other situations, we may be entering an entirely new field and have no theory or prior research to guide us. In this case, we must do our own research to map out the broad domains. For example, we wanted to develop a scale to measure the quality of life of children with epilepsy as they see it (as opposed to how their parents do, which is what existing scales measure). However, we had no idea that what the children felt were the important aspects of their quality of life. To determine this, we first conducted a number of focus groups with the children (Ronen, Rosenbaum, Law, and Streiner, 1999; see Health Research

in Action box 7.1). Unfortunately, drawing on patient expertise in this way is a relatively recent phenomenon; for too long, it was felt that only "experts" had the necessary expertise.

No matter how the domains are derived— and often all of these sources are used—the scale developer or scale user must spell out beforehand what the construct means. This determines the domains that must be captured by the instrument and which ones should be omitted. Bear in mind, though, that the conceptualization of the construct may change in light of what is learned during the focus groups or based on feedback from experts.

The next step is to actually write the items (or "borrow" them from existing scales), which is usually done by the research team. Ideally, this initial pool will contain two or three times the number of items that will ultimately appear on the scale, because many will be weeded out in the subsequent steps. If the scale is to be used by the general public, the items should be written at a Grade 6 reading level (sadly, the reading level of the average high school graduate), and computer programs exist that can check for this.

7.1 Health Research in Action

Because no scale existed that evaluated the quality of life (QOL) of children with epilepsy from their perspective, we had to first determine what the major domains of QOL are. To do so, we used qualitative research techniques, including focus groups and facilitated activities, such as having the children draw environmental maps and use play dough to illustrate what epilepsy felt like. We found that a traditional focus group format was infeasible, as the more verbal children tended to dominate the discussion, so we used a nominal group technique. Here, each child spoke in turn, in answer to direct questions, but they could elaborate on what was said previously. This maximized participation, and prevented a few children from controlling the group. The environmental maps required the children to draw a map of their neighbourhood, including their home, their school, and where they played. For each area, the children talked about any concerns they had regarding their seizures. From this, we identified five major themes: interpersonal/social consequences of epilepsy, worries and concerns, intrapersonal/emotional issues, epilepsy as "my secret," and quest for normality (Ronen et al., 1999).

Checking the Items

Writing items for a scale is not as easy as it may first appear, and they need to be checked for potential problems. One difficulty is the use of jargon. Having spent many years in graduate school and in our work environment, we are unaware of how many of the terms we use are peculiar to our professions (and the term "peculiar" is quite apt in this case). To health care workers, *hypertension* obviously means high blood pressure, but to many in the public, it's part of the continuum, running from *calm*, to *nervous*, through *tense*, and on to *hypertensive*. Similarly, a *stool* is something one sits on and may be painted green; not a polite euphemism for the result of bodily functioning.

Another potential problem is the dreaded **double-barreled question**. This is an item that asks two questions in one, such as "I often feel sad and teary." How should a person answer if she feels sad but is not tearful? The difficulty is that some people will respond "True" because they feel sad, but others will say "False" because they aren't also teary, and we have no way of knowing who is answering each way. The presence of the word "and" in an item is usually a clear sign that the item is double-barreled. A more subtle form of a double-barreled question often shows up in disease-specific quality of life scales, such as "How much has your anxiety interfered with your ability to carry out your usual activities of daily life?" The problem here is that the activities could be affected by many causes. How does the person separate out how much is due to anxiety, how much to arthritis, how much to getting older, and how much to other causes? The question then refers to the degree of interference and its putative cause.

A third issue is the use of vague qualifiers, such as "often" or "rarely." Part of the problem is that the meaning of such terms depends on the context. "Often" connotes a higher absolute frequency for common events, such as shopping, as opposed to rare ones, like contraceptive failure (Parducci, 1968). Similarly, it's dependent on the respondent's own frequency of performing the behaviour; those who watch TV constantly interpret the question, "How often do you watch TV?" very differently from those who watch it infrequently (Wright, Gaskell, and O'Muircheartaigh, 1994). When people were asked to assign a probability to the term "often", it ranged from 0.15 to 0.99; and "cannot be excluded" encompassed the range of 0.07 to 0.98 (Bryant and Norman, 1980; Lichtenstein and Newman, 1967). Whenever possible, these vague terms should be replaced with specific amounts.

When a scale is being developed, or an existing scale is used with a new group of people (e.g., from a different ethnic or cultural background), these and other potential problems can often be identified using **cognitive interviewing**. This can take many forms. In one, people are asked to read the items and then rephrase them in their own terms. In another version, the people first respond to the item, and then the interviewer asks them to explain why they gave that particular answer as opposed to some other one. This accomplishes a number of things. First, we can see if people have difficulty reading any of the words. Second, we can determine if they understand the item as it was intended, or if they are misinterpreting its meaning. Doing this with 10 or 15 people from the target population is usually sufficient to uncover any difficulties.

Biases in Responding

Ensuring that the questions are understood properly doesn't guarantee that they will be answered honestly or correctly. The cognitive processes, from reading the item to responding to it, involve many steps, and things can go wrong at each of them. We cannot go into all of the steps or problems in this brief chapter; they are discussed in more detail in Streiner and Norman (2008). Rather, we will focus primarily on some of the biases that may distort the respondent's answers.

Before mentioning specific biases, it's worthwhile to discuss people's general approaches to responding to scales and questionnaires. We, as researchers administering the questionnaires, hope that the respondents will read each item carefully, think deeply about the various response alternatives, and answer honestly. Borrowing a term from economic theory, Krosnick (1991) calls this **optimizing**—giving the optimal answer to each item. However, this does not always happen. Especially when the person is unmotivated, or the scale is too long, or the items difficult to understand, the respondent may put down an answer that minimally satisfies the demands of the situation: to fill in a response, any response. Krosnick refers to this approach as **satisficing**. This can occur in many ways: endorsing the first or last alternative; agreeing with every statement, irrespective of content; selecting one response (e.g., "mildly agree") and then using it for all subsequent items; saying "I don't know" or using the "neutral" category; or mentally flipping a coin and answering at random. This again argues for items that are easy to understand, and not over-burdening the respondent with lengthy questionnaires.

Of the various factors affecting specific responses, perhaps the most common distortion is **social desirability** (SD) **bias**. It refers to the tendency for people to present themselves to others in a favourable light, by either exaggerating good attributes or minimizing bad ones. If responses to questionnaires are to be believed, everyone attends concerts or goes to the museum on a weekly basis, while dutifully flossing their teeth, donating to charities, exercising regularly, and studiously avoiding junk foods, cigarettes, and "reality" shows on television. One can only wonder why concert halls are empty and dentists' offices are filled.

In fact, there are two forms of SD bias. **Self-deception bias** is seen as an unconscious process of presenting an overly optimistic picture of ourselves, in that we genuinely see ourselves more positively than reality would warrant. If not carried to pathological extremes, this is likely an adaptive strategy, contributing to our self-esteem. (We will not discuss self-deception bias as it applies to politicians, film stars, or university deans, where we refer to it as "malignant hypertrophy of the ego"; see Streiner and Norman, 2009.) On the other hand, with **other-deception bias**, the respondents are aware of the fact that they are distorting their answers in order to create a good impression.

SD bias can occur in a wide variety of situations. People overstate (or overestimate) their compliance with medications; minimize illegal or sanctioned activities, such as drug use or how much they drink; deny prejudice against those from other groups; exaggerate their intelligence and accomplishments, and so on. It is impossible to completely eliminate SD bias from scales and questionnaires, although techniques have been developed over the years to measure (Paulhus, 1991) and minimize it (e.g., Nederhof, 1985).

Another response set that affects responding is the **yea-saying** or **acquiescence bias**, which is the tendency to agree with any statement, irrespective of its content. Thus, people can agree with contradictory items, such as "I am nervous most of the time" and "I generally feel calm and relaxed." This can occur for a number of reasons. The primary reason is satisficing—if the person is not motivated to complete the scale, checking off "Yes" or "Totally Agree" is an easy way to get through the questions. Another factor is cultural, in that people from cultures that tend to avoid disappointing or offending others (e.g., Southeast Asia) are more prone toward this bias (Craig and Douglas, 2005).

The final distortion that we'll discuss (although many others exist; see Streiner and Norman, 2008) is **end-aversion bias**. This is the tendency for people to avoid the extreme ends of scales, and usually occurs when those extremes are absolute categories, such as "Never" or "Always." The reason is that people can usually find an exception or feel that one must exist, even if they can't identify it at the time. This also may be culturally determined to some degree, with people from more emotionally expressive countries (e.g., Italy, Brazil) being more likely to use extremes than their neighbours in countries to the north (Craig and Douglas, 2005).

Scaling the Items

There are many different ways of framing the response options to items. Perhaps the easiest are **categorical judgements**, in which people choose among a number of alternatives. A few examples are shown in Figure 7.1.

Simple as these seem, there are a number of potential problems. Item 1 in Figure 7.1 (religious affiliation) is truly categorical. Item 2 (ability to climb the stairs), though, is really a continuum masquerading as a category. One person may be able to climb the five stairs up to the front porch, but not the 15 stairs to the second floor; while another has no problem walking up to her fifth floor office, but runs out of steam if she has to walk to the tenth floor. The third item (suicidal ideation), as is true for many dichotomous response items, often leaves the person wanting to write in, "It all depends—do you mean fleeting suicidal thoughts or very serious ones?" Respondents usually do not like items requiring Yes/No or True/False answers (Carp, 1989; Jones, 1968) because they are forced to use alternatives that do not apply or left wanting to say "some of the time."

As the name implies, **continuous judgements** require the person to indicate their response along a continuum. There are a number of different response options that can be used. The easiest is probably the **visual analogue scale** (VAS), two of which are shown in Figure 7.2.

The line is usually 10 cm long and may or may not have vertical lines every cm, and the person puts a mark on the line corresponding to their state or belief. VASs are widely used, especially in pain measurement, because of their seeming simplicity. But this simplicity may hide a number of problems. First, a significant proportion of people, particularly the aged or those with limited literacy, have difficulty understanding the concept of translating a feeling into a mark on a line (e.g., Bosi Ferraz

---

(1) What is your religious affiliation:
    ☐ Catholic
    ☐ Protestant
    ☐ Jewish
    ☐ Muslim
    ☐ Hindu
    ☐ Buddhist
    ☐ Other (please specify) _____
    ☐ None

(2) Are you able to climb the stairs?   Yes ___   No ___

(3) I have often felt suicidal.   ( ) True   ( ) False

FIGURE 7.1   Examples of items with categorical judgements

How bad has your pain been during the past week?

No pain |__|__|__|__|__|__|__|__|__|__| Worst pain
at all   imaginable

How much difficulty do you have walking?

No difficulty _____ Unable
  at all   to walk

FIGURE 7.2   Examples of visual analogue scales

et al., 1990; Huskisson, 1974). Second, the person's response is very dependent on the wording of the end-points (Seymour, Simpson, Charlton, and Phillips, 1985). Although the lower end is usually easy to describe (the absence of a state), the upper end is often more problematic; how does the respondent know what is "the most pain imaginable" if the person has never experienced it?

Another version of a continuous scale is the **adjectival scale**, which consists of a series of words, as in Figure 7.3. As with the VAS, the adjectival scale is **unipolar**, in that it describes the least amount of the construct (usually on the left) to the most.

Unlike the previous two continuous judgement scales, a **Likert scale** (pronounced "Lick-urt," not "Like-urt") is **bipolar**; that is, it has extreme values at both ends, most often with a neutral point somewhere in the centre, as in the first example in Figure 7.4. There are times when the scale designer wants to force the respondent to take a stand one way or the other, and the neutral point is omitted, as in the second example.

A variant of the Likert scale is the **Harter scale** (Figure 7.5), which was originally designed to be used with children (Harter, 1982), although it has been successfully used with adults too (Ronen,

Streiner, and Rosenbaum, 2003). The person first decides whether they are better described by the statement on the left or on the right, and then selects which of the two descriptors below that is more appropriate. This format has two advantages. First, by splitting the task in two, it reduces the cognitive demands. Second, it reduces bias by presenting the alternative descriptors as equally normative. Note that there is no neutral point.

For all continuous judgement scales, there are a number of considerations in their construction:

- The ideal number of categories is generally between five and nine (with the exception of the VAS, which usually has 10). Fewer response options results in a loss of information; while people have difficulty discriminating among the alternatives if there are more than about nine (Hawthorne, Mouthaan, Forbes, and Novaco, 2006).

- Whether there should be an odd or an even number of response options in a Likert scale depends on the item. If a neutral point is sensible, then an odd number is preferred; if the person must make a decision, then an even number.

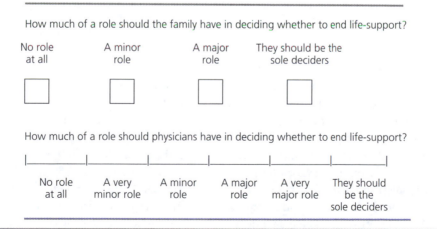

FIGURE 7.3   Examples of adjectival scales

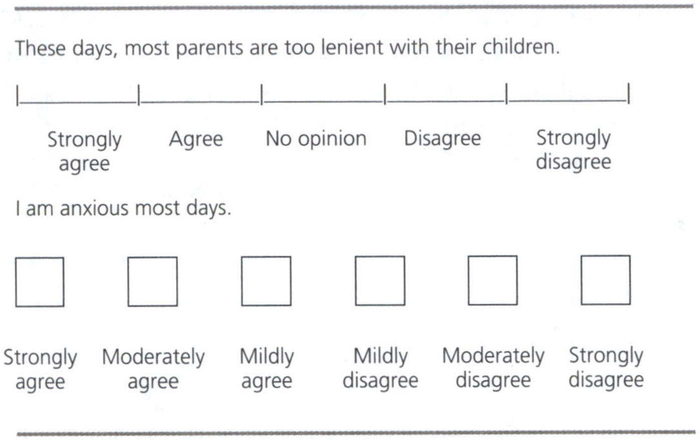

These days, most parents are too lenient with their children.

|_____|_____|_____|_____|_____|

Strongly   Agree   No opinion   Disagree   Strongly
agree   disagree

I am anxious most days.

☐   ☐   ☐   ☐   ☐   ☐

Strongly   Moderately   Mildly   Mildly   Moderately   Strongly
agree   agree   agree   disagree   disagree   disagree

FIGURE 7.4   Examples of Likert scales

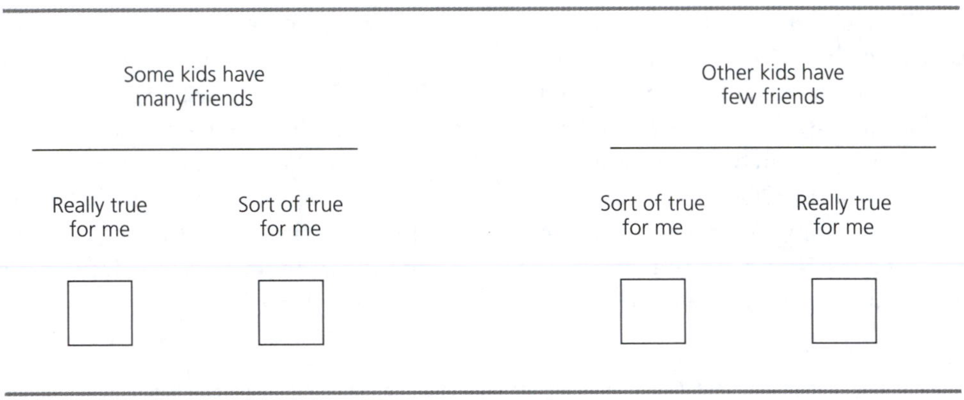

Some kids have   Other kids have
many friends   few friends

Really true   Sort of true   Sort of true   Really true
for me   for me   for me   for me

☐   ☐   ☐   ☐

FIGURE 7.5   Example of a Harter scale

- If there is a neutral point, it does not have to be in the middle. Since there is a positive bias in evaluating students, for example (as in Garrison Keillor's Lake Wobegon, where all the children are above average), it may make sense to place "Average" closer to the left end to allow for mostly positive evaluations.
- It doesn't matter too much whether all of the boxes are labelled, or if every other one is. But in the latter situation, there is a tendency for respondents to use the labelled options.

- The words used in adjectival scales have a moderate influence on the responses, but numbers placed under the options have a very strong effect. If the numbers run from 1 to 7, for example, most of the scale is used; but if they range from −3 to +3, there is a definite bias against using negative ones (Schwarz, Hippler, Deutsch, and Strack, 1991).
- The responses to previous items definitely influence the responses to later items (Schuman and Presser, 1981).

- We have successfully used these scales with children as young as eight (Ronen et al., 2003), though others have also found that younger children have difficulty with them (e.g., Beyer and Aradine, 1988).
- And the question that is most asked: are the data from continuous judgement scales ordinal or interval? The answer is unequivocally "Yes." Strictly speaking, the data are definitely ordinal, but they are often analyzed with parametric statistics as if they were interval. Especially when the sum of a number of items is used, as with total scores, it is fairly safe to treat them as interval.

There are many other response alternatives that are less widely used, such as comparative judgements, econometric methods, goal attainment scaling, and so forth. These are discussed in general books about scale development (e.g., Streiner and Norman, 2008).

Selecting the Items

As we mentioned earlier, we usually write far more items than we hope to end up with. Some will be weeded out because of the considerations we have just discussed—problems with the reading level, the wording, potential for SD bias, and so on. Other problems can be assessed, though, only after we have administered the remaining items to a large number of people. What "large" means depends on the questions we're asking. The first set of questions pertain to the distribution of the responses, and for this we'll need at least 50 respondents, chosen from the **target population**; that is, the ultimate group that will be assessed with the instrument. That means that if the scale is designed for a patient group, it should not be pre-tested on a class of undergraduate students, as handy (and ubiquitous) as this may be.

Ideally, all of the response categories will be used. For dichotomous items, if more than 90 per cent of the respondents choose one option, then the item is not useful because it is not discriminating among people; you might as well assume that everyone will answer that way. For items with more than two response options, it doesn't matter if the responses are skewed (that is, the answers tend to bunch up at one end or the other), especially if the average correlation among the items is above 0.25 (Bandalos and Enders, 1996; Enders and Bandalos, 1999; Feldt, 1993), but most of the response options should be used by at least some of the people.

The usual next step is to factor analyze the scale. **Factor analysis** (FA) is an advanced statistical procedure used to determine if a large number of variables (such as items on a scale) can be grouped into a number of subgroups, in which the variables correlate highly with each other, and poorly with other items (see Norman and Streiner, 2008, for details about this procedure). Even if the scale is designed to measure one construct (as it is in most instances), we often expect to find domains within it (e.g., an anxiety scale having subscales that tap the effect of anxiety on the person's mood, behaviour, thoughts, and physiological state). For FA, we will need a ratio of about 10 respondents to each item on the scale.

With FA, we are looking for three things. First, the grouping of the items should make clinical sense; all of the somatic items, for instance, should correlate with (or "load") on one factor, and that factor shouldn't have items from unrelated domains. Second, the loading of each item should be at least 0.35. (Because a factor loading is a correlation, its absolute value can range between 0 (no relationship) and 1 (a perfect correlation); 0.35 reflects a moderate correlation.) Third, the item should load on only one factor. If any of these conditions is not met, then it means that the item should be either scrapped or rewritten.

Now that a pool of potentially useful items has been formed, it's time to assess them as a scale. The first job is to assess its reliability.

Reliability

Try as we might, we can never eliminate random error. People may misread or misinterpret an item; circle a 3 when they really meant to circle a 2; be influenced by fluctuating changes in their condition; and so on. Furthermore, some scales may be more affected by this than others; and even the same scale may be affected to varying degrees depending on the group to which it is being administered or the conditions under which it is given. One index that captures this is the **reliability** of the scale, which is its ability to produce consistent results under consistent conditions. Reliability is measured on a scale from 0 to 1, where 0 indicates absolutely no consistency, and 1 means perfect consistency; this is the **reliability coefficient**. In mathematical terms, one way to define reliability is:

$$Reliability = \frac{\sigma^2_{True}}{\sigma^2_{Observed}}$$

where σ^2 means the **variance** of the true and observed scores. That is, reliability is the proportion of variance that we observe in relation to the true variance; the greater the proportion, the closer the reliability is to 1.0. Note that reliability is affected only by **random error** (i.e., unpredictable errors that have a mean of 0), not **systematic error** (a bias that affects all scores in one direction; that is, its mean is above or below 0). If everybody misinterprets one item the same way; or if conditions are such that everyone distorts their responses in a similar manner (e.g., because of SD bias), then the reliability may still remain high.

Another way to define reliability, on a conceptual level, is that it is the degree to which "measurements of individuals on different occasions, or by different observers, or by similar or parallel tests, produce the same or similar results" (Streiner and Norman, 2008, p. 7). There are a number of different ways that reliability can be determined.

If a person completes a scale measuring satisfaction with life on one day, and then fills it out again two weeks later, then we would want the two scores to be similar, assuming nothing has changed in the interim. This is referred to as **test-retest reliability**. Usually, the interval between the two assessments is around 10 to 14 days. If it were longer, there's the possibility that the person may have changed; if it were shorter, the person may be able to recall his or her answers and try to repeat them, rather than responding to the content of the items. Needless to say, the interval can be longer if we are measuring a stable trait (e.g., anxiety or extraversion), and must be shorter if we are assessing a short-lived state, such as pain. The reason that test-retest reliability should be high (and we will discuss what we mean by "high" shortly) is that if the scores differ from one administration to another, but the person hasn't changed, we wouldn't trust either score as being an accurate reflection of the person's state.

There are times when the scale is completed, not by the person themselves, but by another individual doing an evaluation. This may occur when a supervisor evaluates a student, or a clinician rates the degree of psychosis in a patient. In these cases, we want the evaluators to have comparable scores; what is called **inter-rater reliability**. The main requirement is that the raters do their evaluations *independently* from one another; otherwise, we are simply capturing how well one can copy the results from the other. Again, we need the reliability to be high, because if the raters don't agree with one another, we wouldn't know which one to trust—or neither one.

Thirdly, two versions of the same scale should yield nearly identical scores: **parallel forms**

reliability. We sometimes encounter parallel forms with intelligence tests, so that the person doesn't "learn" the test. Parallel forms are usually constructed as one very long scale, and then randomly divided into two or three versions. Reliability assesses the degree to which the different forms yield comparable values when measuring the construct.

These types of reliability are often assessed with a Pearson correlation coefficient (r) between the two administrations of the scale. A better index, though, is the **intra-class correlation** (ICC; Shrout and Fleiss, 1979), which gives a more conservative estimate. The reason is that if one rater is consistently higher than the other, or if people consistently respond higher on the second administration of a scale, it does not affect r but it will make the ICC lower.

A fourth form of reliability, **internal consistency**, is somewhat different from the first three. It assesses the degree to which the items in the scale are correlated with one another. The rationale for including this as a form of reliability is predicated on the assumption that scales should measure a single construct (e.g., anxiety or satisfaction with care) and therefore all of the items should tap into the single construct to varying degrees. Internal consistency is usually measured with a statistic called **Cronbach's alpha** (α; Cronbach, 1951). It is by far the most widely used index of reliability, likely because it is the easiest to determine, requiring only one administration of the scale. However, there are a number of problems with internal consistency as an indicator of reliability, and with α as a measure of it. The main problem with α is that it is affected by the number of items in the scale. Longer scales, those with more than about 15 items, can yield high values of α, even if the individual items are tapping different constructs (Cortina, 1993). Furthermore, high values of α may simply point to too much redundancy among the items (that is, we're asking

the same question in different ways) or indicate that the items are measuring the construct too restrictively (we're not tapping the full complexity of the construct; Streiner, 2003; Streiner and Norman, 2008). Related to this last point, increasing the reliability of a scale usually increases its validity, a point we'll discuss later. However, if α is too high, it may actually *decrease* the scale's validity because the construct is being measured too narrowly. For example, we can achieve very high internal consistency in an anxiety scale by asking only about somatic symptoms and totally ignoring the other domains (e.g., the cognitive, behavioural, and so forth). Better indices of internal consistency would be the average correlation among the items, and making sure that the correlation of each individual item with the total score is within the range of 0.20 to 0.70.

How high should a scale's reliability coefficient be? As we mentioned, reliability can range between 0 and 1. For test-retest, inter-rater, and parallel-forms reliability, Nunnally and Bernstein (1994) recommend a minimum of 0.70 for scales that are used in new or developing research areas; a minimum of 0.80 in well-developed research fields; and a minimum of 0.90 when the scale is used for making decisions that affect individuals (e.g., for clinical purposes or to determine whether to admit an applicant into a program). For internal consistency, Streiner and Norman (2008) recommend a maximum value of 0.90; as mentioned, higher values may reflect too much redundancy among the items.

There is a final point about reliability that cannot be emphasized enough: reliability is *not* a fixed property of a scale; it depends on the scale *and the group in which it is being used*. Thomas Jefferson used the phrase "All men are created equal" in the US Declaration of Independence, but this statement is anathema in the field of psychometrics, aside from its sexist language. Another definition of reliability is the degree to which a scale can differentiate among people and determine how they are *not* equal. If everyone gets the same score on a test, then the test is useless and has a reliability of zero. This has two implications. The first is that scales often used in graduate or professional schools to evaluate students, where they are rated as Unsatisfactory/Satisfactory/Above Average, are useless, because everyone is put in the same Above Average category. While this may keep students happy, the scale is useless from a psychometric perspective because it does not discriminate.

The second implication is that the reliability of a scale is dependent on the homogeneity of the group being assessed. For example, if a measure of depression has a given reliability when used in a hospital with in- and out-patients, that value will likely be smaller when the scale is used with people walking into a family doctor's office. The reason is that the range of scores will be smaller in the latter situation (people with very high scores will be in hospital), and this will be reflected in the measure of reliability. Thus, one should never talk about *the* reliability of a scale, but rather its reliability *with this particular group of respondents*.

Validity

If you look at textbooks from 40 years ago (or articles written by people who haven't read any textbooks for the past 40 years), you'll see a definition like, "Validity tells us whether the scale is actually measuring what we think it is." However, the definition of **validity** has changed in a subtle but very meaningful way. Now it is defined as "the degree of confidence we can place on the inferences we make about people based on their scores from that scale" (Streiner and Norman, 2008, p. 251). The major difference between the older and newer definitions is that now, validity is not seen as a fixed, immutable property of the test. In

parallel with the description of reliability, validity is an interaction among the scale, the group with which the scale is being used, and the circumstances under which it is administered. A few examples may illustrate these points.

The Minnesota Multiphasic Personality Inventory (MMPI; Hathaway and McKinley, 1940) is a widely used, multi-scale personality test. When used with patients with psychological problems, elevations on certain scales correctly identify those individuals who are overly concerned with physical problems and who tend to develop them in times of stress. However, these scales are also elevated among patients with multiple sclerosis (Meyerink, Reitan, and Selz, 1988). Among individuals with multiple sclerosis, the high scores reflect the neurological effects of the disease itself and are not indicative of psychopathology. Thus, scales that are very useful for one group of people (psychiatric patients) are not that useful with another group (patients with physical disorders), and the scores have a very different interpretation.

Other scales on the MMPI reflect respondents' "test-taking attitude"; that is, the degree to which they are willing to admit to the presence of psychological problems and of even common, everyday shortcomings, such as having worse manners eating at home than in a restaurant. Usually, elevations on these scales reflect a poor prognosis for therapy, in that the respondents are unwilling or unable to acknowledge their difficulties. However, when the MMPI is administered to parents involved in custody and access disputes, not only is it common for these scales to be high, but it is often interpreted in a positive way; that the parent is aware of social norms and expectations (Postuma and Harper, 1998). In this example, it is the circumstances under which the test is administered that change the meaning and interpretation of the results.

At the same time that the definition of validity was changing, so was the conceptualization of how it is assessed. Prior to the 1970s (and again, still found among authors who have not kept up with the field), people spoke of three "types" of validity, referred to as the "three C's"—content validity, criterion validity, and construct validity—and each of these was further divided into various subtypes (e.g., predictive and concurrent criterion validity; convergent and discriminant construct validity; etc.). Much time was spent (or rather, wasted) debating whether a particular study was an instance of one subtype versus another. Following the seminal work of Messick (1989; 1986), Anastasi (1985), and others, validity is now seen as a unitary concept, subsumed under the name **construct validity**. There are many ways of demonstrating construct validity, but these are methods, not subtypes. That is, we can talk about criterion *validation* as a method or process of demonstrating construct validity, but not of criterion *validity*, as if it were a type of validity separate and distinct from the others. With that as background, let's discuss the different ways of establishing construct validity.

Validity begins with the items that comprise the scale, and **content validation** involves assessing them for their completeness and relevance. If a scale is designed to measure some construct such as depression or quality of life, we want the items to satisfy two criteria. First, all aspects of the con-

struct should be assessed; what is referred to as **content coverage**. This brings us back to what we discussed in the beginning of the chapter, when we introduced the notion of hypothetical constructs. The test designer and the test user must have in mind an idea of what is subsumed by the construct. For example, as we have mentioned, one conceptualization of anxiety posits that there are four components of it: somatic symptoms (e.g., sweating, tachycardia), an emotional component (feelings of dread or apprehension), a cognitive component (thoughts of dying), and behavioural manifestations (avoidance of certain fear-inducing situations) (Seligman, Walker, and Rosenhan, 2000). Content coverage ensures that each of these components is represented by a sufficient number of items (a vague term that is difficult to measure). This is usually assessed qualitatively by a panel of experts in the field (usually three to five people). The easiest way to assess content coverage is to construct a matrix, similar to the one in Table 7.1, where the columns reflect the domains of the construct and the rows are the individual items. A checkmark indicates that the item taps the given domain.

The matrix shows that item 1 goes with the somatic domain, item 2 with the cognitive, and so on. Each domain should have three or more items, and each item should have one and only

TABLE 7.1   A Content Coverage Matrix for a Scale of Anxiety

Item	Domain			
	Somatic	Emotional	Cognitive	Behavioural
1	√			
2			√	
3		√		
4				
⋮	⋮	⋮	⋮	⋮
20		√		√

one checkmark (this is analogous to what we discussed earlier regarding factor analysis—an item should load on one and only one item; content validity does this subjectively, and factor analysis does it statistically, but the aim is the same). Item 4 does not map onto any of the domains, and thus should be eliminated because of **content irrelevance**; that is, it is not related to the content of the scale. On the other hand, item 20 can be placed in two domains, and so should be either rewritten or dropped. (To reiterate, the entire process is a judgemental form of factor analysis, which we discussed under the section "Reliability," and complements, rather than replaces, it.)

A more sophisticated approach to content validation is to use the **content validity ratio** (CVR) developed by Lawshe (1975) and modified by Lynn (1986). An expert panel (which may include content experts, theoreticians, and patients) rates each item on a four-point scale: 4 = Highly Relevant; 3 = Quite Relevant or Highly Relevant But Needs Rewording; 2 = Somewhat Relevant; and 1 = Not Relevant. The CVR for each item is defined as:

$$CVR = \frac{n_e - \dfrac{N}{2}}{\dfrac{N}{2}}$$

where n_e is the number of raters who deem the item to be essential (i.e., a rating of 3 or 4) and N is the total number of raters. The CVR can range between -1 and $+1$, and a value of 0 means that half of the panel feel that the item is essential. To ensure that the results are not due to chance, Lawshe recommended a value of 0.99 for five or six raters, 0.85 for eight raters, and 0.62 for 10 raters; items with lower values would be discarded. At the same time that the raters evaluate relevance, they are also asked to comment on whether any aspects of the construct have been omitted. If there are, new items can be written, which further establishes content coverage.

All other methods for assessing the validity of a scale are also subsumed under the rubric of construct validity. As we discussed, a construct is a hypothesis stipulating why certain observable phenomena hang together. But the theory about the construct goes beyond simply stating a relationship exists; it most often indicates how the construct is related to other phenomena. Keeping with the example of anxiety, we can generate a number of hypotheses, such as: (a) patients attending a phobia clinic should present with more symptoms of anxiety than non-phobic individuals; (b) highly anxious people should perform less well on complex tasks than less anxious people; (c) anxiety should decrease after treatment with anxiolytic drugs (i.e., those that treat anxiety) or behaviour therapy; (d) anxiety should increase before a high-stakes examination; (e) anxiety levels should not be related to intelligence; and so forth.

In turn, then, these "mini-theories" tell us how a newly developed scale of anxiety should perform if it is working well. Hypothesis (a) could be tested by giving the scale to patients in an anxiety disorders clinic and to a group of people who have never attended one. The former group should score higher than the latter, using a statistic like a t-test. For hypothesis (b), we could use our scale to define high- and low-anxiety groups, and use a t-test to compare their performance on a complex task; or correlate scores on the test with scores on the complex task. The next two hypotheses would involve testing the same people on two occasions—before and after treatment for hypothesis (c); and a month versus a day before an exam for hypothesis (d). This would be analyzed using a paired t-test or, if we were more sophisticated and used a comparison group, with a Group by Time analysis of variance (ANOVA). Finally, hypothesis (e) would again involve a correlation, this time between the new test and an IQ test, where we hypothesize finding a low correlation. An example of a validation study is found in Health Research in Action box 7.2.

If the studies come out as we hypothesize, it indicates that both the theory is correct and that the test has some degree of validity under these circumstances. However, if the results are not as we expected, it could be that: (1) the theory is correct but the test is functioning poorly; (2) the test is fine, but the theory was wrong in this regard; or (3) both the theory and the test are flawed. We won't know which of these three options is the reason; only further studies can tell us.

These examples highlight a number of points. First, the number of hypotheses we can generate is virtually limitless, meaning that in one sense, the process of validation is never completed. There is always more that we can learn about what the scores mean in different situations and with different groups of people. Second, even studies that are not designed primarily to be validational in nature give us information about how the scale performs with different groups and under various conditions, and therefore can be used to buttress the validity of the scale. Third, while there are two statistical tests that we commonly use in reliability testing (the ICC and Cohen's α), those used in validation are more varied and depend on the type of study: independent t-tests when there are two groups, related t-tests if the same group is assessed under two conditions, ANOVA in its various forms if there are mixed designs or more groups, correlations if the scale is being correlated with another one, and so on.

Feasibility

When evaluating whether or not a given scale is appropriate for your needs, there is one other factor that must be taken into consideration, and that is its feasibility. The first element that influences this is the amount of time necessary to complete the scale. Some are very brief, and can be finished in five to ten minutes, while others, such as various personality inventories, can take hours to complete. A test that takes a

---

7.2   Health Research in Action

The construct of "illness intrusiveness" was developed by Devins et al. (1983) to describe the disruptions to a person's valued interests and activities that impair quality of life and the availability of rewarding experiences caused by chronic disease. It was originally applied to patients suffering from end-state renal disease, but has subsequently been invoked with many other chronic conditions such as epilepsy (e.g., Poochikian-Sarkissian, Sidani, Wennberg, and Devins, 2008) and anorexia nervosa (Carter, Bewell, and Devins, 2008). The construct is assessed by the Intrusiveness Rating Scale (Devins et al., 1983). Devins et al. (1990) tested a number of hypotheses that are derived from the construct: (1) some domains, such as marital and family relations, work, and finances would be more affected than others, such as recreation and social relations; (2) home dialysis would affect marital and family relations more than in-hospital dialysis; and (3) certain illness-related factors, such as fatigue and uremic symptom levels, would affect the degree of intrusiveness. They tested these hypotheses with 99 patients receiving different forms of dialysis, and found support for all of them, which strengthened the validity of the instrument for this group of patients.

long time to complete may not be an issue if the respondents are in-patients and have little else to do with their time; in fact, they may actually welcome the distraction. However, if the scale is to be administered as part of a larger battery, or to people who have other things to do, longer scales may lead to satisficing and therefore invalid results.

A second consideration is whether the scale is self-administered or meant to be completed by an observer. If the latter, then the cost of the study may increase, assuming observers must be paid. Further, additional observer training may be required so that there is adequate inter-rater reliability. A third issue is how simple or complicated it is to score the scale. Most scales require nothing more than adding up the number of endorsed items, but others may require complicated, computer-based scoring algorithms, again leading to cost considerations.

Summary

- Measurement is a process of assigning numbers to phenomena.

- Not all numbers are the same; depending on what they represent, some can be added and divided meaningfully (e.g., ratio and interval scales) and others cannot (nominal and ordinal scales).

- Many of the phenomena we encounter are "hypothetical constructs," and are not directly measureable.

- Scales designed to measure various constructs are often developed in a multi-stage process, involving:

- devising the items;

- checking them for attributes such as reading level, ambiguity, and relevance;

- devising an appropriate response scheme;

- selecting items based on their performance;

- determining the reliability of the scale in different situations; and

- determining the validity with various groups and in different situations.

Review Questions

1. Indicate at what level the following variables are measured (nominal, ordinal, interval, or ratio):

    a. Height

    b. Diagnosis

    c. Degree of pain on a 10 cm visual analogue scale

    d. IQ

    e. The ranking of professions on the basis of income

    f. Stage of breast cancer (i.e., I, IIa, IIb, III, IV)

2. As the variability of scores within a group of people increases, the reliability of a scale:

    a. Increases

    b. Decreases

c. Doesn't change

d. Changes in an unpredictable way

3. Reliability is affected by:

    a. Systematic error

    b. Random error

    c. Both random and systematic error

    d. Neither random nor systematic error

4. The true score is:

    a. The actual score a person obtains on a scale

    b. The score a person would obtain if there were no bias

    c. The score a person would obtain if there were no error

    d. The most accurate score the person could obtain

5. Which of the following is a bipolar scale?

    a. Likert scale

    b. Visual analogue scale

    c. Adjectival scale

    d. Categorical scale

6. Validity is best defined as:

    a. Seeing if the scale measures what it says it does

    b. Determining if the scale is correlated with similar scales

    c. Knowing what the scores tell us about respondents

    d. Seeing if the scale differentiates between groups

Recommended Readings

Streiner, D.L. and Norman, G.R. (2008) *Health Measurement Scales: A Practical Guide to their Development and Use.* 4th ed. Oxford: Oxford University Press.

This book explains to the reader how to construct and evaluate scales used in the health sciences. The chapters are in the order that the topics are confronted by people developing their own instruments.

Streiner, D.L. (1993) A checklist for evaluating the usefulness of rating scales. *Canadian Journal of Psychiatry,* 38(2), 140–8.

This article is aimed at people who will use, rather than develop scales, and points to what they should look for in articles describing potentially useful instruments.

Anastasi, A. and Urbina, S. (1997) *Psychological Testing.* 7th ed. Upper Saddle River, NJ: Prentice Hall.

One of the essential books surrounding test construction. Although oriented more toward achievement and aptitude tests, it provides a solid foundation of the underlying theories.

Fischer, J. and Corcoran, K.J. (2007) *Measures for Clinical Practice: A Sourcebook.* 4th ed. New York: Oxford University Press. (Two volumes)

McDowell, I. and Newell, C. (1996) *Measuring Health.* 2nd ed. Oxford: Oxford University Press.

Foddy, W.H. (1994) *Construction Questions for Interviews and Questionnaires.* Cambridge: Cambridge University Press.

A guide to writing questions.

These books give critical reviews of existing scales used in health research, and provide copies of the scales themselves.

References

Allen, M.J. and Yen, W.M. (1979) *Introduction to Measurement Theory*. Monterey, CA: Brooks/Cole.

American Psychiatric Association. (1968) DSM-II. *Diagnostic and Statistical Manual of Mental Disorders*. 2nd ed. Washington, DC: Author.

Anastasi, A. (1985). Psychological testing: Basic concepts and common misconceptions. In Rogers, A.M. and Sheirer, C.J. (Eds.). *G. Stanley Hall Lecture Series*, Vol. 5 (pp. 87–120). Washington, DC: American Psychological Association.

Anastasi, A. and Urbina, S. (1997) *Psychological Testing*. 7th ed. Upper Saddle River, NJ: Prentice Hall.

Bandalos, D.L. and Enders, C.K. (1996) The effects of non-normality and number of response categories on reliability. *Applied Measurement in Education*, 9, 151–60.

Barrera, M. (1986) Distinctions between social support concepts, measures, and models. *American Journal of Community Psychology*, 14, 413–45.

Beck, A.T., Steer, R.A., and Brown, G.K. (1996) *Manual for the Beck Depression Inventory-II*. San Antonio, TX: Psychological Corporation.

Beyer, J. and Aradine, C. (1998) Convergent and discriminant validity of a self-report measure of pain intensity for children. *Child Health Care*, 16, 274–81.

Bosi Ferraz, M., Quaresma, M.R., Aquino, L.R.L., Atra, E., Tugwell, P., and Goldsmith, C.H. (1990) Reliability of pain scales in the assessment of literate and illiterate patients with rheumatoid arthritis. *Journal of Rheumatology*, 17, 1022–4.

Bryant, G.D. and Norman, G.R. (1980) Expressions of probability: Words and numbers. *New England Journal of Medicine*, 302, 411.

Carp, F.M. (1989) Maximizing data quality in community studies of older people. In Lawton, M.P. and Herzog, A.R. (Eds.). *Special Research Methods for Gerontology* (pp. 93–122). Amityville, NY: Baywood Publishing.

Carter, J.C., Bewell, C., and Devins, G.M. (2008) Illness intrusiveness in anorexia nervosa. *Journal of Psychosomatic Research*, 64, 519–26.

Cortina, J.M. (1993) What is coefficient alpha? An examination of theory and applications. *Journal of Applied Psychology*, 78, 98–104.

Craig, C.S. and Douglas, S.P. (2005) *International Marketing research* (3rd ed.). Chichester, UK: Wiley.

Cronbach, L.J. (1951). Coefficient alpha and the internal structure of tests. *Psychometrika*, 16, 297–334.

Cronbach, L.J., and Meehl, P.E. (1955) Construct validity in psychological tests. *Psychological Bulletin*, 52, 281–302.

Devins, G.M., Binik, Y.M., Hutchinson, T.A., Hollomby, D.J., Barré, P.E., and Guttman, R.D. (1983) The emotional impact of end-state renal disease: Importance of patients' perceptions of intrusiveness and control. *International Journal of Psychiatry in Medicine*, 13, 327–43.

Devins, G.M., Mandin, H., Hons, R.B., Burgess, E.D., Klassen, J., Taub, K., Schorr, S., Letourneau, P.K., and Buckle, S. (1990) Illness intrusiveness and quality of life in end-state renal disease: Comparison and stability across treatment modalities. *Health Psychology*, 9, 117–42.

Enders, C.K. and Bandalos, D.L. (1999) The effect of heterogeneous item distributions on reliability. *Applied Measurement in Education*, 12, 133–50.

Feldt, L.S. (1993) The relationship between the distribution of item difficulties and test reliability. *Applied Measurement in Education*, 6, 37–48.

Goldman, B.A. and Mitchell, D.F. (2008) *Directory of Unpublished Experimental Measures*. Washington, DC: American Psychological Association.

Harter, S. (1982) The perceived competence scale for children. *Child Development*, 53, 87–97.

Hathaway, S.R. and McKinley, J.C. (1940) A multiphasic personality schedule (Minnesota): I. Construction of the schedule. *Journal of Psychology*, 10, 249–54.

Hawthorne, G., Mouthaan, J., Forbes, D., and Novaco, R.W. (2006) Response categories and anger measurement: Do fewer categories result in poorer measurement? Development of the DAR5. *Social Psychiatry and Psychiatric Epidemiology*, 41, 164–72.

Huskisson, E.C. (1974) Measurement of pain. *Lancet, ii*, 1127–31.

Jones, R.R. (1968) Differences in response consistency and subjects' preferences for three personality response formats. In *Proceedings of the 76th Annual Convention of the American Psychological Association*, (pp. 247–8). Washington: APA.

Krosnick, J. (1991) Response strategies for coping with the cognitive demands of attitude measures in surveys. *Applied Cognitive Psychology*, 5, 213–36.

Lawshe, C.H. (1975) A quantitative approach to content validity. *Personnel Psychology*, 28, 563–75.

Lichtenstein, S. and Newman, J.R. (1967) Empirical scaling of common verbal phrases associated with numerical probabilities. *Psychonomic Science*, 9, 563–4.

Lynn, M.R. (1986) Determination and quantification of content validity. *Nursing Research*, 35, 362–5.

Messick, S. (1989) Validity. In Linn, R.L. (Ed.), *Educational Measurement*, 3rd ed., (pp. 13–103). New York: Macmillan.

Messick, S. (1996) Validity of performance assessment. In Philips, G. (Ed). *Technical Issues in Large-Scale Performance Assessment*. Washington, DC: National Center for Educational Statistics.

Meyerink, L.H., Reitan, R.M., and Selz, M. (1988) The validity of the MMPI with multiple sclerosis patients. *Journal of Clinical Psychology*, 44, 764–9.

Murphy, L.L., Impara, J.C., and Plake, B.S. (*1999*) *Tests in Print V: An Index to Tests, Test Reviews, and Literature on Specific Tests*, Vol. 5. Lincoln, NB: Buros Institute of Mental Measurement.

Nederhof, A.J. (1985) Methods of coping with social desirability bias: A review. *European Journal of Social Psychology*, 15, 263–80.

Norman, G.R. and Streiner, D.L. (2008) *Biostatistics: The Bare Essentials*, 3rd ed. Shelton, CT: PMPH USA.

Nunnally, J.C. and Bernstein, I.H. (1994) *Psychometric Theory*. 3rd ed. New York: McGraw-Hill.

Parducci, A. (1968) Often is often. *American Psychologist*, 25, 828.

Paulhus, D.L. (1991) Measurement and control of response bias. Measures of personality and social psychological attitudes. In J.P. Robinson, P.R. Shaver and L.S. Wrightsman (Eds.). *Measures of Personality and Social Psychological Attitudes, Measures of Social Psychological Attitudes*, Vol. 1 (pp. 17–59). San Diego, CA: Academic Press.

Poochikian-Sarkissiana, S., Sidani, S., Wennberg, R.A., and Devins, G.M. (2008) Psychological impact of illness intrusiveness in epilepsy: Comparison of treatments. *Psychology, Health and Medicine*, 13, 129–45.

Postuma, A.B. and Harper, J.F. (1998) Comparison of MMPI-2 responses of child custody and personal injury litigants. *Professional Psychology: Research and Practice*, 29, 437–43.

Ronen, G.M., Rosenbaum, P.L., Law, M., and Streiner, D.L. (1999) Health-related quality of life in childhood epilepsy: The results of children's participation in identifying the components. *Developmental Medicine and Child Neurology*, *41*, 554–9.

Ronen, G.M., Rosenbaum, P.L., and Streiner, D.L. (2003) Health-related quality of life in childhood epilepsy: The development of self-report and proxy-response measures. *Epilepsia*, *44*, 598–612.

Schuman, H. and Presser, S. (1981) *Questions and Answers*. New York: Academic Pres.

Schwarz, N., Hippler, H.J., Deutsch, B., and Strack, F. (1985) Response scales: Effects of category range on report behavior and subsequent judgments. *Public Opinion Quarterly*, *49*, 388–95.

Seligman, M.E.P., Walker, E.F. and Rosenhan, D.L. (2000) *Abnormal Psychology*. 4th ed. New York: Norton.

Seymour, R.A., Simpson, J.M., Charlton, J.E., and Phillips, M.E. (1985) An evaluation of length and end-phrase of visual analog scales in dental pain. *Pain*, *21*, 177–85.

Shrout, P.E. and Fleiss, J.L. (1979) Intraclass correlations: Uses in assessing rater reliability. *Psychological Bulletin*, *86*, 420–8.

Stevens, S.S. (1946) On the theory of scales of measurement. *Science*, *103*, 677–80.

Streiner, D.L. (2003) Starting at the beginning: An introduction to coefficient alpha and internal consistency. *Journal of Personality Assessment*, *80*, 99–103.

Streiner, D.L. and Norman, G.R. (2008) *Health Measurement Scales: A Practical Guide to their Development and Use*. 4th ed. Oxford: Oxford University Press.

Streiner, D.L. and Norman, G.R. (2009) Randomized controlled trials. *Community Oncology*, *6*, 83–85.

Uchino, B.N. (2009) Understanding the links between social support and physical health: A life-span perspective with emphasis on the separability of perceived and received support. *Perspectives on Psychological Science*, *4*, 236–55.

Wright, D.B., Gaskell, G.D., and O'Muircheartaigh, C.A. (1994) How much is "Quite a bit"? Mapping between numerical values and vague quantifiers. *Applied Cognitive Psychology*, *8*, 479–96.

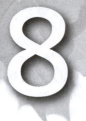

8 Sampling

Jean Dumais

CHAPTER OUTLINE

Introduction

Populations are large. Studying them requires a lot of tedious work, a lot of careful people, a lot of time, and a lot of money. However, in many situations, studying a population does not mean that the researcher needs to see and talk to each individual: a spoonful of soup tells you what kind of soup it is. In the earliest written accounts of "studies of populations" one finds census taking as a means to collect information about a population. States have used census taking to establish taxation and collect taxes, raise armies and wage wars, or plan public services like electoral representation, schooling and health care.

In the late nineteenth and early twentieth centuries, mathematicians (who had devised probability theory in the mid-seventeenth century) and statisticians (who compiled data on populations) converged and realized that probability theory could be applied to the study of large populations through the selection of relatively small samples, and that this sampling mechanism could be used to obtain population-level estimates.

Probabilistic sampling (also called statistical sampling, random sampling or even scientific sampling) relies on probability theory to describe (or compute) the odds of an individual being selected in a sample, much like it can be used to compute your odds at winning a lottery, at roulette, or at poker. This is how one can compute how much one can expect to win (or lose) should one play for a very long time. And using similar reasoning, survey statisticians can compute the average contribution of a selected individual to the estimated population parameter (average income, prevalence of high blood pressure, incidence of AIDS).

When the decision is taken to conduct a survey to answer data needs, the researcher needs to plan how to select the sample. *Sampling is a means of selecting a subset of units from a population for the purpose of collecting information from those units to draw inferences about the population as a whole.* There are two broad classes of sampling techniques: non-probability, and **probability sampling**. The one chosen depends primarily on whether reliable inferences are to be made about the population.

Non-probability sampling uses a subjective method of selecting individuals or units from a population. It provides a fast, easy, and inexpensive way of selecting a sample. However, in order to make inferences about the population from the sample, the researcher must assume that the sample is somehow representative of the population. This is often a risky assumption to make in the case of non-probability sampling.

Probability sampling involves the selection of individuals or units from a population based on the principle of randomization or chance. Probability sampling is more complex, time-consuming, and usually more costly than non-probability sampling. However, because individuals from the population are randomly selected and each individual's inclusion probability can be calculated, reliable estimates can be produced along with estimates of the sampling error, and inferences can be made about the population.

There are several different ways in which a probability sample can be selected. The design chosen depends on the availability of a **sampling frame**—that is, an extensive and up-to-date list of all members of the population—on the variability among members of the population and how costly it is to survey them.

The purpose of this chapter is to present different probability sample designs and factors to consider when determining the appropriate design for a specific survey. Some aspects of sample size computation, weighting, and estimation are also briefly covered.

One intuitive way to consider the various sampling strategies is to examine the behaviour of two newspaper food columnists at some "All-you-can-eat Chinese buffet." How can a restaurant critic speak of the available food there? On what pieces of information can he base his judgement on the quality, the variety, the flavours, the aroma, the colours, the savoury, and the sweet? And then, how many pieces of food does he need to eat before he can write his column?

One columnist could be guided by his senses of sight and smell: "this looks or smells good; I'll have some; this looks bland, I'll skip" or "never mind the vegetables, they're always the same. Show me the sweets!" He could also be constrained by the deadline: "I only have time for a soup and a few dumplings." These strategies are based on judgement, personal preferences, or convenience.

Using a different strategy, another columnist may decide to pick something from every third dish, from the left end of the buffet table to the right end. Or say something like "There are soups, seafood, fowl and poultry, meats, vegetables, rice dishes, dumplings and rolls, fruit, cakes, and other sweets. I'll have from every category." But, clearly, that critic need not eat the full bowl of steamed broccoli to form an opinion; a few bites will be enough.

Which columnist would be in the better position to speak of what that buffet has to offer? Sampling is after unbiased choices of respondents, and after variety of responses. In sampling, there is something as "too much of a good thing."

Non-Probability Sampling

Non-probability sampling is a method of selecting individuals from a **population** using a subjective (i.e., non-random) method. (Probability sampling is examined in the next section.) Since non-probability sampling does not require a complete sampling frame, it is a fast, easy, and inexpensive way of obtaining data. The problem with non-probability sampling is that it is unclear whether or not it is possible to **generalize** the results from the sample to the population. The reason for this is that the selection of individuals from the population for a non-probability sample can result in large biases.

For example, a common design is for the interviewer to subjectively decide who should be sampled. Since the interviewer is most likely to select the most accessible or friendly members of the population, a large portion of the population has no chance of ever being selected, and this portion of the population is likely to differ in a systematic manner from those selected members. Not only can this **bias** the results of the survey, it can falsely reduce the apparent variability of the population due to a tendency to select "typical" individuals and eliminate extreme values.

Due to **selection bias** and (usually) the absence of a frame, an individual's inclusion probability cannot be calculated for non-probability samples, so there is no way of producing reliable estimates or estimates of their **precision (sampling error)**. Inferences about the population can only be made by assuming that the sample is representative of the population. This usually requires assuming that the characteristics of the population follow some model or are evenly or randomly distributed over the population. This is often dangerous due to the difficulty of assessing whether or not these assumptions hold.

Non-probability sampling is often used by researchers as an inexpensive and quick alternative to probability sampling, but it is not a valid substitute for probability sampling for the reasons delineated above. So, why bother with non-probability sampling? Non-probability sampling can be used to generate ideas; as a preliminary step toward the development of a probability sample survey; or as a follow-up step to help understand the results of a probability sample survey.

For example, non-probability sampling can be used for exploratory or diagnostic studies to gain insights into people's attitudes, beliefs, motivations, and behaviours. Sometimes non-probability sampling is the only viable option—for example, sampling volunteers may be the only way of obtaining data for medical experiments, drug trials, or psychological tests.

Non-probability sampling is often used to select individuals for focus groups and in-depth interviews. For example, at Statistics Canada, non-probability sampling is used to test Census of Population questionnaires, to ensure that the questions asked and concepts used are clear to respondents. In addition, if the content of a question is deemed to be controversial, subpopulations may be selected and tested.

Six different types of non-probability sampling schemes are described in the next few paragraphs: **haphazard sampling**, **judgement sampling**, **volunteer sampling**, **quota sampling** and **modified probability sampling**, and finally, **network** or **snowball sampling**.

In *haphazard sampling*, individuals are selected in an aimless, arbitrary manner with little or no planning involved. Haphazard sampling assumes that the population is homogeneous: if the population units are all alike, then any individual may be chosen for the sample. An example of haphazard sampling is the "man in the street" interview where the interviewer selects any person who happens to walk by. Unfortunately, unless the population is truly homogeneous, selection is subject to the biases of the interviewer and whoever happened to walk by at the time of sampling.

With *volunteer sampling*, the respondents are volunteers, as the name suggests! Generally, volunteers must be screened so as to get a set of characteristics suitable for the purposes of the study (e.g., smokers, diabetics, people with sleep disorder). This method can be subject to large selection biases, but is sometimes necessary. For example, for ethical reasons, volunteers with particular medical conditions may have to be solicited for some medical experiments or drug testing.

Judgement sampling is done based on previous ideas of population composition and behaviour. An expert with knowledge of the population decides which individuals in the population should be sampled. In other words, the expert purposely selects what is considered to be a representative sample. Judgement is perhaps even more biased than haphazard sampling. However, it can be useful in exploratory studies, for example in selecting members for focus groups or in-depth interviews to test specific aspects of a questionnaire.

Quota sampling is one of the most common forms of non-probability sampling. Sampling is done until a specific number of units for various subpopulations (the quotas) has been selected. Quota sampling is a means for satisfying sample size objectives for the subpopulations, for example by fixing the proportions of men and women in the sample to be those in the population. Quota sampling can be considered preferable to other forms of non-probability sampling (e.g., judgement sampling) because it forces the inclusion of members of different subpopulations. Quota sampling is somewhat similar to stratified sampling in that similar individuals are grouped together (see below). However, it differs in how the individuals are selected. Contacted individuals that are unwilling to participate are simply replaced by individuals that are, in effect ignoring nonresponse bias. Market researchers often use quota sampling (particularly for telephone surveys) instead of stratified sampling to survey individuals with particular socioeconomic profiles. This is because compared with stratified sampling, quota sampling is relatively inexpensive and easy to administer, and it has the desirable property of satisfying population proportions. However, it disguises potentially significant selection bias.

Quota sampling can easily be improved by using a combination of probability and nonprobability sampling. The first stages are usually based on probability sampling (see the following section). The last stage is a non-probability sample, usually a quota sample. For example, geographical areas may be selected using a probability design, and then within each region, a quota sample of individuals may be drawn. This technique is called *modified probability sampling* or *quasi probability sampling*.

Now, when the researcher needs to find and contact rare individuals in the population, they may already know of the existence of some of these individuals. One approach is to contact those individuals and simply ask them if they know anyone like themselves, contact those people, etc. The sample grows like a snowball rolling down a hill to hopefully include virtually everybody with that rare characteristic. *Snowball sampling* is useful for small or specialized populations such as blind, deaf, or other persons who may not belong to an organized group or not readily identified on a survey list frame. However, some individuals or subgroups may have no chance of being sampled. In order to make inferences, strong modelling assumptions (which are usually not met) are required.

Probability Sampling

Probability sampling is a method of sampling that allows inferences to be made about the population based on observations from a sample. In order to be able to make inferences, the sample should not be subject to selection bias. Probability sampling avoids this bias by randomly selecting individuals from the population (using a computer or table of random numbers). It is important to note that random does not mean arbitrary. In particular, the interviewers do not arbitrarily choose respondents since then sampling would be subject to their personal biases. Random means that selection is unbiased—it is based on chance. With probability sampling, it is never left up to the discretion of the interviewer to subjectively decide who should be sampled.

There are two main criteria for probability sampling: one is that the individuals be randomly selected, the second is that all individuals in the **survey population** have a non-zero inclusion probability in the sample and that these probabilities can be calculated. It is not necessary for all individuals to have the same inclusion probability, indeed, in most complex surveys the inclusion probability varies from individual to individual.

There are many different types of probability sample designs. The most basic is **simple random sampling** and the designs increase in complexity to encompass **systematic sampling**, **probability-proportional-to-size sampling**, **cluster sampling**, **stratified sampling**, **multi-stage** (and **multiphase**) **sampling**, and **replicated sampling**. Each of these sampling techniques is useful in different situations. If the objective of the survey is simply to provide overall population estimates, simple random sampling should be sufficient. If the cost of survey collection is high and the resources are available, cluster sampling may be an option. If subpopulation estimates are also desired (such as estimates by province, age group, or size of community), stratified sampling is usually performed.

Most of the more complex designs use auxiliary information on the sampling frame to improve the efficiency of the sampling strategy (see stratified sampling later). If the frame has been created from a previous census or from administrative data, there may be a wealth of supplementary information that can be used for sampling. For example, for a survey of people, demographic information (e.g., age, sex, ethnic origin, socioeconomic status) may be available for everyone from the last population census. In order for the auxiliary information to improve sampling efficiency, there must be a correlation between the auxiliary data and the survey variables (see stratified sampling).

The main advantage of probability sampling is that since each individual is randomly selected and each individual's inclusion probability can be calculated, reliable estimates of interest such as prevalence, incidence or association, and an estimate of the sampling error of each estimate can be produced. Therefore, inferences can be made about the population. In fact, with a probability design, a relatively small sample can often be used to draw inferences about a large population.

The main disadvantages of probability sampling are that it is more difficult, takes longer, and is usually more expensive than non-probability sampling. In general, the expense of creating and maintaining a good quality sampling frame is substantial. And because probability samples tend to be more spread out geographically across the population than non-probability samples, sample sizes are generally much larger and data collection is often more costly and difficult to manage.

Simple random sampling (SRS) is used as a benchmark for evaluating the **efficiency** of other sampling strategies. In order to understand the concept of efficient sampling, some definitions are presented here.

PRACTICAL TIP

Why Such a Fuss with Survey Statistics?

In elementary statistics, populations are infinite and samples are made up of independent and identically distributed observations. The *Central Limit Theorem* rules and samples of size $n = 30$ are "large enough."

In survey statistics, populations are *finite* and samples are made up of *dependent* units of unknown distributions. The original *Central Limit Theorem* no longer holds; sample sizes of $n = 100$ are "bare minimum." Basically, most of the statistics we learn in introductory statistics classes have to be re-written.

In elementary statistics, the values are random; in survey sampling, the values are fixed (albeit unknown) and the composition of the sample is the random element.

We call the mean and variance of the infinite population μ and σ^2; the finite-population equivalents of these parameters are $\overline{Y}$ and S^2, and their estimates are respectively σ^2 and s^2. Those parameters are defined as

$$\overline{Y} = \frac{1}{N} \sum_{i \in U} Y_i$$

and

$$S^2 = \frac{1}{N} \sum_{i \in U} \left(Y_i - \overline{Y}\right)^2,$$

where the sum is taken over all units comprising the finite population U. In survey statistics, the convention is to use capital Roman letters to denote the (finite) population parameters and values, and lower case letters to represent their estimates or sample values; alternatively a "hat" crowning a parameter denotes its estimate, as in this symbolic expression for "the estimator of the population mean is the sample mean", or $\hat{\overline{Y}} = \overline{y}$. The mathematical form of the estimators $\overline{y}$ and s^2 will depend on the sampling method used.

Bernoulli Sampling

Bernoulli sampling is the easiest sampling method, modelled on the toss of a coin. This technique is useful when sampling moderate to large size samples from very large electronic files. To draw a Bernoulli sample of size n from a file of size N, it is sufficient to draw a random number r between 1 and the sampling fraction $f = n / N$. Then, if r is less than or equal to f the individual is selected, otherwise, it is not included in the sample. With this process, the sample size is random and can vary quite a lot from the nominal n. This is a very quick, cheap,

and effective method, but it is likely the least precise of the methods reviewed here. Using Bernoulli sampling when collection and processing budgets are an issue is ill-advised. When the problem at hand is merely to have a random ("representative") sample of cases from a large administrative database "to get a feel," Bernoulli sampling might be quite appropriate. For example, the Ministry of Health may be interested in auditing annually, say, 1 per cent of health insurance card holders. There are millions of health insurance card holders (the population size "N") and 1 per cent (the sampling fraction "f") of them may still be a substantial

TABLE 8.1 Bernoulli Sample (*N* = 45, *n* = 7)

Unit	Random Number	Selected?	Unit	Random Number	Selected?	Unit	Random Number	Selected?	Unit	Random Number	Selected?
1	0.006	**yes**	12	0.569	no	23	0.058	**yes**	34	0.915	no
2	0.869	no	13	0.985	no	24	0.082	**yes**	35	0.954	no
3	0.722	no	14	0.198	no	25	0.722	no	36	0.802	no
4	0.431	no	15	0.624	no	26	0.087	**yes**	37	0.997	no
5	0.408	No	16	0.064	yes	27	0.931	no	38	0.151	**yes**
6	0.922	no	17	0.323	no	28	0.288	no	39	0.003	**yes**
7	0.150	**yes**	18	0.001	yes	29	0.394	no	40	0.410	no
8	0.808	no	19	0.678	no	30	0.553	no	41	0.567	no
9	0.077	**yes**	20	0.075	yes	31	0.383	no	42	0.718	no
10	0.724	no	21	0.898	no	32	0.577	no	43	0.598	no
11	0.902	no	22	0.596	no	33	0.033	**yes**	44	0.391	no
									45	0.508	no

sample. A "computerized coin" could be tossed by the computer (e.g. using the command "=RAND()" in Microsoft Excel) selecting the records for which the "coin toss" gives a value less than 0.01. The following table illustrates Bernoulli sampling on a population of *N* = 45 units; the desired (or nominal) sample size is *n* = 7. Note that, in this example, the achieved sample is of size 12.

In most applications controlling the sample size, that is controlling collection and processing costs, is an important aspect of the survey management. The next two sampling methods allow for better control of the sample size, barring **non-response**, of course.

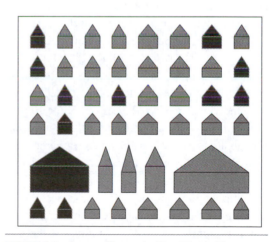

FIGURE 8.1 Bernoulli sample (*N* = 45, *n* = 7)

Simple Random Sampling (SRS)

The starting point for all probability sampling designs is simple random sampling (SRS). SRS is a one-step selection method that ensures that every possible sample of size *n* has an equal chance of being selected. As a consequence, each individual in the sample has the same inclusion probability. This probability, π, is equal to *n/N*, where *N* is the number of units in the population. The idea of drawing names out of a hat is the best image one can have of SRS.

Sampling may be done with or without replacement. Sampling with replacement allows for an individual to be selected more than once. Sampling without replacement means that once an individual has been selected, it cannot be selected again. Simple random sampling with replacement (SRSWR) and simple random sampling without replacement (SRSWOR) are practically identical if the sample size is a very small fraction of the population size. This is because the possibility of the same unit appearing more than once in the sample is small. Generally, sampling without replacement yields more precise results and is operationally more convenient. For the purpose of this chapter, sampling is assumed to be without replacement unless otherwise specified.

Consider a population of five people and suppose that a sample of three is to be selected (SRSWOR). Label the people in the population 1, 2, 3, 4, and 5 and denote the population as the set {1, 2, 3, 4, 5}. There are ten possible samples of three people: {1, 2, 3}, {1, 2, 4}, {1, 2, 5}, {1, 3, 4}, {1, 3, 5}, {1, 4, 5}, {2, 3, 4}, {2, 3, 5}, {2, 4, 5} and {3, 4, 5}. Each of these samples has an equal chance of being selected and each individual is selected in six out of the 10 possible samples, thus each individual has an inclusion probability of $p = n / N = 3/5$. If this enumeration is possible with $N = 5$, it is impractical to do with life-size human populations.

Simple random sampling supposes that a sampling frame is available. On the frame, the units are numbered 1 to N, although the method of assigning a unique number to each unit is not important. Next, a computer-generated random number is assigned to each of the N entries of the list, and the list sorted in, say, ascending order by the random number; then the first n units make up the sample. See the illustration below.

SRS is the simplest sampling technique and requires no additional (auxiliary) information

on the frame in order to draw the sample. The theory behind SRS is well established so there are standard and easy to use formulas to determine the sample size, population estimates, and variance estimates. However, because it makes no use of auxiliary information that may exist, SRS can result in estimates being less statistically efficient than if another sample design had been used. SRS can be expensive if personal interviews are used, since the sample may be widely spread out geographically. Some consider it is possible to draw a "bad" SRS sample. Since all samples of size n have an equal chance of being included in the sample, it is possible to draw a sample that is not well dispersed and that poorly represents the population. Now, there are so many different SRSWOR of size n that the chances of hitting a "bad" sample are slim. For example, from a population of 1000 people, the chances of drawing *the* simple random sample of $n = 100$ that is comprised of the 100 richest persons are less about 1 in 10^{139} (10 followed by 138 zeroes!). . . and that sample is just as likely to be drawn as any other SRS of size $n = 100$.

Systematic Sampling (SYS)

In systematic sampling (SYS), individuals are selected from the population at regular intervals. A sampling interval and a random start are required. When the population size, N, is a multiple of the sample size, n, every kth individual is selected, where the interval k is equal to N / n. The random start, r, is a single random number between 1 and k, inclusively. The individuals selected are then: $r, r + k, r + 2k, \ldots r + (n - 1)k$. Like SRS, each individual has an inclusion probability, p, equal to n / N but, unlike SRS, not every combination of n individuals has an equal chance of being selected: SYS can only select samples in which the units are separated by k. Thus, under this method, only k possible samples can be drawn from the population.

TABLE 8.2　Simple Random Sample (N = 45, n = 7)

Unit	Random Number	Selected?	Unit	Random Number	Selected?	Unit	Random Number	Selected?	Unit	Random Number	Selected?
24	0.022	**yes**	41	0.307	no	27	0.517	no	8	0.776	no
12	0.040	**yes**	1	0.326	no	6	0.527	no	10	0.810	no
16	0.105	**yes**	7	0.356	no	3	0.539	no	33	0.817	no
18	0.106	**yes**	32	0.357	no	34	0.605	no	40	0.844	no
17	0.124	**yes**	11	0.374	no	29	0.643	no	31	0.853	no
23	0.157	**yes**	28	0.403	no	25	0.661	no	19	0.856	no
43	0.189	**yes**	21	0.424	no	45	0.661	no	4	0.858	no
38	0.192	no	37	0.502	no	20	0.700	no	9	0.862	no
26	0.253	no	14	0.505	no	13	0.713	no	15	0.896	no
5	0.284	no	35	0.506	no	22	0.715	no	30	0.919	no
2	0.302	no	42	0.515	no	36	0.773	no	44	0.923	no
									39	0.988	no

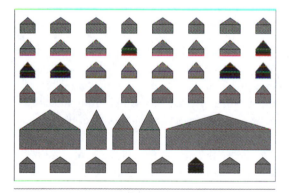

FIGURE 8.2　Simple random sample (N = 45, n = 7)

To illustrate SYS, suppose a population contains N = 36 individuals, and a sample of size n = 12 individuals is to be drawn. The sampling interval would be k = N / n = 36/12 = 3. Next, a random number between 1 and k = 3, say 1, is chosen. The population units selected for the sample are then numbered: 1, 4, 7, . . . , 31 and 34.

With a sampling interval of 3 and a population of size 36, there are only three possible SYS samples, while for a simple random sample of size 6, there are over 1.9 million possible samples.

One advantage of systematic sampling is that it can be used when no list of the population units is available in advance. In this case, a conceptual frame can be constructed by sampling every kth person until the end of the population is reached. But then, the sample size is not known until after the sample has been selected.

If N cannot be evenly divided by n, the sampling interval for SYS is not a whole number. In this case, k could be set equal to the nearest whole number, but then one of the possible samples would have one extra individual. For example, suppose that N = 45 and n = 7, then k = 45 / 7 = 6.428. If k is rounded down to 6 and if r = 4, the sample contains those individuals numbered: 4, 10, 16, 22, 28, 34 and 40. If the random start is $r = 1$ and every sixth unit is selected, then the sample consists of individuals: 1, 7, 13, 19, 25, 31, 37, and 43 and now the sample size is 8.

Alternatively, if N cannot be evenly divided by n then, to avoid a variable sample size, *circular systematic sampling* could be performed. With this method, the population units are thought to exist on a circle and modular counting is used. The value of k is set equal to the whole number nearest to N/n, but now the random start, r, can be between 1 and N, rather than 1 and k (i.e., the first unit can be anywhere on the list). The individuals are selected as before and when the end of the list is reached, sampling continues at the beginning of the list. The advantage of the circular method is that each individual has an equal chance of being in the sample. For example, using the previous example, suppose that $N = 45$ and $n = 7$ and $k = 6$. A random start, r, between 1 and 45 is selected, say $r = 26$. Then the selected population units are: 26, 32, 38, 44, 50 (corresponding to 5), 11, 17, and finally 23, because 25 is now the end of the list.

SYS is often used as a proxy for SRS when no frame exists but direct access to individuals is possible (e.g., by walking city blocks); much like

SRS, SYS relies on sound theory. SYS can be more dispersed than SRS, which can be a bonus when this dispersion can be somehow controlled by clever fieldwork and file sorting. However, it can result in a "bad" sample if the sampling interval matches some periodicity in the population (e.g., always selecting the corner house of a city block face, selecting hospital admissions based on time periods but always selecting "rush hours"). Much like the SRS, SYS has no use for auxiliary information, which makes it comparatively inefficient.

SRS, SYS, and Bernoulli sampling have all been applied to individual elements of the population. In the next section, we look at sampling groups or clusters of individuals.

Statistics Canada's General Social Survey (GSS), an ongoing annual survey with a different focus every year based on a five-year rotation cycle, uses the equivalent of SRS drawing from a sampling frame of telephone numbers: the GSS uses a technique called Random Digit Dialling.

Cluster Sampling

The three sampling methods described above assume that a frame of individual units exists and is available to the researcher. It may not always be practical or possible to sample individuals directly. Sometimes, sampling groups of the population units is much easier (e.g., entire households). *Cluster sampling* is the process of randomly selecting complete groups (clusters) of population units from the sampling frame. It is usually a less statistically efficient sampling strategy than SRS of individuals but it can greatly reduce the cost of collection, particularly if the population is spread out and personal interviews are conducted. Moreover, it allows the production of estimates for the clusters themselves (e.g., average revenue per household).

Cluster sampling is a two-step process. First, the population is grouped into clusters; clusters may be

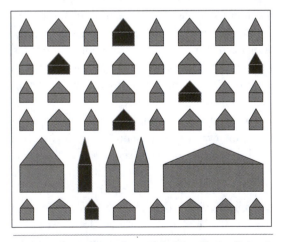

FIGURE 8.3   Systematic sample ($N = 45$, $n = 7$, $k = 6$, $r = 4$)

decided by the researcher (e.g., all the admissions to a hospital department in a day) or they may be natural features of the environment (e.g., city blocks, households, schools, hospital wards). The second step is to select a sample of clusters and interview all individuals within the selected clusters.

The sampling frame may dictate that cluster sampling be used. In the case of household surveys, many countries do not have complete and up-to-date lists of the people or households available to non-governmental agencies, but they do have maps. In this case an area frame could be created, with the geographical areas divided into regions (clusters), the regions sampled, and everyone within the region interviewed.

In order for estimates to be statistically efficient, the units within a cluster should be as different as possible. Otherwise, if the units within a cluster are similar, they all provide similar information and interviewing one individual would be sufficient.

Unfortunately, individuals within a cluster frequently have similar characteristics and therefore are more homogeneous than individuals randomly selected from the general population. This results in a sampling procedure that is less efficient than SRS. For example, suppose that for a city of 100,000, two samples are drawn. For the first sample, cluster sampling is used and one city block, containing 400 residents, is selected at random. For the second sample, SRS is used to select 400 people from the list of 100,000 residents. The 400 residents in the SRS sample are likely to be far more diverse in terms of income, age, occupation, and educational background (to name only a few variables) than the 400 people in the cluster sample who all live on the same city block.

The **statistical efficiency** of cluster sampling depends on how homogeneous the units within the clusters are, how many population units are in each cluster, and the number of clusters sampled. When neighbouring units are similar, it is more statistically efficient to select many small clusters rather than a few, larger clusters. However, when personal interviews are conducted, the more dispersed the sample is, the more expensive the survey. The researcher must strike a balance between the optimal number and size of clusters, and the cost.

Cluster sampling can greatly reduce the cost of data collection by having a less dispersed sample than SRS. This is particularly important when the population is spread out and personal interviews

8.1   Health Research in Action

Does Anyone Really Use Cluster Sampling?

The monthly Labour Force Survey uses cluster sampling of dwellings to collect information on labour market activity, rent, and ad hoc survey topics. Similarly, the Ontario Survey on the Prevalence and Control of Hypertension (Leenen et al., 2008) used cluster sampling of households to increase the chances of collecting enough information from targeted ethno-cultural groups. In both surveys clusters are determined by drawing a line down the middle of the street. This makes it easy to decide whether a dwelling is in the sample or not.

Both the National Population Health Survey (NHPS) and the Canadian Community Health Survey (CCHS) rely on Labour Force Survey (LFS) clusters and lists of dwellings to draw their respective samples; the LFS changes one sixth of their clusters every month and the "rotated-out" clusters become available to other Statistics Canada surveys.

are conducted since savings can be achieved by reducing the travel time of interviewers, especially for rural populations. Cluster sampling is also easier to apply than SRS or SYS to populations that are naturally clustered (e.g., households, schools) and for certain conceptual populations, such as people crossing a border during a specific time interval. For such populations, it may be difficult, expensive, or impossible to construct a list of all individual units of the population, required by SRS.

However, cluster sampling can be less statistically efficient than SRS if the units within the clusters are homogeneous with respect to the study variables. The final sample size is not usually known in advance, since it is not usually known how many individuals are within a cluster until after the survey has been conducted. Computing estimates and estimating their precision can be much more difficult than with individual element sampling schemes seen earlier. (This topic is discussed in detail in more advanced textbooks like Kish's (1965), Lohr's (1999), or Särndal's (1992), given in the references.)

SRS and SYS are both equal probability sample designs, and they can be used to sample individual units or clusters of units. Not all sampling techniques result in equal probabilities. The sample designs described in the following sections can result in unequal probabilities. It is important to remember that in probability sampling, the criterion is not that all units have the same inclusion probability but that all units have a known non-zero inclusion probability. Often, sampling with unequal probabilities can improve the statistical efficiency of the sampling strategy.

Probability-Proportional-to-Size (PPS) Sampling

Contrary to SRS and SYS, *probability-proportional-to-size* (PPS) sampling is one technique that uses auxiliary data and yields unequal probabilities of inclusion. If population units vary in size and these sizes are known such information can be used during sampling to increase the statistical efficiency.

PPS can yield dramatic increases in precision if the size measures are accurate and the variables of interest are correlated with the size of the unit. For less accurate size measures, it is better to create size groupings and perform stratified sampling (see Stratified Sampling below).

Examples of size variables are area and population. Agricultural surveys often use PPS, where the size measure is the size of the farm in hectares. Admittedly, the size of a farm can grow (or shrink) if the farmer buys or sells land, but for the most part, farm size is constant from year to year. In addition, typical questions for farm surveys, such as income, crop production, livestock holdings, and expenses are often correlated with land holdings. Similarly, most variables on surveys of human populations tend to be correlated with the size of the community where those populations live, e.g., day care needs, medical expenses, prevalence of certain diseases.

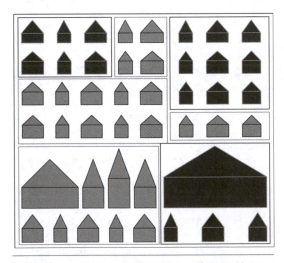

FIGURE 8.4   Cluster sampling (three of seven clusters are sampled)

To illustrate, assume that there is a population of six families and that the researcher is interested in estimating the total family health-related expenses by sampling only one family. (A sample of size one is used for the purpose of illustration; in practice, one hardly ever selects only one unit.). Suppose that there is a stable size measure for each health unit (the size of the families) and, to illustrate the efficiency gains over SRS, assume that each family's expenses are known. (Obviously, in real life, if the expenses were known, there would be no need to conduct the survey.)

Consider the following (very small) population of families:

For this population of six families, the true total expenses are $2807. A simple random sample could be selected, where each sample contains one unit and each unit has an inclusion probability of 1/6. Six different SRS samples of size $n = 1$ are possible. Consider the results from SRS (see table below). (For now, a population total is estimated by multiplying the sampled unit's value by the unit's weight. This **weight** is the average number of units in the survey population that the sampled unit represents and is the inverse of the inclusion probability.)

Here, for the SRS strategy, estimates range from $1464 to $3882; for the PPS strategy the range of values shrinks to $2696 to $3050. For the PPS sample, the sampling variability is much lower.

Clearly, the main advantage of PPS sampling is that it can improve the statistical efficiency of the sampling strategy by using auxiliary information. This can result in a dramatic reduction in the sampling variance compared with SRS or even stratified sampling. Notice how the SRS estimates range from 1464 to 3882 (range of 2418) while the PPS estimates range from 2696 to 3050 (range of 354).

However, the advantages of PPS come at a price: (1) a sampling frame that contains good quality, up-to-date auxiliary information for all units on the frame that can be used as a meas-

TABLE 8.3 Population Values

Family	Auxiliary Frame Information: Family Size	Survey Variable of Interest: Health-related Expenses
1	5	$ 556
2	3	353
3	4	445
4	2	244
5	6	647
6	5	562
Total	25	2807

ure of size (MOS) is required; an inaccurate or unstable MOS may render PPS counterproductive; (2) when the MOS is not well correlated with the main survey variables, there may be no statistical gain in efficiency; and (3) because the selection probabilities differ with each unit, the estimation of the sampling variance of an estimate is more complex than with equal probability models.

There are many PPS sampling schemes, much like there are many equal probabilities sampling schemes. However, three commonly used techniques are the random method, the systematic method, and the randomized systematic method. (The following assumes that the size measures are integer values.) The two simplest are the *random PPS* and *systematic PPS* methods.

The random method of PPS sampling

This is the equivalent to drawing names from a hat, except that units have as many pieces of paper in the hat as their size indicates. Hence, for each unit in the population, cumulate the size measures for units up to and including itself; determine the range corresponding to each unit in the population, that is, from (but not including) the cumulative sum for the previous unit to the

TABLE 8.4 All Possible SRS and PPS Samples of Size $n = 1$

Sample (Selected Family)	SRS Sampling			PPS Sampling		
	Expenses ($)	Inclusion Probability (π)	Population Estimate of Total Expenses ($)	Family Size	Inclusion Probability (π)	Population Estimate of Total Expenses ($)
1	556	1 / 6 = 0.16667	3336	5	5/25 = 0.200	2780
2	353	0.16667	(353 × 6 / 1=) 2118	3	0.120	(353 × 25/3 =) 2942
3	445	0.16667	2670	4	0.160	2781
4	244	0.16667	**1464**	2	0.080	**3050**
5	647	0.16667	**3882**	6	0.240	**2696**
6	562	0.16667	3372	5	0.200	2810
	2807	**Average[1]:**	**2807**	**25**	**Average:**	**2807**

1. The average is taken over all possible samples of size n. When drawing SRS, all samples have the same probability of being selected; when drawing PPS, all samples have different probabilities of being selected; these have to be used when computing the average of the sample estimates.

cumulative sum for the current unit; select a random number between 1 and the total cumulative size and select the unit whose range contains the random number; and repeat previous step until n units have been selected.

Using again the population of $N = 6$ families, a sample of $n = 3$ three units can be obtained by drawing three random numbers between 1 and 25. Suppose these numbers are: 8, 5, and 21. Then the selected families are: family 1, family 2, and family 6.

In the case of the random method for PPS sampling without replacement, if more than one unit is selected, complications arise both in attempting to keep probabilities directly proportional to size and in estimating the sampling variances of survey estimates. This becomes even more complicated when more than two or three units are selected with PPS without replacement, and in fact, is the subject of considerable research (see Lohr, 1999, Levy and Lemeshow, 1999; or Statistics Canada, 2010).

TABLE 8.5 PPS Sampling Using the Random Method

Family	Auxiliary Frame Information: Family Size	Cumulative Size	Range	Random Selection
1	5	5	1–5	2nd draw
2	3	8	6–8	1st draw
3	4	12	9–12	
4	2	14	13–14	
5	6	20	15–20	
6	5	25	21–25	3rd draw

The systematic method

This is the equivalent to the equal probability SYS seen earlier. Again, for each unit in the population, the MOS are cumulated and running totals are recorded. The procedure now requires (1) computation of a sampling interval, k = (total cumulative size)/n; and (2) determination of a random start, r, between 1 and k; and selection of those units whose range contains the random numbers r, $r+k$, $r+2k$, ... $r+(n-1)k$. Here, we have a sampling step k = (total cumulative size) / n = 25 / 3 = 8 and a random start of r = 8.

When the MOS is less reliable, basing sampling and estimation on that very MOS might not be the wisest statistical strategy. Gains in precision, if this was the goal of sampling with PPS, can also be achieved by a less stringent method known as stratification. This is not a selection method but rather a way to reorganize the frame so its utility can be maximized.

Stratified Sampling

Stratification is not a selection method, it is a way to organize the population in homogeneous, mutually exclusive groups called strata. Then, independent samples are selected from each stratum. Any of the sample designs mentioned in this chapter can be used to sample within strata,

from the simpler methods such as SRS or SYS to the more complex methods such as PPS, cluster, multi-stage, or multi-phase sampling (discussed later in this chapter). For example, with cluster sampling, it is very common to first stratify, and then draw the cluster sample. This is called stratified cluster sampling.

A population can be stratified by any variables that are available *for all units* on the frame prior to the survey being conducted. For instance, this information may simply be the address of the individual, allowing stratification by province, or there may be income data on the frame, allowing stratification by income group. Commonly used stratification variables include: age, sex, geography (e.g., province), income, revenues, household size, socioeconomic status, ethnic origin, reason for hospital admission, use of health services over previous year, etc.

There are two main reasons for stratification. The first is to make the sampling strategy more efficient than SRS or SYS. The second is to ensure adequate sample sizes for specific domains of interest for which analysis is to be performed. As a consequence, efficiently stratified samples will rarely be found to be one of the "bad" samples referred to earlier (see section on SRS).

First, for a given sample size n and estimator, e.g. a mean or a ratio, stratification may lead to lower sampling error or, conversely, for

TABLE 8.6 PPS Sampling Using the Systematic Method

Family	Auxiliary Frame Information: Family size	Cumulative Size	Range	Random Selection
1	5	5	1–5	
2	3	8	6–8	1st draw = start = 8
3	4	12	9–12	
4	2	14	13–14	
5	6	20	15–20	2nd draw = start + step = 16
6	5	25	21–25	3rd draw = 2nd draw + step = 24

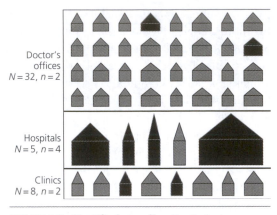

Doctor's offices
$N = 32, n = 2$

Hospitals
$N = 5, n = 4$

Clinics
$N = 8, n = 2$

FIGURE 8.5   Stratified sampling $H = 3$ strata

a given target sampling error, to a smaller sample size. Note that while both cluster sampling and stratification group units in the population, with stratified sampling, samples of individuals are drawn within each stratum, while for cluster sampling, samples of clusters are drawn and everyone in the cluster surveyed. And while stratification generally increases the precision of estimation with respect to SRS, clustering generally decreases it (since neighbouring units are usually similar).

In order to improve the statistical efficiency of a sampling strategy with respect to SRS, there must be strong homogeneity within a stratum (i.e., individuals within a stratum should be similar with respect to the variable of interest) and the strata themselves must be as different as possible from one another (with respect to the same variable of interest). Generally, this is achieved if the stratification variables are correlated with the survey variable of interest.

Stratification is particularly important in the case of *skewed populations* (i.e., when the distribution of values of a variable is not symmetric, but leans to the right or the left). For example, the sizes of the various cities and towns of a province have a skewed distribution—few large cities and

many small to moderate size towns. In such cases, a few population units can exert a large influence on estimates—if they happen to be selected in the sample, they can greatly increase the estimate, and if they are not selected, the estimate will be much lower. In other words, these units can increase the sampling variability of the estimate. Therefore, such units (e.g., Vancouver, Toronto, Halifax) should be placed in a stratum by themselves to ensure that they do not represent other, potentially much smaller, units in the population (e.g., Mission, Cornwall, Truro).

The second reason for stratification is to ensure adequate sample sizes for known domains of interest. When designing a survey, often the overall goal is to estimate a total. For example,

PRACTICAL TIP

Stratification: Are There Limits?

Strata can be defined using categorical variables (e.g., gender, province) and they can also be defined on continuous variables (e.g., age, income). When defining strata on continuous variables, experience shows that there is little precision to be gained after six strata per stratification variable.

Any number of stratification variables can be used, but each new variable, crossed or nested within the previous one(s) increases the minimum sample size required. For example, stratification on gender, province, and community size can easily lead to gender (2) × community size (4) × province (10) = 80 strata; this translates to a minimum sample of 160 individuals before accounting for nonresponse. If estimates of (even) moderate quality are required for each of those cells, then the minimum sample easily grows to 80 × 100 = 8000 individuals.

Clearly, the limit on stratification is not imagination, but rather the budget.

"How many people were unemployed last month? What were the total expenses for prescribed and over-the-counter drugs last month?"

In addition to overall totals, stratification is often required to produce reliable estimates for subgroups of the population, called domains. For example, you may wish to know how many men were unemployed and compare this with the number of women who were unemployed. Similarly, the researcher may want to know the sales last month for broad classes of drugs: e.g., pain killers, medications for the control of blood pressure or cholesterol. Creating estimates for subgroups is called domain estimation. If domain estimates are required, the ability to calculate them with a large enough sample in each domain should be incorporated into the sample design. If the information is available on the frame, the easiest way to do this is to ensure that strata exactly correspond to the domains of interest.

Stratification is also often used for operational or administrative convenience. It can enable the researcher to control the distribution of fieldwork among its field offices. For example, if data collection is conducted by province, then stratification by province is appropriate, in which case the provincial field office can recruit their portion of the sample.

Once the population has been divided into strata, the researcher needs to determine how many units should be sampled from each stratum. This step is referred to as allocation of the sample and is covered in textbooks on survey sampling (Lohr, 1999) or survey methods (Statistics Canada, 2010).

Inclusion probabilities usually vary from stratum to stratum; they depend on how the sample is allocated to each stratum. To calculate the inclusion probabilities for most sample designs, the size of the sample and the size of the population in each stratum must be considered. To illustrate, consider a population with $N = 1000$

units stratified into two groups: one stratum has $N_1 = 250$ units and the other has $N_2 = 750$ units. Suppose that SRS is used to select $n_1 = 50$ individuals from each stratum. The respective probabilities of selection are $p^1 = 50 / 250 = 1 / 3$ and $p_2 = 50 / 750 = 1 / 15$. Individuals thus have different probabilities of inclusion—an individual in the first stratum is more likely to be selected than one in the second.

In summary, stratification can improve the precision of the estimates at a very low cost, ensure that important subgroups are adequately covered, and that field procedures can be managed efficiently. However, these gains come at the price of much work to be done on the quality, completeness and "up-to-dateness" of the frame information, slightly more complex estimators (which specialized software can handle), and the illusion that stratification on administrative criteria (e.g., geography, gender, age group) will dramatically improve the precision of weakly related subject matter variables.

Multi-stage Sampling

Thus far, the discussion has centred around one-stage sample designs. *Multi-stage sampling* is the process of selecting a sample in two or more successive stages. The units selected at the first stage are called primary sampling units (PSUs) while units selected at the second stage are called second stage units (SSUs), etc. The units at each stage are different in structure and are hierarchical (for example, people live in dwellings, dwellings make up a city block, city blocks make up a city, etc.). In two-stage sampling, the SSUs are often the individual units of the population.

A common multi-stage sample design involves two-stage cluster sampling using an area frame (geographical maps) at the first stage to select regions (the PSUs) and then a systematic sample of dwellings

8.2   Health Research in Action

Is This Really Used?

Until 2006, census enumeration of rural areas took place as follows: census enumerators were given tasks consisting of a map covering a few square kilometres of land and the responsibility to "walk" all the roads, find, and list all the dwellings within the boundaries of their assigned area. Then, the enumerator would pick a random start from the first five dwellings and select every fifth dwelling for the "2B" questionnaire (the so-called long form). The remaining dwellings were given the "2A" questionnaire (the so-called short form). Looking at the "2B," this is a peculiar two-stage design with complete enumeration of clusters and systematic sampling of SSUs.

The Labour Force Survey uses a similar approach on a sample of census areas (the actual design involves various strategies of stratification, administrative frames, different approaches for urban cores, etc.).

Multi-stage sampling was also adopted by the Ontario Survey on Prevalence of Hypertension and is described in detail in Stratychuk and Dumais (2007). Basically, in a sample of cities (first stage), census areas were stratified according to the largest ethnic group they comprised, then areas were sampled (second stage) within those strata, and lists of dwellings were prepared by field enumerators; finally, a sample of dwellings (third stage) was drawn for interviews.

The late NPHS and the National Canadian Health Survey (NCHS) both drew from stratified multi-stage designs.

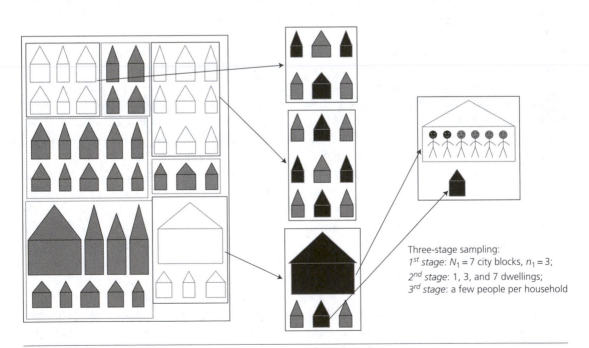

Three-stage sampling:
1st stage: $N_1 = 7$ city blocks, $n_1 = 3$;
2nd stage: 1, 3, and 7 dwellings;
3rd stage: a few people per household

FIGURE 8.6   Three-stage sampling

(the SSUs) within a region at the second stage. With the one-stage cluster sampling presented earlier, every unit within a sampled cluster is included in the sample. In two-stage sampling, only some of the units within each selected PSU are sampled.

Multi-stage sampling is commonly used with area frames to overcome the inefficiencies of one-stage cluster sampling. If the neighbouring units within a cluster are similar, then it is more statistically efficient to sample a few SSUs from many PSUs than to sample many SSUs from fewer PSUs.

Multi-stage samples can have any number of stages, but since the complexity of the design (and estimation) increases with the number of stages, designs are often restricted to two or three stages. It should be noted that the frame for the first stage is generally quite stable. For example, an area frame covering large geographical areas does not change rapidly over time.

Each stage of a multi-stage sample can be conducted using any sampling technique. Consequently, one of the chief advantages of a multi-stage sample is its flexibility. For example, within one PSU drawn at the first stage, an SRS sample may be drawn. For another PSU, there may be a measure of size that is correlated with the key survey variables, so PPS may be used within this PSU.

Finally, note that although the examples provided thus far use an area frame at the first stage this is by no means a requirement for multi-stage sampling. An example of a multi-stage sample using a different kind of frame is a travel survey conducted at an airport. The primary sampling unit could be time, days in a month, while the second stage unit could be actual travellers. For a more complex travel survey, the second stage unit could be arriving passenger planes, while the third stage unit could be actual seats on the plane.

While multi-stage sampling is usually not as statistically efficient as SRS, it can be a more efficient sampling strategy than a one-stage cluster design when clusters are homogeneous with respect to the variables of interest (i.e., a sample size reduction). Multi-stage sampling can greatly reduce the travel time and cost of personal interviews as a result of the sample being less dispersed than for other forms of sampling, such as SRS. Still, organizing field work remains a daunting task and the total sample size will only be known at the end of the collection campaign. It is important to note that the complexity of the sampling design and that of estimation of population parameters and of their sampling errors grow simultaneously.

8.3 Health Research in Action

The sample for the LFS, as the Labour Force Survey is often referred to (see Statistics Canada (2008)) is an example of a multi-stage stratified sample. The country is divided into over 1100 strata. Each stratum consists of a group of enumeration areas (EAS). EAS are geographic areas defined by the Census of Population such that the area covered can be canvassed by one census representative (they were created by keeping in mind the size of territory and the density of the population). The first stage of sampling is a stratified sample of clusters (EAS or groups of EAS) from within these strata. At the second stage, the clusters are mapped, all dwellings in them are listed, and the LFS enumerator selects a systematic sample of dwellings from each list. All persons within a selected dwelling are then interviewed for the survey.

Other Topics

In this very brief exposition, it was assumed that a sufficient sample was available or affordable, and all problems related to determining sample size were assumed "solved." Allocation of a fixed sample size to optimize sampling in strata, and conversely, determining the sample size that will ensure meeting some criterion of precision have not been discussed either. There are many more possible sampling designs, some with rather unique characteristics, some adapted to specific problems of accounting, auditing, wildlife preservation, or opinion polling. Most are beyond the scope of this book. Interested readers would benefit from consulting the references given below.

Weights and Estimation

Estimation is a technique for producing information on a population of interest based on data gathered from a sample of that population. It is intimately connected to sampling. The first step in estimation is to assign a weight to each sampled unit or to each of the responding sampled units. The *design weight* can be thought of as *the average number of units in the survey population that each sampled unit represents* and is determined by the sample design.

Whether the weights are important or not in the analysis is a matter of analytic purpose. Imagine that you conduct a study involving 20 volunteers, 10 men and 10 women, with 10 suffering from diabetes and 10 normal (control cases) to be taken equally from the men and women. In essence, you have a sample of 20 persons. While you may safely pretend that the sexes are "well represented" in your sample, and you might also be safe in saying that half the population is comprised of men. However, you would probably not dare say that half the population suffers from diabetes (an unweighted estimate).

The importance of using proper estimation weights and estimation procedures when analyzing data from complex survey designs (that is, not SRS) cannot be stressed enough.

Summary

- Sampling is a means of selecting a subset of individuals or units from a population of interest for the purpose of collecting information from those units to draw inferences about the population as a whole.

- There are two broad classes of sampling techniques: non-probability, and probability sampling. The one chosen depends primarily on whether reliable inferences are to be made about the population.

- Non-probability sampling is a method of selecting individuals or units from a population using a non-random method.

- Non-probability samples cannot be assumed to be representative of or generalizable to the population of interest. Given this, inferences about the population cannot be made when a study draws from non-probability based sampling approaches.

- Non-probability based sampling approaches include: haphazard sampling, judgement sampling, volunteer sampling, quota sampling, modified probability sampling, and network or snowball sampling.

- Non-probability sampling is often used to select individuals for focus groups and in-depth interviews.

- Probability sampling involves the selection of individuals or units from a population based on the principle of randomization or chance.

- Because probability sampling avoids selection bias by randomly selecting individuals from the population, it can be assumed that the sample is representative of or generalizable to the population of interest. Given this, inferences about the population can be made when a study draws from probability based sampling approaches.

- There are two main criteria for probability sampling:

  - Individuals or units must be randomly sampled

- Every individual unit in the population much have a non-zero probability of being included in the sample; further, the probability for inclusion must be calculable.

- Probability based sampling approaches include: Bernoulli sampling, simple random sampling, systematic sampling, probability proportionate to size sampling, cluster sampling, stratified sampling, multi-stage sampling and replicated sampling.

- Weights are intimately connected to sampling and are often used when making estimates about a population of interest.

- A weight can be thought of as the average number of individuals or units in the population that each sampled unit represents and is determined by the sampling design used.

Review Questions

1. Give two key advantages and two key disadvantages of non-probability sampling.

2. Suppose you need to survey teenagers (13- to 18-year-olds) living in the city where you live. A colleague suggests using school registers as a sampling frame. How is that a good suggestion? How is that a bad suggestion? What would you suggest as an alternative frame?

3. How do *with* replacement and *without* replacement sampling differ? Which is more precise? And why?

4. Use the systematic random sampling method explained in the section on systematic sampling (and perhaps the random number function of your calculator), draw a sample of size $n = 4$ from this population of $N = 12$ families; the number of family members and the number of seasonal colds are given for each family. With your sample, what is your estimate for the total number of colds suffered by that population?

Family	1	2	3	4	5	6	7	8	9	10	11	12
No. of members	2	3	2	4	2	2	4	5	2	1	2	3
No. of colds in family	3	3	1	6	1	1	1	3	3	0	0	2

Recommended Readings

Bethlehem, J. (2009) *Applied Survey Methods: A Statistical Perspective*. New York: John Wiley and Sons.

This is a comprehensive guide to survey methods, including both theoretical and practical applications, with an emphasis on statistical perspectives.

Droesbeke, J.-J., Fichet, B., and Tassi, P. (1987) *Les Sondages*. Paris : Economica.

This book, written in French, presents the essential features of survey methods and theory.

Kish, L. (1965) *Survey Sampling*. New York: John Wiley and Sons.

Leslie Kish's 1965 book should be compulsory reading for anyone interested in developing and conducting a sample survey. The mathematics is serious but the text is rich with lessons drawn from real-life surveys from all fields of economic and social research, and surprisingly easy to read.

Lavallée, P. and Rivest, L.–P. (2006) *Méthodes d'Enquêtes et Sondages: Pratiques Européenne et Nord-Américaine*. Paris : Dunod.

Lavallée and Rivest (2006) is a compendium of papers presented at a conference. Chapter 3 is dedicated to health—in the broader sense—surveys.

Lohr, S. (1999) *Sampling: Design and Analysis*. Pacific Grove, USA: Duxbury Press.

Sharon Lohr's book is an introductory textbook on survey sampling, aimed principally at students in mathematics departments; Levy and Lemeshow's, also an introductory textbook, concentrates on sampling human populations and covers a narrower field than Lohr's.

Statistics Canada. (2010) *Survey Methods and Practices*, Catalogue Number 12-587-X, Ottawa. Retrieved from www.statcan.gc.ca/pub/12-587-x/12-587-x2003001-eng.pdf.

Statistics Canada's 2010 textbook lies at the opposite end of the spectrum. It covers "survey methodology" rather than merely sampling and estimation theory. Management of field operations, questionnaire design, data collection and processing, data analysis, and other survey-related topics are also covered in that book. The target audience comprises graduates of social and economic studies.

Additional References

Leenen, F., Dumais, J., McInnis, N., Turton, P., Stratychuk, L., Nemeth, K., Moy Lum-Kwong, M., and Fodor, G. (2008) Results of the Ontario survey on the prevalence and control of hypertension. *Canadian Medical Association Journal*, 178, 1441–9.

Levy, P.S. and Lemeshow, S. (1999) *Sampling of Populations: Methods and Applications*. 3rd ed, New York: John Wiley and Sons.

Särndal, C.E., Swensson, B. and Wretman, J. (1992) *Model Assisted Survey Sampling*. New York: Springer-Verlag.

Statistics Canada. (2008) *Methodology of the Canadian Labour Force Survey*, Catalogue number 71-526-X, Ottawa. Retrieved from www.statcan.gc.ca/pub/71-526-x/71-526-x2007001-eng.pdf.

Stratychuk, L. and Dumais, J. (2007) Ontario survey on the prevalence of hypertension (OSPH): Practical aspects in sample allocation and collection. In *Proceedings of the Survey Methods Section*, Statistical Society of Canada Annual Meeting, June 2007.

9

Qualitative Health Research

Rachelle Hole

CHAPTER OUTLINE

Introduction

This chapter is concerned with qualitative health research. Of important note, however, the field of qualitative inquiry is very broad and diverse; there are numerous qualitative methods each with a theoretical framework, a history, and a literature. As such, this chapter can only provide an introduction to select key concepts. Readers are encouraged to consult the vast and extensive methodological literature for fuller instruction in particular qualitative methods and the respective philosophical underpinnings of different qualitative approaches. This chapter introduces the following key concepts in qualitative research:

- the nature of qualitative health research;
- some of the main approaches used when conducting qualitative health research (ethnography, institutional ethnography, autoethnography, phenomenology, grounded theory, narrative inquiry, qualitative description, and interpretive description);
- the variety of ways theory is employed in qualitative research using examples of critical theory, critical race theories, and feminist theories; and
- central aspects of qualitative research design, including:
  - sampling,
  - data collection (observational methods, interviews, focus groups, photovoice, and community mapping),
  - data analysis (constant comparison, thematic, and discourse analysis),
  - rigour, and
  - use of computer assisted qualitative data analysis software.

What is Qualitative Health Research?

Qualitative inquiry is a burgeoning field of inquiry crossing disciplinary boundaries and subject matters. It is often characterized by its naturalistic and interpretive practices (e.g., Flick, 2009; Marshall and Rossman, 2011; Mayan, 2009). **Naturalistic** refers to the practice that many qualitative approaches take place in the natural environment rather than in set-

tings such as labs where control is an important factor in research design. **Interpretive** refers to the practice of constructing meaning from data (interpreting) with the aim of explaining the phenomenon of study. And while numerous definitions exist, at its core **qualitative research** is a practice of empirical inquiry focused on naturally occurring phenomena. The qualitative researcher attempts to make sense of or interpret phenomena in terms of the meanings people bring to them (Denzin and Lincoln, 2011: 3); they seek in-depth understanding, although not exclusively, through people's own accounts. The contextual, in-depth procedures aligned with qualitative inquiry lend themselves to rich exploration and excavation of the complex social experiences and phenomena in health research. Thus, while quantitative research seeks to measure, predict, and explain relationships, qualitative research focuses on the contexts and meanings of health, illness, and disease. For example, qualitative health researchers have studied: the identification of health care needs; the patterns in health seeking behaviours/practices; the illness experience; the experiences and practices of professional care providers; the experiences of recovering from illness; the cultural practices of nursing and healthcare professions; and health care evaluation (Morse, 2011).

The unique context of health and health care in Canadian society is complex, and it has been argued that qualitative health research is a distinct form of qualitative inquiry (Morse, 2011). This chapter introduces the complex landscape of qualitative inquiry with a specific focus on health research. Thus, this chapter discusses some of the major approaches to qualitative health research and presents some of the main characteristics of qualitative research design including sampling, data collection, data analysis, evaluative criteria, and future/emerging trends in qualitative research.

Approaches to Qualitative Health Research

The practice of qualitative research is diverse, encompassing numerous approaches, theoretical orientations/perspectives, and interpretive practices (Denzin and Lincoln, 2011). Qualitative researchers use multiple systems of inquiry including, but not limited to, ethnography, phenomenology, grounded theory, narrative, qualitative description, and interpretive description. In fact, it can be argued that there exists a growing variety of qualitative approaches and methods to choose from, and it is not uncommon for researchers to develop and implement new qualitative methods (e.g., emerging virtual, online methods). For this reason, it is impossible to provide a description of every method (Mayan, 2009); as such, traditional approaches used in health research are discussed in this section.

Ethnography

Ethnography is one of the oldest qualitative approaches with its historical origins in anthropology. Its main focus is the exploration of culture and it is both a method and product: ethnographic practices direct an approach to research (a method/process) that generates/produces a description of a culture studied from the perspective of the individuals belonging to that culture (a product). The purpose is to provide a detailed, in-depth description of everyday life and practice—a "thick description" (Geertz, 1973)—grounded in the "insider's point of view" or what is called an *emic* perspective.

Cultures and subcultures are everywhere. They are found among people in specific places (e.g., a health clinic, a hospital) or among people who share a similar experience but might not know each other (e.g., street kids, graduate students, parents who have adopted) (Mayan, 2009). Thus,

ethnography implemented as a research method is diverse and can be practised in health research in a variety of ways. For example, with a focus on understanding the cultural beliefs and practices of a group, ethnography can inform our understandings of the cultural perceptions and experiences—the matrix of meaning—surrounding illness. Further, in a related way, ethnography can aid greater understanding of behaviour surrounding health and illness (Savage, 2000). "Ethnography can show, for example, how the effectiveness of therapeutic interventions can be influenced by patients' cultural practices and how ethnocentric assumptions on the part of professionals can impede effective health promotion" (Savage, 2000: 1401). Further, ethnographers also use a variety of strategies to conduct research: a researcher may use participant observation, interviews, focus groups, field notes, video, photography, art, and/or other documents when conducting research. Finally, because of diverse research interests and theoretical orientations, multiple kinds of ethnographies have developed over time—e.g., institutional ethnography, autoethnography.

Institutional ethnography

Institutional ethnography (IE) is a theorized way of seeing and knowing that orients the researcher in particular kinds of ways (Campbell and McGregor, 2002). Developed by Smith (2005), a feminist sociologist, IE begins with a particular set of theoretical assumptions: institutional practices and cultures are replete with relations of power that affect social relations; unequal social relations within institutional cultures condition/proscribe people's everyday lives; and, examining the institutional culture from the everyday experiences of people affected by these relations of power can illuminate these practices and inform transformative change. Thus, as Mayan (2009) states, "IE enables the researcher to examine organizational text and language as a form of power and to address how this externally organized text, in turn, organizes social relations" affecting people's everyday lives (p. 40).

IE has been used in health research in Canada and internationally. For example, IE health researchers have examined the ways in which the activities, knowledge, and concerns of health care recipients have been shaped by their involvement within the health care system (e.g., Lane, McCoy, Ewashen, 2010). Other studies have examined the work experiences of a professional group (e.g., nurses) within the hospital setting with a particular focus on how hospital culture shapes nurses' everyday experiences (e.g., Rankin and Campbell, 2009). Finally, with a focus on health promotion and health disparities, Sinding (2010) investigated the work that women did to receive care and treatment for cancer. For example, she looked at the work women do when responding to the costs of cancer care: (re)allocating money between competing needs, figuring out what can be done without, sustaining paid work in the face of fatigue and treatment symptoms, arranging affordable transportation for appointments and treatments, and organizing around responsibilities at home or in paid workplaces to make time for treatments. Using IE, Sinding was able to link the barriers and difficulties participants experienced to specific features of the health systems she studied demonstrating how these institutional processes could be linked to cancer disparities experienced by the women in the study.

Autoethnography

Autoethnography draws on ethnographic practices linking the personal to the cultural through a self-narrative (Mayan, 2009): the focus is on the individual's (the researcher's) experiences understood within the social and cultural context for the purposes of extending understanding (Muncey,

2010). In autoethnography the researcher becomes not only a "participant in the social context in which their experience takes place, but they are also an observer of their own story and its social location" (Muncey, 2010: 3). Although a relatively new qualitative method, health researchers are beginning to use autoethnography to further our understandings: for example, Uotinen (2011) focused on her illness experience with HIV and her experiences within an ICU; Malthouse's (2011) autoethnography focused on the family's experience of dementia and relational aspects of these experiences.

Phenomenology

Phenomenology is a research method which seeks to explore, describe, and analyze the "lived experience." The purpose of this approach is to gain "a deeper understanding of the nature or meaning of our everyday experiences" (van Manen, 2001: 9). With strong philosophical underpinnings, various schools of phenomenology (e.g., existential phenomenology, hermeneutic phenomenology, transcendental phenomenology) have emerged based on the interpretations of different philosophers' works (e.g., Husserl, Heidegger, Merleau-Ponty) (Mayan, 2009). That said, the different philosophical orientations do rest on some common grounds: primarily, phenomenology is the study of the lived experiences of persons and aims to develop rich descriptions of the essence of these experiences (Creswell, 2007). This aim requires two commitments. First, phenomenology requires "radical reflection" on the "pre-reflective" lived experience (van Manen Phenomenology Online, June 4, 2013): "the experience, not as it is *thought* to be but as it is *lived*" (Mayan, 2009: 49). Second, phenomenology requires the expression/writing of the lived experience. The researcher produces textual portrayals that resonate with the kinds of meanings that are recognized in pre-reflective experience (van Manen, 2001). With this aim in mind, the researcher identifies an object of human experience (e.g., pain). Participants are recruited who have experienced the phenomenon and the researcher works to develop a description of "'what' they experienced and 'how' they experienced it" (Creswell, 2007: 58): a description of the essence of the experience for all individuals. Important to these descriptions is the concept of **the phenomenological nod** (Munhall, 1994): the audience should experience a resonance, a ring of truth, upon hearing and/or reading the portrayal of the lived experience thus pointing to the merits and rigour of the findings. Van Manen's (2012) research studying parents' experiences carrying their neonatal baby during transfers between hospital and home environments is an example of a phenomenological study in the hospital setting. While a seemingly common practice, parents transferring their new baby between environments can give rise to unsuspected anxieties, pain, and worries in the patient (van Manen, 2012). This phenomenological study has implications for health care teams who provide care to neonatal infants and their families.

Grounded Theory

Grounded theory (GT) is a qualitative methodology for developing theory that is based in the data, where the theory is developed inductively (Glaser and Strauss, 1967). Thus, it is a method that maximizes the explanatory power of qualitative research as it aims to explain the "basic social processes" and "underlying social structures" of a phenomenon in theoretical terms (Dey, 1999; Glaser, 2001). As Strauss and Corbin (1998) state, "process and structure are inextricably linked, and unless one understands the nature of their relationship[s] . . . it is difficult to truly grasp what is going on" (p. 127).

GT shares some common practices with other qualitative methods. Similar to much qualitative research, in GT research data col-

lection and data analysis occur concurrently. However, of importance to GT research are a number of interrelated concepts: **constant comparison**, **theoretical sampling**, and **saturation** (Boeije, 2002). Together these concepts combine data collection and analytic techniques utilizing induction, deduction, and verification. There are many iterations and descriptions of different technical approaches to constant comparison (e.g., Strauss and Corbin, 1998), but at its core it is a method of comparing and contrasting data in order to establish the boundaries of categories and the relationships among the categories to develop a theory that explains the phenomenon of study. As the researcher moves through the analysis, they decide what data will be gathered next on the basis of provisionary theoretical ideas allowing for ongoing comparison of data, emerging ideas, and verification of analytic hunches (Boeije, 2002). This process continues until the process reaches saturation: saturation is reached when new cases do not bring any new information to light and can be assigned to one of the already existent categories in the growing theory (Boeije, 2002: 393). What is interesting to note is that some of the research practices are taken up in other qualitative methods, but what makes GT distinctive is the centrality of these to the inductive development of an explanatory theory. Because of the explicit commitment to theory development and explanation, qualitative health researchers have utilized GT in many ways. For example, Watt et al. (2012) used grounded theory to explain Chinese immigrant parents' perceptions about complementary and alternative medicine for their children who had been diagnosed with cancer.

Narrative Inquiry

Narrative inquiry is an interdisciplinary approach to qualitative research that manifests itself in many guises, depending on the theoretical orientation of the researcher and the research question (see Health Research in Action box 9.1). Narrative researchers base their inquiries on different theoretical and philosophical views of the stories people tell, and how they live and think. Often it is a method where stories are understood as a social process and where individuals make (construct) meaning of their experiences in the stories they tell (Hole, 2007). "Humans are constantly engaged in the activity of construing meaning (Bruner, 1990) and narrative is the primary means through which humans organize their experience and ascribe meaning to human existence" (Hole, 2007: 38). Thus, narrative inquiry aims to study life experience but places primary emphasis on narrative materials or stories (Riessman, 1993). For example, Medved and Brockmeier (2011) used a narrative-discursive methodology to explore the views of men and women about cardiovascular disease and the emotions and social relations that were involved in their personal experiences of cardiovascular disease. Their findings point to the

gendered and social influences on participants' efforts to negotiate healing and rehabilitation.

Qualitative Description

Not all qualitative research fits into traditional qualitative methods such as ethnography, grounded theory, or phenomenology. When this is the case, Sandelowski (2000) and others (e.g., Caelli, Ray, and Mill, 2003) caution researchers from inappropriately forcing their research into an ill-fitted method. Instead, the research question and purpose should direct the method; thus, if the researcher's aim is to understand a phenomenon through description, then **qualitative description** may be the most appropriate method.

The basic tenets of qualitative description are drawn from naturalistic inquiry where the phenomenon of interest is studied in its natural setting/state. Qualitative description "offer[s] a comprehensive summary of an event in the everyday terms of those events" (Sandelowski, 2000: 336). The findings represent an accurate

9.1   Health Research in Action

A Narrative Study

Ross, Epstein, Anderson, and Eady employed narrative inquiry to explore **LGBTQ** (lesbian, gay, bisexual, transgender, queer) people's experiences of adoption in Ontario after the Ontario Child and Family Services Act was amended in 2000 to permit same-sex adoption. Using a semi-structured interview guide, 43 LGBTQ individuals'/couples' narratives of successful adoption experiences were collected by the researchers. The narrative interview sought "to elicit participants' stories of adoption, beginning with their decisions to pursue adoption and closing with their experiences

since the adopted child(ren) joined their family" (p. 276). Through analysis of the narratives, the researchers found three prominent themes: negative/unsupportive experiences (e.g., experiences and expectations of homophobia/heterosexism), positive/supportive experiences (e.g., experiences with knowledgeable adoption workers), and identity-based experiences (e.g., experiences as a bisexual or trans-identified person or as an LGBTQ person living in a small town). The findings illustrate strengths and limitations of the adoption system in Ontario, Canada and provide "recommendations for further improvements to facilitate access for LGBTQ people" (p. 272).

accounting of the event and/or phenomenon studied such that others observing the event/phenomenon would agree that the description is accurate. Thus, researchers utilizing qualitative description aim for descriptive validity. This approach may be the method of choice when an unencumbered description or summary of a phenomenon is required (Sandelowski, 2000; 2010). This method of inquiry is distinct yet equal to other qualitative methods, and is frequently employed in practice disciplines such as nursing, social work, and other allied health disciplines (Sandelowski, 2000).

Interpretive Description

Similar to the re-valuing of qualitative description described above, **interpretive description** emerged in response to the growing trend of qualitative health researchers looking beyond the traditional qualitative approaches (e.g., ethnography, grounded theory, phenomenology) (Thorne, 2008). In fact, the emergence of interpretive description was a direct response to growing interest and desire for methodological approaches that explore meanings and provide explanations that yield clinical understandings and practice applications (Thorne, 2008). Thus, interpretive description aims to answer clinical questions and places the "analysis back into the context of the practice field, with all of its inherent social, political, and ideological complexities" (p. 50)—clinical application in practice and policy is paramount.

Interpretive description originally emerged within the field of nursing, and was developed with the aim to meet the disciplinary needs of nursing researchers. Given its emphasis on clinical application, interpretive description is finding ground within practice-based disciplines and health based disciplines. As Thorne et al. (2004b) assert, "interpretive description offers the qualitative health researcher an opportunity to work outside of the disciplinary confines of the more traditional methodological approaches and create a design logic that is consistent with the aims of an investigation of clinical health and illness phenomenon" (p. 18). For example, Thorne et al. (2004a) used interpretive description to study health care communication among patients living with multiple sclerosis (MS) and their health care providers. The researchers identified communications that were perceived as helpful or unhelpful to those living well with this chronic illness. From these findings, the authors drew interpretations regarding what might be considered communication competencies for individuals who care for patients with MS.

The Role of Theory in Qualitative Research Design

The role of theory in qualitative research differs from the use and role of theory in quantitative methods, and the ways and degree to which theory is explicitly engaged varies across researchers and approaches. A researcher may choose a method and not identify a particular theoretical position/perspective; she may choose a theoretical position/perspective and not select a method; and, alternatively, she may choose a theoretical position/perspective and identify a method (Mayan, 2009). For example, a researcher may engage in a descriptive qualitative study without identifying a theoretical perspective. A researcher may design a qualitative project using Foucauldian analysis rooted in the theoretical works of Michel Foucault (e.g., Foucault, 1973). Or, a researcher may choose to engage in a feminist ethnography where she explicitly identifies a qualitative method and her theoretical perspective. This choice would focus her study on culture and society (ethnography) while employing feminist theory; for example, she would include a gender-based analysis in her research. Thus, researchers are cautioned to be thoughtful about the role of theory in their research and its influence in qualitative research design. As Mayan (2009) aptly captures:

> Method is important, yet we cannot become so preoccupied with it that we disregard ontology, epistemology, theoretical positions/perspectives, or the ideas of great thinkers, which direct us and our research in more profound ways than we can ever fully know. Similarly, theoretical position is important, but not to the point where we can dismiss well-established methods with their accompanying strategies, procedures, and protocols. Regardless, what is fundamental is making thoughtful, wise decisions through the course of the research so that at the end you will have something to conclude or "problematize" about the data you collected (p. 32).

Increasingly, qualitative scholars acknowledge the ever-present influence of theory, whether explicitly named or not. As the history of qualitative research has unfolded, a critical, interpretive turn has taken place in qualitative inquiry which now acknowledges the influence of social theory (e.g., critical theory, feminist theories, poststructural theories) in qualitative practices. As such, there is a growing practice of theoretically informed qualitative studies. The following section will briefly discuss three examples of theoretical perspectives that might influence and inform a qualitative study: critical theory, critical race theory, and feminist theories; other perspectives include poststructural approaches, (e.g., see Cheek, 2000), queer theory (e.g., see Browne and Nash, 2010) and cultural studies (Giardina and Newman, 2011).

Critical theory, an overarching umbrella term that encompasses numerous theories, is concerned with power and how power produces structural inequalities in society. Thus, research informed by critical theories aims to critique and transform existing social relations that produce such inequalities; restitution and transforma-

tion become the research goals (Denzin and Lincoln, 2011). Thus, as Denzin and Lincoln explain, "research [employing critical theory] is driven by the study of social structures, freedom and oppression, and power and control. Researchers believe that the knowledge that is produced can change existing oppressive structures and remove oppression through empowerment" (p. 103). Because of this, critical theory (e.g., Friere, 1970; 2007) often informs participatory action research and also may inform qualitative health research studies. For example, drawing on a qualitative methodology framed by critical theory, Greenspan et al. (2011) studied self-directed harm reduction strategies among drug using ethno-racially diverse gay and bisexual men. They found that drug users' awareness of possible harm and a personal investment in harm reduction have direct implications for community-based and public health organizations' practice in promoting and strengthening harm reduction among gay and bisexual men from ethno-racially diverse backgrounds. Health Research in Action box 9.2 gives an example of a critical ethnography.

Critical race theory is linked to critical theory generally and to postcolonial theory. As such, critical race theorists focus on issues of racism, racial oppression, and racial discrimination as the core focus of their analysis (Marshall and Rossman, 2011). For example, Dhand (2009), employing a critical race theoretical perspective, investigated and analyzed the legal barriers faced by ethno-racial psychiatric consumer/survivors in Ontario, Canada.

Feminist research is informed by many diverse feminist theories—e.g., standpoint theorists, transnational perspectives, poststructural perspectives. In spite of these differences, feminist research is generally committed to a gender-based analysis of social relations and dedicated to research that challenges unequal social relations while promoting social change

9.2   Health Research in Action

A Critical Ethnography

DeForge, Wyk, Hall, and Salmoni (2011) condu-cted a critical ethnography in an urban long-term care home exploring the (un)intended consequences of health care policy that regulates provision of care through standardization. Informed by critical theory, critical ethnography "can be conceptualized as alternative or disruptive in that it is poised as openly ideological and interested in identifying how oppressive situations are (re)produced and reified within the cultures they study" (p. 416). The researchers collected data related to staff perceptions of the (un)met care needs of residents living in long-term care homes and sought to better understand the role that socio-political/structural conditions play in reshaping staff relationships with residents. The findings reveal how policy-driven mechanisms aimed at standardization of practice (re)produced conditions that resulted in care staff being afraid and unable to care.

(Ramazanoglu and Holland, 2007). And, because of the social diversity of gender rela-tions—gender, sexuality, race, religion, abilities, sexualities are fluid and interlocking—feminist researchers increasingly advocate for an intersec-tional analysis when researching gender relations (Marshall and Rossman, 2011). Thus, feminist researchers politicize their theoretical orien-tations and employ them to direct all aspects of their research practices from the questions asked, design, and ethical practice, to dissemina-tion activities (e.g., how will the research be used to effect social change?) Numerous examples of feminist researchers conducting qualitative health research exist. For example, using fem-inist post-structuralist perspectives, Shea and Beausoleil (2012) examined how 15 Canadian immigrant youths' ideas of health and fitness were influenced by cultural and institutional discourses. Donnelly et al. (2011) used femin-ist qualitative research to explore the challen-ges influencing immigrant and refugee women's mental health. And, Van Herk, Smith, and Andrew (2011) explored nurses' experiences of privilege and oppression in health care settings utilizing a feminist intersectional approach.

Summary

Choosing a method is a central task of designing a qualitative research study. It involves a choice about how the researcher best believes the phe-nomenon can be revealed, problematized, or described. Fundamentally, the aim of the study and the research question directs the qualita-tive approach taken and the overall design. For example, a researcher interested in emergency room practices might approach this topic using different qualitative methods depending on their aim. If they were interested in understanding how the cultural practices of the emergency department shape patient experiences, they would most likely use a form of ethnography. Another researcher may want to understand the lived experiences of emergency patients waiting for admission in a hospital where a shortage of beds is a mitigating factor. In such a case, phenomenology would be a possible research approach. A researcher inter-ested in explaining the social processes at work influencing family members' decisions to access the emergency ward upon experiencing chest pains might turn to grounded theory. Another researcher interested in how patients make meaning of their experiences of accessing the emergency department during an acute illness episode might turn to narrative methods as a research approach. Though not exhaustive, the above examples point to the diversity of approaches possible when considering qualitative methods in health research. Thus, the research question posed directs the qualitative approach taken and the overall design; however, it is important to note that the theoretical orientation of the researcher has profound impact. Readers are encouraged to explore the vast methodological literature for further instruction regarding the specific qualitative methods.

Research Design—The "How" of the Study

Research design in qualitative research is a non-linear process; it is emergent and the stages are interdependent informing one another in a non-linear manner (Flick, 2009). In fact, design decisions can and usually should be revisited and reconsidered throughout the project (Richards, 2009): the researcher continues to make design decisions and revisions based on what they are learning and what additional data is needed in order to answer the research question. That said, "you need to start with a plan" (Richards, 2009: 14), and this plan must answer the following three questions: (1) What are you asking (the research question)? (2) How are you asking it (the method and/or theoretical position/perspective)? (3) What data will you need in order to provide a good answer? The following section provides an introduction to design issues in qualitative research, including sampling, creating data (data collection), data analysis, criteria for evaluating the quality of the research, and strategies for sharing findings (knowledge translation).

Sampling

As with other elements of research design, issues of sampling occur throughout the stages of the research and sampling decisions are influenced by the qualitative approach/method being utilized. In qualitative designs, participants are selected based on their relevance to the research topic/question, the conceptual framework, and the method being employed. Thus, rather than informed by a commitment to statistical representation, sampling decisions are driven by selecting participants or relevant material that promises the greatest insights regarding the phenomenon of interest (Flick, 2009). "Sampling proceeds according to the relevance of cases instead of their representativeness" (p. 128), and sample composition often evolves in the course of the research as the researcher makes decisions on sample size and who else (or what else) needs to be included in the sample. Based on this, there are a number of different sampling procedures. Four common sampling protocols are (Morse and Richards, 2002):

- Purposeful sampling—the researcher selects the best participants based on the quality of their insights about and willingness to reflect upon the phenomenon of interest: "who (or what data) can give me the most and the best information about my topic?"
- Snowball (or chain) sampling—participants in the study are asked to invite others who meet the sampling criteria to contact the researcher if they are interested in participating.
- Convenience sampling—participants are selected based on their availability to participate.
- Theoretical sampling—participants are selected based on the researcher's emerging theoretical framework; participants are selected to elaborate and refine the emerging categories and the theory. This strategy is a core aspect of grounded theory.

What sample size is needed in a qualitative study?

Frequently, students and new qualitative researchers question the sample size needed in a qualitative study. Richards replies, "The only safe answer is, 'when I have the data needed to answer my research question and all subsequent pertinent questions arising from the data'" (Richards, 2009: 19). That said, the question of sample size is a complex one. Some useful criteria include (Morse, 2000):

- quality of the data;
- scope of the study;
- nature of the topic;
- amount of useful information from each participant (or source);
- number of interviews per participant (some designs propose to interview participants more than once); and
- qualitative method and study design.

In addition, a traditional criterion informing the decision to stop sampling is referred to as saturation. Saturation occurs when each category is rich and thick, and no new information is coming to light: "[it] provides the researcher with certainty and confidence that the analysis is strong and the conclusions will be right" (Morse and Richards, 2002: 174).

Creating Data

Related to sampling decisions (i.e., who and/or what you need in order to answer your question), finding and collecting data is integral to the research design. Qualitative data collection is a flexible approach that aims to understand a complex situation in context (Richards, 2009). Qualitative data are found in a variety of empirical sources; these may be people, policy documents, maps, movement, image, text, sound, etc. However, qualitative data often involve human participants and the data can be created in a variety of ways: in-depth interviews, semi-structured interviews, participant observation, photovoice, videography, etc. What is unique to qualitative data collection is the concept that the researcher is the research instrument: the researcher actively makes decisions throughout the research as to what to select and interpret based on the research topic or question. Making data is a collaborative, ongoing, and complex process, occurring in a dynamic environment (Richards and Morse, 2013: 119). Thus, "[m]aking data is not a passive process; rather, it is an active, cognitive process that requires tremendous investment on the part of the researcher and requires extraordinary concentration" (p. 122). Some of the more prominent methods of "creating" data are presented in the following section. Of note, when choosing among the numerous data collection strategies, the researcher must be sure to select strategies that will produce data that are sufficiently rich, complex, and contextual to address the research question and to support the required analysis (Richards and Morse, 2013).

Observation and participant observation

Observational methods of data collection are often used in conjunction with other methods of data collection; researchers enter the research site (the field) and observe what is happening around them (e.g., physical surroundings, behaviours of people present, interactions among people) while recording their observations and interpretations, most frequently, in the form of field notes. That said, "observing is a special skill" (Creswell, 2007: 134) and involves careful forethought regarding an observational protocol that ensures the data are collected systematically and that they are valuable as they relate to addressing the research question. For example, the researcher needs to carefully think about what kind of information should be collected and how it should be described: the researcher should consider how descriptive notes are made and how analytic notes are documented. Creswell (2007) describes observational data collection as a series of steps that requires the researcher to: select a site and gain permission to access the site (when necessary); determine who or what is the focus of observation including when and for how long; consider the role of the observer (will they participate actively or be a complete observer); develop observational protocols for documenting notes in the field; and plan for how to enter and leave the site (e.g., will someone introduce you?) While these steps provide a useful starting point, they highlight that "there are myriad ways of watching and listening" (Morse and Richards, 2002: 96).

The variety of approaches to observational methods is captured explicitly in the literature relating to participant observation. As the name aptly portrays, the researcher can be both a participant in the field and/or an observer. Thus, terms such as the complete observer, the observer as participant, the participant as observer, and the complete participant are the four most frequently identified types of participant observation (Mayan, 2009). These labels aim to capture the degree to which the researcher is actively (or not) participating in the research setting, or the degree of involvement on the part of the researcher. For example, the emphasis for the observer as participant is on the researcher's role as an observer (as separate from the group) whereas for the participant observer, the researcher is more involved as a participant in the group while still maintaining a focus on observing the group dynamics and cultural processes; in the case of the complete participant, the researcher is a fully involved participant in the group that they are studying. While listed as discrete categories (or ways of participating in the field), in practice the type of participation can vary depending on the length of time spent in the setting, the purpose of the observation, and the unfolding nature of the observation as it relates to the research question (Mayan, 2009). For example, if the researcher is engaged in participant observation, they must continually assess the quality of the data they are collecting and determine what additional data may be required to answer the research question.

Observational techniques and participant observation have been used frequently in qualitative health research. Participant observation is often employed for the purpose of learning about the often unexamined practices and beliefs, taken for granted in a particular setting (Morse and Richards, 2002). Lee and Bell (2011) used participant observation of family group meetings to study the impact of cancer on family relationships among Chinese patients. Based on their findings, the researchers highlight the need for practitioners to focus on the entire family when designing interventions to help patients cope with cancer. Adams et al. (2010) used multiple methods of data collection (observational techniques, interviews, and analysis of textual and visual data) to elicit children's views about the hospital environment at the Hospital for Sick Children in Toronto. These researchers' findings "begin to address the significant gap in understanding the relationship between the perceptions of children and the settings where their healthcare occurs" (p. 658).

Interviewing

As mentioned previously, qualitative data can take many forms. One very common form is the interview. "Qualitative interviewing is a kind of guided conversation in which the researcher carefully listens 'so as to hear the meaning' of what is being conveyed" (Warren, 2002: 85). However, as Richards and Morse (2013) warn, "[b]eware of the assumption that any good listener can interview" (p. 127). Although there are a variety of interview strategies (e.g., the narrative interview), there are three main interview designs discussed in the literature: the structured interview, the semi-structured or focused interview, and the unstructured or open-ended interview.

A **structured interview** follows a sequence of exactly the same questions that are asked in exactly the same order. The questions may include both open and closed-ended questions. Close-ended questions elicit short or single-word answers such as yes/no answers. Open-ended questions are designed to encourage reflection and discussion about the topic frequently starting with "what," "how," "why," and "describe." The predetermined questions and wording in structured interviews reduces the risk that interviewers may introduce their own biases and offers consistency across interviews. This can be particularly valuable in research involving multiple interviewers. However, the highly structured nature of the interview leaves little freedom to draw fully on the participants' knowledge through an exploration of their responses or through encouragement of the participant to expand on their responses through the use of probes. Further, while being more expensive and time-consuming, there are few advantages to a structured interview administered by an interviewer over a mailed survey.

Semi-structured interviews include specific predetermined items/questions, but latitude is given to interviewers to explore participant responses pertaining to the research questions of interest. The questions centre on selected topics and hypotheses, often from the researcher's knowledge of the literature, but the interviews are not entirely predetermined.

The **unstructured/open-ended interview** is the most common type of qualitative interview. Although frequently researchers plan an interview guide consisting of planned topics for exploration, the aim of the unstructured interview is to allow the participant the opportunity to tell their story with minimal interruption from the interviewer (Richards and Morse, 2013). Skill is required to guide the research conversation without interrupting or skewing the participant's story (Richards and Morse, 2013), thus once the participant has told their story, the interviewer is given the freedom to explore any other relevant avenues that may have emerged during the interview. The interviewer uses probes to seek in-depth clarification of the participant's experiences and is encouraged to follow analytic hunches based on the goals of the research. Thus, in an unstructured/open-ended interview, participants should be given as much latitude as possible to provide their perspectives on the research topic.

When deciding among the different interview protocols, several factors may inform the researcher's decisions. First, the researcher must consider the degree of detail required to fully answer the research question. An unstructured/open-ended interview provides the most opportunity to elicit in-depth detail; however, the interviewer needs to be trained and well-prepared in order to take advantage of the benefits of the unstructured interview. The researcher should consider the extent to which the interviewers are trained, prepared, and able to elicit data on their own from the research participants. Further, in deciding the kind of interview process, it is important to be cognizant of how much is already known about the topic and what is to be learned through the current project in light of the existing knowledge. Finally, the researcher might take into consideration the extent to which simplicity in data analysis (coding) is a determining factor; the more unstructured the gathered data (e.g., open-ended interviews), the more complex the analytic process.

A number of practical issues also need to be considered. The researcher should consider how the interview will be recorded: Will it be digitally recorded? Is the interviewer familiar with the recording device? Will the interviewer keep field notes? In addition, the researcher should keep in mind process issues: Will the interview guide be pilot tested? In what order should the questions be asked? Are there issues with language that need to be considered when developing the interview questions? Another issue pertains to data management: Where will the recordings be kept? Where will the field notes and/or demographic information be stored? Finally, will the researcher be providing an honorarium for the participants? What form will the honorarium be in (cash, a gift card, a gift)? What if the participant withdraws from the interview/study? What will happen with respect to the honorarium and what will happen with the participant's data? As one can see, decisions about interview protocol require careful consideration. There are direct implications relating to ethical issues (e.g., voluntary withdrawal from the research), to the quality of the data, and to the validity of the research findings. As Morse and Richards (2002) assert, "it is the nature of the questions asked and the attention that the researcher gives to the par-

ticipants and to detail that determine the quality of the data collected" (p. 89).

Focus groups

Focus groups are the most common type of group interview used in qualitative research (Mayan, 2009). As the name suggests, it is a focused interview involving more than two participants, and most often consisting of six to ten participants (Mayan, 2009). It is "a research technique that collects data through group interaction on a topic determined by the researcher" (Morgan, 2002: 130). Given the obvious presence of group dynamics and interaction, group interaction is a necessary focal point of both data generation and data analysis (Mayan, 2009); the purpose of a focus group is to better understand how people think or feel about the designated topic (Krueger and Casey, 2000) and to analyze this while considering the context of the group interaction. Thus, the researcher must be vigilant

---

PRACTICAL TIP

As you prepare your interview questions, it important to evaluate them before being used in an interview situation. Here are some sample questions to consider when evaluating each of your interview questions (adapted from Flick, 2009: 167).

1. Why did you ask this specific question?
    a. What is the link to the research question?
    b. What is its theoretical relevance?
2. Why did you formulate the question in this way and not differently?
    a. Is the question easy to understand?
    b. Does the question invite dialogue? (e.g., open ended?)
3. Why did you position this question (or block of questions) at this specific place in the interview guide?
    a. How does it fit into the rough (or detailed) structure of the interview guide?
    b. What is the distribution of questions across the interview guide?
    c. What is the relationship between single questions?

in examining how the participants operate as a group (Mayan, 2009).

Focus groups are described as a flexible data gathering technique and are thought to be time and cost efficient (e.g., Creswell, 2003). In addition, focus groups can generate more ideas and issues about a topic than an individual conversation might because participants can build on each other's ideas and shared experiences. Thus, a qualitative researcher may decide to use focus groups if they are looking for a range of ideas that people have about a topic and they want the ideas to emerge in the context of a group. Other reasons why researchers may use focus groups include: pilot testing ideas, obtaining information to design a larger quantitative study (e.g., finding appropriate language to use in an instrument), or seeking insight into quantitative data already obtained (Morgan, 2002). Finally, focus groups may also be used as a research strategy in participatory action research as a tool to engage in decision making and consensus seeking (Morgan, 2002).

There are potential limitations with focus groups. Some participants may be uncomfortable expressing their views or describing their experiences in a group setting, particularly for more sensitive topics; the researcher will spend less time overall with the total number of participants than when conducting individual interviews; group influences can distort individual opinion; and, there are limits to confidentiality—i.e., members of the group may disclose aspects of the group process outside of the group (Creswell, 2007).

Visual Methods—Photovoice, Community Mapping

Visual methods are a growing dimension to a rapidly expanding repertoire of qualitative research techniques. Photovoice is one such visual method that is growing in popularity. Utilizing cameras, participants are asked to take pictures relating to the research question. This process provides individuals with the opportunity to identify, reflect, and convey their everyday lives and challenges through photographs that are culturally and contextually relevant. The photographs can be conceived of as data themselves and/or they can be data in addition to a more traditional form of data collection strategy. For example, Oliffe and Bottorff (2007) used photovoice in their study examining men's experiences of prostate cancer. Not only were the pictures data, but they were used during an interview to elicit/explore the participants' stories and meanings associated with the photographs.

Photovoice is often conceived as a strategy of value to participatory action research (PAR) (Wang and Burris, 1994). PAR is a research approach that places collaboration with community partners at its core. The explicit aim of PAR is social change that benefits the community. In a PAR project, photography and stories may provide access to the all too silent themes associated with the lives of under-represented individuals, families, and communities. "Through photography, participants act as recorders of their own experience and are in control of how they represent themselves and their lives" (Mayan, 2009: 44). There are three main goals of photovoice PAR according to Wang and Burris (1994): to empower people to document the strengths and weaknesses of their community by photographing daily life; to facilitate group communication and dialogue in the identification of important community issues; and, to appeal to policymakers and other people of influence in the interest of change. Thus, in a PAR framework, photovoice is conceptualized as a multi-step process that combines equal parts photography, research, group process, storytelling, social action, and development of awareness of personal and community issues (see Health Research in Action box 9.3).

9.3   Health Research in Action

Health Research Using Photovoice

Oliffe and Bottorff (2007) used photovoice in a study aimed at understanding 19 men's experiences of surviving prostate cancer. The men were asked "to imagine that they were being paid to mount a photographic exhibition entitled *Living with My Prostate Cancer*, an exhibition that would show prostate cancer from their unique perspective" (p. 850). Through photo elicitation the researchers found that the process of deciding what pictures to take promoted planning, introspection, and reflection in the men about their experiences of prostate cancer, and the photos (and photo elicitation process) contributed depth in description and detail in subsequent interviews with the participants. In addition to the contribution of photos to the interview process, the pictures also provided a rich source of data and were highly valuable in knowledge translation activities (presentation of the findings). They offered a visual representation that showed rather than told about the participants' experiences.

Community mapping is another qualitative technique that can contribute to PAR practices. In community mapping, community members pool their knowledge and experiences of their community, and represent this knowledge and these experiences in a graphic form, or map (Mayan, 2009). Community members identify important aspects of community life. For example, these may include physical, cultural, and social dimensions of the community. As with all participatory approaches, it is as much about the process of engaging the community as it is about the product—the map (Mayan, 2009: 47).

All strategies of data collection are complex and involve a variety of processes as such data "inevitably vary in quality" (Richards and Morse, 2013: 122). In spite of the wide range of techniques for making data, Richards and Morse describe some general principles as to what constitutes good data:

- Records are rich, thick, and dense, offering enough detail to allow someone to comprehend the situation or understand the setting without asking additional questions.

- The data are relevant and focused, but not focused so tightly that the context is omitted from or restricted within the description.
- Good data are developed in careful recognition of participants' perspectives. (p. 122–3)

Finally, of utmost importance when deciding what kind of data to generate is the research topic and/or question. Each of the above strategies for making data has extensive literature detailing instructions of how to go about creating quality data.

Data Analysis

Data analysis and data collection are directly linked and interdependent. In fact, "the quality of the analysis is dependent on the quality of [the researcher's] data records and [her/his] skills in working up from them to ideas and explanations" (Richards, 2009: 73). Thus, data collection and data analysis are frequently carried out concurrently with each informing the other as the project unfolds.

Similar to other aspects of qualitative inquiry, there are many approaches to data analysis: i.e., thematic analysis, narrative analysis, discourse analysis, conversational analysis, and constant comparison. That said, there are some commonalities across the varied approaches. Starks and Brown Trinidad (2007) describe qualitative data analysis as an iterative inductive process of decontextualization and recontextualization:

> During decontextualization the analyst separates data from the original context of individual cases and assigns codes to units of meaning in the texts. In recontextualization he or she examines the codes for patterns and reintegrates, organizes, and reduces the data around central themes and relationships drawn from across all the cases and narratives (p. 1375).

Thus, data analysis is a process of sorting, categorizing, grouping, and regrouping data into chunks that are meaningful (Rossman and Rallis, 2003). The process is not linear and data are grouped and regrouped several times; each grouping allows the researcher to see different aspects of the data, enriching understanding and insight into the phenomenon of interest (Rossman and Rallis,

2003). The researcher is not a passive agent in the process of analysis; they always play an active role "in identifying patterns/themes, selecting which are of interest, and reporting them to the readers" (Braun and Clarke, 2006). Below, three prominent data analysis methods used in qualitative research are described followed by a brief discussion of the importance of transcription.

The **constant comparative** method is the core of grounded theory analysis. It involves: (1) open coding where the researcher examines, compares, conceptualizes, and categorizes the data; (2) axial coding where the researcher reassembles the data into groups based on relationships and patterns within and among the categories identified; and (3) selective coding where the researcher identifies and describes the central phenomenon, or "core category" (Starks and Brown Trinidad, 2007). Relationships between conceptualized categories are tested through a comparison and contrast of emerging analytic ideas, the data, and new data being collected—a constant comparison—with

---

PRACTICAL TIP

Qualitative Data Analysis Tips

1. Practise good data management skills. Qualitative data software is very useful for data management.
2. Keep your research question(s) in the foreground as well as the interview questions, topics, and probes.
3. Continue to ask analytic questions such as, "What does she mean by that?," "How does this relate to other findings?"
4. Document all the time. Note hunches, thoughts, impressions, write descriptive and analytic memos. Keep an audit trail of research decisions and the rationale for these decisions.
5. Read and re-read what the literature says and check your data: do your participants say similar things and/or different things?
6. Be creative in the use of metaphors, images, and conceptual maps. Think about how you might characterize what you are learning: What images does it evoke?

(Adapted from Rossman and Rallis, 2003)

the aim of developing an explanatory theory of the phenomenon of interest (Boeije, 2002). Data analysis and data collection occur concurrently, and ideally, each interview is analyzed prior to proceeding to the next interview. Theoretical sampling (choosing subsequent participants based on emerging findings) and negative case sampling (seeking examples where the findings do not fit) are integral to constant comparative analysis as these strategies help to refine the developing theory and aid in determining the limits of the theory (e.g., when don't these findings apply in the case of negative case sampling).

Thematic analysis "is a method for identifying, analysing and reporting patterns (themes) within data" (Braun and Clarke, 2006: 79). A theme captures something important pertaining to the research question and represents a pattern within the data set; this does not mean that the theme must be prevalent across the entire data set, but ideally there will be a number of instances of a theme across the data. Thus, the question of prevalence of a theme cannot be reduced to quantifiable measures; rather it is dependent upon whether it captures something of relevance to the overall research question(s) (Braun and Clarke, 2006).

Discourse analysis is an analytic framework that examines how language "both shapes and reflects dynamic cultural, social, and political practices (Starks and Brown Trinidad, 2007: 1374) where "the researcher aims to understand how people use language to create and enact identities and activities" (p. 1373). The analysis focuses on what discourses are used and how they shape identities, activities, and relationships. Thus, the researcher focuses on how understanding is produced through the words, images, and ideas used by participants, and how meaning is shaped through language.

Finally, an often overlooked component of data analysis is the process of **transcription**. If data are digitally recorded and/or video recorded,

transcription is a necessary step in the process of interpretation (Flick, 2009). As Flick notes, "the documentation of data is not only a technical step in the research process. It also has an influence on the quality of the data you can use for interpretations" (p. 293). As such, it is important to explicitly plan in advance the transcription decisions and protocols.

Quality and Rigour

The issue of validity in qualitative research has garnered much debate. However, it is generally agreed that quantitative criteria cannot be used when evaluating the quality and rigour of qualitative research (Tobin and Begley, 2003). This, however, does not mean that qualitative researchers do not have to be accountable to the quality and rigour of their research. "[R]igour is the means by which we demonstrate the integrity and competence . . . a way of demonstrating the legitimacy of the research process" (p. 390). Controversy surrounding how to address rigour in qualitative research continues with numerous stances being advanced (see Chapter 10 of Creswell, 2007; and Tobin and Begley, 2003). In 1981, Guba argued that the **trustworthiness** of qualitative research could be evaluated using the concepts of credibility, transferability, dependability, and confirmability. These four constructs replaced traditional criteria used in quantitative research: credibility in preference to internal validity; transferability in preference to external validity/generalizability; dependability in preference to reliability; and confirmability in preference to objectivity. This approach to the issue of validity is still used but is fervently contested and debated by many qualitative researchers including Lincoln, Lynham and Guba (2011) (other examples include: Denzin and Lincoln, 2011; Lather, 1993; Lincoln, 1995; Polkinghorne, 2007; Richardson, 2000). Despite these debates,

PRACTICAL TIP

Tips for Transcription Protocol

- If analyzing the data manually (without computer assisted qualitative data analysis software), set up a three-column format. The left/first column will be used to record any analytic notes/thoughts/questions. In the middle column, type the interview dialogue. The right column will be used for analysis (open coding, thematic analysis, discourse analysis/analytic readings). Number each line continuously and insert page numbers.

- Begin the interview transcript by typing all relevant identifying information (e.g., name of interviewer and transcriber).

- Assign pseudonyms and then introduce each speaker with the pseudonym or identification code (e.g., JANE SMITH, PRINCIPAL 17).

- Start a new line each time the speaker changes.

- Type everything as you hear it. Do not correct grammar or pronunciation (e.g., if a word is mispronounced, spell it phonetically to indicate that).

- Determine what transcription conventions you will use to explain interruptions, pauses, or unclear words e.g., [laughing], [PR17 stopped tape so that she could answer the phone], [unclear phrase].

- Indicate non-word sounds and pauses ("umm," "huh-huh," "gee") if it helps convey the speech patterns and thinking of the speaker. For example, "phew" often indicates relief.

what is clear is that qualitative researchers need to plan how they are going to address issues of rigour and legitimation and commit to explicating these practices in the reports drawn from their findings. Therefore, after a researcher has determined the criteria by which they want the research to be evaluated, they must describe the strategies used to meet these criteria. Several strategies that may be used include:

- keeping an audit trail—documenting and recording all research decisions and the rationale for these decisions;
- reflexivity—the practice of examining one's place, biography, self, and others to understand how they shape the analytic exercise (Macbeth, 2001).

- prolonged engagement—spending extended time in the field to learn or understand the phenomenon of interest;
- member checking—the activity of exploring one's findings with participants. This can be done after the interview has been analyzed, by sharing findings with participants to obtain their input and feedback;
- triangulation—a means of checking the integrity of the inferences one draws involving the use of "multiple data sources, multiple investigators, multiple theoretical perspectives, and/or multiple methods" (Schwandt, 2007: 298); and/or,
- peer debriefing—the process of checking one's interpretations and analytic findings with a colleague or peer.

Computer Assisted Qualitative Data Analysis Software

Increasingly, qualitative researchers are using qualitative data analysis software to assist with research. It is important for researchers to note, however, that "software . . . cannot do the analysis for you, not in the same sense in which a statistical package such as SPSS or SAS can do, say multiple regressions" (Weitzman, as cited in Marshall and Rossman, 2011: 181). The researcher must do the analytic thinking including the coding and theorizing. Further, computer programs do not reduce bias or increase reliability. And, finally software does not improve the quality of the analysis on its own. The researcher is the instrument guiding the analytic process. Qualitative software, however, does have strategic benefits. As the website *Online QDA* (n.d.) states, quali-

tative software can help to structure work and provide data management and organization, an essential aspect of qualitative research design. In addition, qualitative software allows one to interact closely with the data where the software facilitates the researcher(s)' ability to explore the data, to code and retrieve sections of text, to search and interrogate the created database (i.e., by searching for relationships between codes), to create memos, comments, and annotations about the data and the analytic process. Further, the software has abilities related to research output (i.e., generating reports, conceptual models). As such, it is valuable for researchers to assess the advantages and disadvantages of using qualitative software, and it is important for researchers to be familiar with the strengths and weaknesses of the various qualitative software packages as this is an incredible burgeoning industry.

Summary

- Qualitative research is a complex and intentional craft whose specialists use diverse methods with rich theoretical traditions, histories, and literatures. In-depth attention to these vast literatures is beyond the scope of this chapter. It is hoped that readers are motivated to engage the diverse resources available to further expand their understanding and appreciation of qualitative health research.

- Qualitative research is frequently characterized as naturalistic, interpretive, and inductive, seeking in-depth understanding of phenomena in terms of the meanings people bring to them.

- There are many approaches to qualitative health research:

  - Ethnography focuses on the exploration of culture and generates a thick description from the perspective of the individuals

    belonging to that culture. Phenomenology aims to explore, describe, and analyze the essence of the *lived experience*.

  - Grounded theory aims to develop an explanatory theory of the phenomenon of interest with the goal of explaining the basic social processes and underlying social structure. Narrative inquiry is focused on narrative materials or stories and how people use narratives in their day-to-day lives to make meaning of their experiences.

  - Qualitative description aims to depict a phenomenon through a comprehensive summary.

  - Interpretive description emphasizes research that produces meanings and explanations that yield clinical understandings and practical applications.

- Theory may play multiple roles in qualitative research. A researcher may adopt a particular method and not name a theory, a researcher may adopt a method and explicitly name a theoretical perspective, or a researcher may develop a methodology specifically located within a theoretical orientation.

- When engaging in qualitative research, the research question and the method (e.g., ethnography or a theoretically informed methodology) are paramount in informing practical issues and design decisions.

- Qualitative research design is emergent and non-linear where the study plan informs design but the researcher must re-visit design decisions as the study unfolds. Sampling, data collection, and data analysis are intricately tied to one another.

Review Questions

1. The emergent and non-linear qualities of qualitative research have been presented in this chapter. What implications do these qualities have for qualitative research design (e.g., sampling, data collection, and data analysis)?

2. What kinds of roles does theory play in qualitative research?

3. Interpretive description emerged within nursing. What is its particular focus and what are the implications for health research?

4. If you were conducting a qualitative study, how might you determine the sample size for your project?

5. What practical issues need to be considered when conducting qualitative interviews?

Recommended Readings and Websites

Mayan, M. (2009) *Essentials of Qualitative Inquiry.* Walnut Creek, CA: Left Coast Press.

Maria Mayan offers a book that is particularly useful to newcomers to qualitative inquiry. It is very accessible and she covers the important, "essential" elements of qualitative research including the relationship between theory and qualitative research design.

Richards, L., and Morse, J. (2013) *Read Me First for a User's Guide to Qualitative Methods.* 3rd ed. Thousand Oaks, CA: Sage Publications Inc.

This work offers a map to researchers relating to methodological choices. Although an introductory text, the authors offer clear practical discussions about qualitative techniques; a useful text to assist in designing a qualitative study that ensures methodological congruence.

Richards, L. (2009) *Handling Qualitative Data: A Practical Guide.* Thousand Oaks, CA: Sage Publications.

This is an excellent resource directly dealing with qualitative data analysis. As one of the creators of NVivo[qsr] the book nicely complements computer assisted data analysis software.

Online QDA: Learning qualitative data analysis on the web. Retrieved from http://onlineqda.hud.ac.uk/index.php.

This website focuses on providing resources that teach an array of qualitative data analysis strategies/techniques. Materials include tutorials along with audio and video materials.

International Institute for Qualitative Methodology. Retrieved from www.iiqm.ualberta.ca/.

The IIQM offers a wide variety of training and networking opportunities through annual conferences (e.g., Qualitative Health Research, Advances in Qualitative Methods), courses, and workshops. It is based at the University of Alberta.

The CAQDAS Networking Project: Computer Assisted Qualitative Data Analysis Software. Retrieved from www.surrey.ac.uk/sociology/research/researchcentres/caqdas/resources/index.htm.

This website offers information on computer assisted qualitative data analysis software.

References

Adams, A., Theodore, D., Goldenberg, E., McLaren, C., and McKeever, P. (2010) *Social Science and Medicine*, 70(5), 658–67.

Boeije, H. (2002) A purposeful approach to the constant comparative method in the analysis of qualitative interviews. *Quality and Quantity*, 36, 391–409.

Braun, V. and Clarke, V. (2002) Using thematic analysis in psychology. *Qualitative Research in Psychology*, 3, 77–101.

Browne, K. and Nash, C.J. (Eds.) (2010) *Queer Methods and Methodologies: Intersecting Queer Theories and Social Science Research*. Burlington, VT: Ashgate Publishing.

Bruner, J. (1990) *Acts of Meaning*. Harvard University Press: United States.

Caelli, K., Ray, L., and Mill, J. (2003) "Clear as mud": Toward a greater clarity in generic qualitative research. *International Journal of Qualitative Methods*, 2(2), Article 1.

Campbell, M. and McGregor, F. (2002). *Mapping Social Relations: A Primer in Doing Institutional Ethnography*. Toronto, Ont: Broadview Press.

Cheek, J. (2000) *Postmodern and Poststructural Approaches to Nursing Research*. 2nd ed. Thousand Oaks, CA: Sage.

Creswell. J.W. (2007) *Qualitative Inquiry and Research Design: Choosing Among Five Approaches*. 2nd ed. Thousand Oaks, CA: Sage.

DeForge, R., van Wyk, P. Hall, J., and Salmoni, A. (2011) Afraid to care; unable to care: A critical ethnography within a long-term care home. *Journal of Aging Studies*, 25(4), 415–26.

Denzin, E.G., and Lincoln, Y.S. (2000) The discipline and practice of qualitative research. In Denzin N.K. and Lincoln Y.S. (Eds.), *Handbook of Qualitative Research*. 2nd ed. (pp. 1–28). Newbury Park: Sage.

Denzin, N.K. and Lincoln, Y.S. (Eds.) (2011) *The Handbook of Qualitative Research*. 4th ed. Thousand Oaks, CA: Sage.

Dey, I. (1999) *Grounding Grounded Theory: Guidelines for Qualitative Inquiry*. San Diego, CA: Academic Press.

Dhand, R. (2009) Challenging exclusion: A critique of the legal barriers faced by ethnoracial psychiatric consumer/survivors in Ontario. Dissertation/Thesis. University of Toronto.

Donnelly, T.T., Hwang, J.J., Ste, D., Ewashen, C., Adair, C., and Clinton, M. (2011) If I was going to kill myself, I wouldn't be calling you. I am asking for help: Challenges influencing immigrant and refugee women's mental health. *Issues in Mental Health Nursing*, 32(5), 279–90.

Flick, U. (2009) *An Introduction to Qualitative Research*. 4th ed. Thousand Oaks, CA: Sage.

Foucault, M. (1973) *The Birth of the Clinic: An Archeology of Medical Perception*. London: Routledge.

Friere, P. (2007) *Pedagogy of the Oppressed*. New York: Continuum.

Geertz, C. (1973) *Interpretation of Cultures*. New York: Basic Books.

Giardina, M. D. and Newman, J.I. (2011) Cultural studies: Performative imperatives and bodily articulations. In Denzin N.K. and Lincoln Y.S. (Eds.) *The Handbook of Qualitative Research*, 4th ed. (pp. 179–207). Thousand Oaks, CA: Sage.

Glaser, B. (2001) *The Grounded Theory Perspective: Conceptualization Contrasted with Description*. Mill Valley, CA: The Sociology Press.

Glaser, B. and Strauss, A.L. (1967) *The Discovery of Grounded Theory: Strategies for Qualitative Research*. New York: Aldine de Gruyter.

Goldberg, L., Harbin, A., and Campbell, S. (2011) Queering the birthing space: Phenomenological interpretations of the relationships between lesbian couples and prenatal nurses in the context of birthing care. *Sexualities*, 14(2), 173–92.

Greenspan, N.R., Aguinaldo, J.P., Husbands, W., Murray, J., Ho, P., Sutdhibhasilp, N., Cedano, J., Lau, C., Gray, T., and Maharaj, R. (2011) "It's not rocket science, what I do": Self-directed harm reduction strategies among drug using ethno-racially diverse gay and bisexual men. *International Journal of Drug Policy*, 22(1), 56–62.

Guba, E.G. (1981) Criteria for assessing the trustworthiness of naturalistic inquiries. *Educational Communication and Technology Journal*, 29, 75–91.

Hole, R. (2007) Narratives of identity: A poststructural analysis of three Deaf women's life stories. *Narrative Inquiry*, 17(2), 259–78.

Lincoln, Y.S., Lynham, S.A. and Guba, E.G. (2011). Paradigmatic controversies, contradictions, and emerging confluences, revisited. In Denzin, N.K. and Lincoln Y.S. (Eds.) *The Handbook of Qualitative Research* 4th ed. (pp. 97–128). Thousand Oaks, CA: Sage.

Koro-Ljungberg, M. (2004) Impossibilities of reconciliation: Validity in mixed theory projects. *Qualitative Inquiry*, 10(4), 601–21.

Krueger, R.A. and Casey, M.A. (2000) *Focus Groups: A Practical Guide for Applied Research*. 3rd ed. Thousand Oaks, CA: Sage.

Lane, A., McCoy, L., and Ewashen, C. (2010) The textual organization of placement into long-term care: Issues for older adults with mental illness. *Nursing Inquiry*, 17(1), 2–13.

Lather, P. (1993) Fertile obsession: Validity after poststructuralism. *Sociological Quarterly*, 34(4), 673–94.

Lee, J. and Bell, K. (2011) The impact of cancer on family relationships among Chinese patients. *Journal of Transcultural Nursing*, 22(3), 225–234.

Lincoln, Y. S. (1995) Emerging criteria for quality in qualitative and interpretive research. *Qualitative Inquiry*, 1, 275–89.

Macbeth, D. (2001) On reflexivity in qualitative research: Two readings, and a third. *Qualitative Inquiry*, 7(1), 35–68.

Malthouse, M. (2011) An autoethnography on shifting relationships between a daughter, her mother and Alzheimer's dementia. *Dementia*, 10(2), 249–56.

Marshall, C. and Rossman, G.B. (2011) *Designing Qualitative Research*. 5th ed. Thousand Oaks, CA: Sage.

Mayan, M. (2009) *Essentials of Qualitative Inquiry*. Walnut Creek, CA: Left Coast Press.

Medved, M.I. and Brockmeier, J. (2011) Heart stories: Men and women after cardiac incident. *Journal of Health Psychology* 16(2), 322–31.

Morgan, D.L. (2002) Focus group interviewing. In Gubrium, J.F. and Holstein, J.A. (Eds.) *The Handbook of Interview Research: Context and*

Method (pp. 141–60). Thousand Oaks, CA: Sage.

Morse, J. (2011) Molding qualitative health research. *Qualitative Health Research*, 21(8), 1019–21.

Morse, J. (2000) Determining sample size. *Qualitative Health Research*, 10, 3–5.

Morse, J., Bottorff, J., and Hutchinson, S. (1994) The phenomenology of comfort. *Journal of Advanced Nursing*, 20, 189–95.

Morse, J. and Richards, L. (2002) README FIRST *for a User's Guide to Qualitative Methods*. 2nd ed. Thousand Oaks, CA: Sage.

Muncey, T. (2010) *Creating Autoethnographies*. Thousand Oaks, CA: Sage.

Munhall, P. (1994) *Revisioning Phenomenology: Nursing and Health Science Research*. New York: National League for Nursing.

Oliffe, J.L. and Bottorff, J.L. (2007) Further than the eye can see? Photo elicitation and research with men. *Qualitative Health Research*, 17(6), 850–8.

Polkinghorne, D.E. (2007) Validity issues in narrative research. *Qualitative Inquiry*, 13(4), 471–486.

Riessman, C.K. (1993) *Narrative Analysis*. Newbury Park, CA: Sage

Ramazanoglu, C., and Holland, J. (2007) *Feminist Methodology: Challenges and Choices*. Thousand Oaks, CA: Sage.

Rankin, J. M. and Campbell, M. (2009) Institutional ethnography, nursing work, and hospital reform: IE's cautionary analysis. *Forum: Qualitative Social Research*, 10(2), 1–20.

Richards, L. (2009) *Handling Qualitative Data: A Practical Guide*. 2nd ed. Los Angeles, CA: Sage.

Richards, L. and Morse, J. (2013) *Read Me First for a User's Guide to Qualitative Methods*. 3rd ed. Thousand Oaks, CA: Sage.

Richardson, L. (2000) Evaluating ethnography. *Qualitative Inquiry*, 6(2), 253–5.

Ross, L.E., Epstein, R., Anderson, S., and Eady, A. (2009) Policy, practice, and personal narratives: Experiences of LGBTQ people with adoption in Ontario, Canada. *Adoption Quarterly*, 12, 272–93.

Rossman, G.B. and Rallis, S.F. (2003) *Learning in the Field: An Introduction to Qualitative Research*. 2nd ed. Thousand Oaks, CA: Sage.

Sandelowski, M. (2000) Whatever happened to qualitative description? *Research in Nursing and Health*, 23, 334–40.

Sandelowski, M. (2010) What's in a name? Qualitative description revisited. *Research in Nursing and Health*, 33, 77–84.

Savage, J. (2000) Ethnography and health care. *British Medical Journal*, 2(321), 1400–2.

Schwandt, T.A. (2007). *The Dictionary of Qualitative Inquiry*. 3rd ed. Thousand Oaks, CA: Sage.

Shea, J.M. and Beausoleil, N. (2012) Breaking down "healthism": Barriers to health and fitness as identified by immigrant youth in St. John's, NL, Canada. *Sport, Education and Society*, 17(1), 97–112.

Sinding, C. (2010) Using institutional ethnography to understand the production of health care disparities. *Qualitative Health Research*, 20(12), 1656–63.

Smith, D. (2005) *Institutional Ethnography: A Sociology for People*. New York: AltaMira Press.

Starks, H. and Brown Trinidad, S. (2007) Choose your method: A comparison of phenomenology, discourse analysis, and grounded theory. *Qualitative Health Research*, 17(10), 1372–80.

Strauss, A., and Corbin, J. (1998) *Basics of Qualitative Research: Techniques and Procedures for Developing Grounded Theory*. Thousand Oaks, CA: Sage.

Thorne, S. (2008) *Interpretive Description*. Walnut Creek, CA: Leftcoast Press.

Thorne, S., Con, A., McGuinness, L., McPherson, G., and Harris, S.R. (2004a) Health care communication issues in multiple sclerosis: An interpretive description. *Qualitative Health Research*, 14(1), 5–22.

Thorne, S., Reimer, S.K., O'Flynn-Magee, K. (2004b) The analytic challenge in interpretive description. *International Journal of Qualitative Methods*, 3(1), 1–21.

Tobin, G.A., and Begley, C.M. (2003) Methodological rigour within a qualitative framework. *Journal of Advanced Nursing*, 48(4), 388–96.

Uotinen, J. (2011) Senses, bodily knowledge, and autoethnography: Unbeknown knowledge from an ICU experience. *Qualitative Health Research*, 21(10), 1307–15.

Van Herk, K.A., Smith, D., and Andrew, C. (2011) Examining our privileges and oppressions: Incorporating an intersectionality paradigm into nursing. *Nursing Inquiry*, 18(1), 29–39.

van Manen, M. (2001) *Researching Lived Experience: Human Science for an Action Sensitive Pedagogy*. London, Canada: Althouse.

van Manen, M. (2012) Carrying: Parental experience of the hospital transfer of their baby. *Qualitative Health Research*, 22(2), 199–211.

van Manen, M. (2013) Retrieved from Phenomenology Online, June 4.

Wang, C. and Burris, M.A. (1994) Empowerment through photo novella: Portraits of participation. *Health Education and Behavior*, 21(2), 171–86.

Warren, C.A.B. (2002) Qualitative interviewing. In Gubrium, J.F. and Holstein, J.A. (Eds.) *The Handbook of Interview Research: Context and Method* (pp. 83–102). Thousand Oaks, CA: Sage.

Watt, L., Gulati, S., Shaw, N., Sung, L., Dix, D., Poureslami, I., and Klassen, A. (2012) Perceptions about complementary and alternative medicine use among Chinese immigrant parents of children with cancer. *Supportive Care in Cancer*, 20(2), 253–60.

10

Measures of Frequency, Effect, and Outcome

David L. Streiner

CHAPTER OUTLINE

Introduction

Although we may think of "health care" simply as the delivery of services to those in need, a significant component of it also involves counting—how many people require those services; how effective (or ineffective) are the interventions; what proportion of people benefit from them; if the disorder is potentially life-threatening, how many people die from it; and so on. Increasingly, clinicians are being asked—or compelled—to justify what they do in terms of targeting those most in need and by using therapies that have been shown to be effective, and again this involves counting. Many of the counting measures that are used come from the field of **epidemiology**. To clarify one area of confusion, epidemiology has nothing to do with skin problems; that's dermatology, the treatment of disorders of the epidermis. Rather, the term epidemiology comes from the Greek words *epi*, meaning among, and *demos*, which refers to the population; and it refers to the study of the distribution and patterns of health-related states and factors that affect these (Streiner and Norman, 2009a).

To provide a context for learning about these measures, we will discuss a disorder that has plagued many people over the centuries: *photo-numerophobia* (PNP), which is the fear that one's fear of numbers will come to light. Although we first described this dread disease nearly two decades ago (Norman and Streiner, 1994), it has not yet been listed in the major diagnostic manuals, for reasons that still defy understanding. Despite that serious omission, we will begin by trying to determine just how many people are afflicted.

Measures of Frequency— Incidence and Prevalence

In order to determine how widespread PNP is, it is necessary to do a survey of the general population. To keep our example manageable, we will limit our sample size to 100 people, randomly selected from the population. Bear in mind, though, that in order to get accurate estimates, most surveys are considerably larger than this, often numbering thousands or tens of thousands of individuals (see Health Research in Action Box 10.1). Each person will be interviewed to determine (1) if the person has ever suffered from PNP, and (2) if so, when it began, and (3) if and when it ended. Let us assume that we find 12 people, and the time-course of their disorder is shown in Figure 10.1.

The first decision we have to make is to determine as of when to count the cases. If we do the counting at Time 1, we would capture six cases; eight at Time 2; and there will be only three cases at Time 3. Unless we are studying a condition that depends on the time of year, such as the flu or seasonal affective disorder, it shouldn't matter too

---

10.1   Health Research in Action

The Canadian Community Health Survey 1.2— Mental Health and Well-Being (CCHS 1.2; Gravel and Béland, 2005) was the first national survey of the prevalence of mental disorders in Canada. Data collection began in May of 2002, and extended over eight months. Nearly 37,000 people over the age of 15 chosen to be representative of the general population (excluding the three territories) were included. Computer-assisted interviewing was used; about 85 per cent of people were seen in person and the rest interviewed over the telephone. The overall response rate was 77 per cent. An expert panel selected the disorders to be covered, which included various anxiety and mood disorders, substance abuse, gambling, and eating disorders. Other questions asked about service use, psychological well-being, stress, physical activities, and spiritual values. Despite the size of the survey, serious and persistent mental disorders such as schizophrenia and obsessive-compulsive disorder were not included, because their very low prevalence in the general population precluded accurate estimates when the data were analyzed by province. The study was repeated in 2013, using a smaller sample of approximately 20,000 individuals.

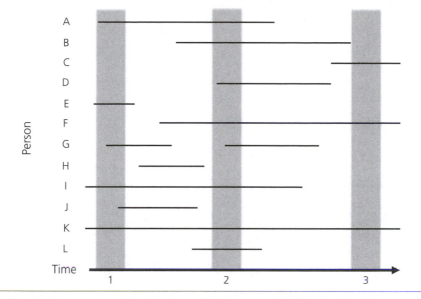

FIGURE 10.1 **Results from a cross-sectional survey of photonumerophobia, showing that counts may vary at different points in time**

much when we do the counting if the survey is sufficiently large (a deliberately vague term, that usually means over 1000 or so respondents). In CCHS 1.2 (Health Research in Action 10.1), sampling was spread out over an entire year, in part to minimize any such time-dependent effects. The second decision is how wide to make the window; those grey areas in the figure during which time we will determine if a case exists. Ideally, it would be very narrow, so that we can say, "These many cases exist at this time." A narrow window also eliminates the problem of whether or not to count disorders of a very short duration (e.g., the flu) that may start and end within its time frame. However, there are a few problems with very narrow windows. First, a person may recall that they were first affected some time in March, for example, but would be hard-pressed to remember the exact day. Second, many disorders, such as depression, multiple sclerosis, or irritable bowel syndrome, have a very slow and insidious onset, so that it would be extremely difficult, if not impossible, for a person

to say exactly when it began. Similarly, problems may resolve slowly and giving an exact date when they ended would be equally difficult.

For these reasons, windows are generally one month, six months, or one year wide, depending on the condition we are studying. If the condition is rare relative to the size of our sample, we would need a wider window in order to find a sufficient number of cases, so there is often a trade-off between the sample size and the window size. Another window that is sometimes used is the person's entire life; later, we will discuss why this can be problematic. As a reader of research, you should be aware of the window that was used in a particular article; results may seem to vary from one study to the next, and this may be due to the fact that they used windows of different sizes.

Prevalence Rate

The **prevalence rate** refers to the proportion of people at risk who have a specific condition at a given time. If we use Time 2 in Figure 10.1 as our window, we see eight people who have PNP, so the prevalence is:

Prevalence Rate =

$$\frac{\text{Number of people with the disorder}}{\text{Number of people at risk in a given interval}} = \frac{8}{100} = 0.080.$$

[10-1]

If the window was six months wide, we would say that the six-month prevalence was 0.08, or 8 per cent, or 8 per 100. For very rare conditions, we could express this as the number of people per 10,000 or even per 100,000.

Sometimes, it is possible to have a very narrow window, one day or one week in duration. For example, we can use administrative databases to determine how many people with a specific disorder were in hospital in a province on a particular date. We would call this a **point prevalence**. In contrast, when the window is wider—one month, six months, or a year—we would call these estimates **period prevalences**. The dividing line between what is deemed to be a point prevalence versus a period prevalence is quite arbitrary.

At the opposite end of the continuum from point prevalence is **lifetime prevalence**, which counts the number of people who have ever had the disorder at any time in their lives. When this can be determined through administrative data (e.g., hospital admission or laboratory records) or based on diagnostic tests, it can be a useful measure of how many people have ever been affected. However, especially in psychiatry, it is usually estimated by asking people to recall if they have ever had symptoms that would be diagnostic of a disorder. This assumes that people are able to recall past events accurately, and we know this is not the case. Indeed, almost all studies of lifetime prevalence in psychiatry have shown paradoxical results, in that the prevalences seem to decrease

with age (e.g., Henderson et al., 1998; Kessler et al., 2005; Streiner, Cairney, and Veldhuizen, 2006). The paradox is that lifetime prevalence can never decrease as people get older; it can only increase or remain the same (Robins et al., 1984), because once a person has a disorder, he or she should have it for life. The apparent decline seems to be due to people forgetting earlier episodes, and this is in direct proportion to how long ago the episode was (Patten et al., 2012). Our recommendation is that lifetime prevalence should never be used if the data are based on patient recall (Streiner et al., 2010).

Incidence Rate

Note that the prevalence rate that we just calculated consists of a mix of different types of cases. Some people already had the condition at the start of the interval (Persons A, B, F, I, K, and L) and others developed it during the time frame (D and G). The **incidence rate** looks at only the new cases; those who came down with PNP within the window. But even here we have a problem. Person G had a previous episode of PNP, so is she counted as an incident case? The answer is a very definite, "It all depends." What it depends upon has nothing to do with epidemiology or statistics, but rather on our knowledge or conceptualization of the disorder. If we believe, based on these, that a person can have the disorder and be cured of it, as with a specific phobia or a broken leg, then this would be considered to be a new case of PNP. On the other hand, if we feel that PNP is a disorder that waxes and wanes but that is never cured, much like multiple sclerosis, then this episode would be deemed a reemergence of an already-existing condition and would not be counted. Often, as with the case of schizophrenia or depression, we don't know, so we make an arbitrary decision: "If the previous episode ended less than X months ago, we will consider this to be an existing case. If it ended more than X months ago, it will be counted as a new case." Bear in mind, though, that the choice of X is an arbitrary one, and may vary from one study to the next. In our study, we will set X to be six months. Now our sampling time looks like Figure 10.2: there's a window that's six months wide, and an interval, also six months wide, for each person who had an episode of PNP that starts at the end of the previous episode. Note that the start date for the interval is different for each person, and depends on when the previous episode ended.

According to our definitions, then, Person G meets the criterion to be counted as a new case. Then, the six-month incidence is:

Incidence Rate =

$$\frac{\text{Number of new cases}}{\text{Number of people at risk in a given interval}} = \frac{2}{94} = 0.021$$

$$[10\text{--}2]$$

or 2.1 per cent. The question that arises is why the denominator is 94 rather than 100. The answer is that there are six people who had the disorder at the start of the window. Because they have PNP, they cannot be at risk of developing it, so they are excluded from the denominator. Persons E and G would be considered at risk of having a new episode, since their previous ones ended more than six months before the current one. H and J are also at risk, because there's a possibility that they could have an episode before the window closes, although they are at risk for less than six months.

It is obvious that all incident cases are also prevalent ones, but not all prevalent cases are incident ones.

Incidence Density

The data for our study came from a **cross-sectional survey**, which means that we sampled people at one point in time. A much more useful, albeit far more expensive, study design is a **longitudinal survey**, in which people are inter-

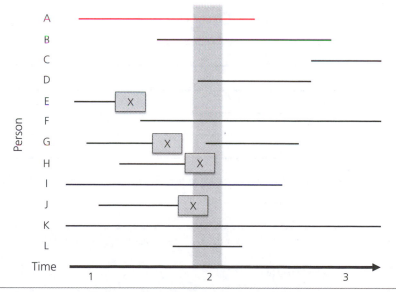

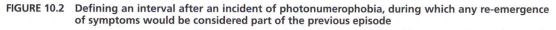

FIGURE 10.2 **Defining an interval after an incident of photonumerophobia, during which any re-emergence of symptoms would be considered part of the previous episode**

viewed repeatedly over time. It is more useful because we can determine with greater certainty when a disorder began and ended; but more expensive because the survey has to be done a number of times, and people's moves have to be tracked in the intervals between the surveys. In a longitudinal survey, we can also derive a more accurate estimate of incidence because it is based on more data.

In Figure 10.3, we see the results from the first eight people in such a survey. The D indicates when they developed PNP, and the C means that the data are **right censored**. This does not mean that conservative activists shut the project down; rather, it means that the study ended before the people developed PNP, and we do not know what happened to them subsequently. They could have developed PNP the very next day, or have gone on to lead phobia-free lives until they died; but the point is that we will never know. Despite this, though, they will have each contributed a varying number of years without PNP, and we can make use of their data.

Person A contributes about 2.25 person-years to the study; Person B just under 4 person-years; and so forth. If we add these up for all of the people in the survey, we can calculate the **incidence density** (ID), which is defined as:

$$ID = \frac{\text{Number of new cases in a given time}}{\text{Total person} - \text{time of observation}} = \frac{3}{22} = 0.136,$$

[10-3]

which here is 3 per 22 person-years, or about 13.6 cases per 100 person-years of observation.

So which is more important, incidence or prevalence? The answer is that both are useful because they tell us different things. If we were interested in the natural history of a disorder—how it changes over time—then incidence is much more informative. Figure 10.4 shows the number of new cases of HIV/AIDS in Canada over time. We see the sudden increase starting in the mid-1980s, a dramatic drop in 1996, and then a more gradual decline. This could lead to hypotheses for future research regarding why it started when it did, why

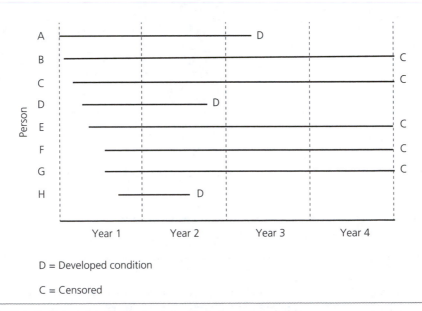

D = Developed condition

C = Censored

FIGURE 10.3   Results from a longitudinal survey of photonumerophobia

there was a sudden drop, why the decline is continuing, and why the rate of decline changed.

On the other hand, if you were an administrator of a health care facility or a clinician working in a clinic, you would be more concerned about the number of patients seeking service, and this would be given by the prevalence rates. That is, prevalence reflects the burden of the disorder on society (see Health Research in Action Box 10.2).

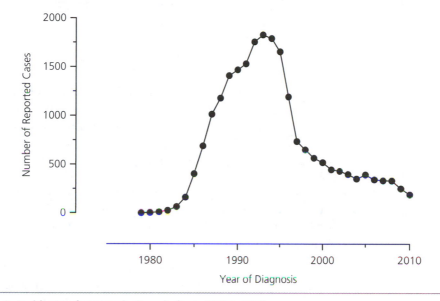

FIGURE 10.4   Incidence of HIV/AIDS in Canada from 1979 to 2010

Source: Data from Public Health Agency of Canada (n.d.)

10.2   Health Research in Action

The CCHS 1.2 data (see Health Research in Action Box 10.1) were used by Cairney, Corna, and Streiner (2010) to determine the proportion of people 55 and older who met the criteria for having at least one mental disorder within the past year and who used mental health services. There were nearly 13,000 older adults, of whom approximately 4.25 per cent met criteria. Among this group, only 37 per cent sought help; of these, most saw their family physician, and a smaller proportion saw a psychiatrist, psychologist, or social worker. The only factor that predicted service use was psychological distress. Surprisingly, gender did not influence who did or did not seek services, nor did education or social support. Having more medical problems was positively associated with service use, and limitations in activities of daily living was negatively correlated with use. However, because the sample size was relatively small ($n = 513$), neither of these predictors was statistically significant. This illustrates one major problem with trying to study disorders with low prevalence: despite the fact that the original survey included nearly 37,000 people, by the time we focused on a narrower range in age and a relatively low prevalence condition, the sample size was insufficient for some analyses.

Duration

If we know the incidence and prevalence of a disorder, we can easily determine its duration—how long the disorder lasts. They are related by the formula:

$$Duration = \frac{Prevalence}{Incidence}, \qquad [10\text{-}4]$$

which means that:

$$Prevalence = Incidence \times Duration \qquad [10\text{-}5]$$

and

$$Incidence = \frac{Prevalence}{Duration}. \qquad [10\text{-}6]$$

Thus, disorders such as schizophrenia and HIV/AIDS, that have a low incidence but long duration, have a high prevalence; while for the common cold, which has a very short duration, the prevalence may be low, but the incidence high.

Measures of Mortality

Troubling as it is for sufferers of PNP, the disorder is not life-threatening. Consequently, in order to look at measures of mortality, it is necessary for us to look at a different problem; one that has a significant degree of mortality associated with it. For that, we must turn to yet another disorder discovered by your intrepid author, *malignant hypertrophy of the ego* (MHE; Streiner and Norman, 2009b). As the name implies, MHE is marked by a pathological enlargement of the person's ego, and is especially prevalent among movie and sports "personalities," politicians, university deans, and neurosurgeons. It can be easily detected by counting the number of times the person uses the pronoun "I" in a sentence; the inability to pass by a mirror without stopping to look at and admire the reflection; and endorse-

ment of statements such as "The world revolves around me." Early deaths are often due to engaging in high-risk behaviours, as these people believe they are immune from the laws of nature; and homicide at the hands of others around them who become increasingly irritated by these egotists' self-centredness.

Mortality Rate

Incidence rate tells us how many people develop a disorder in a given time span. In an analogous manner, **mortality rate** (MR) reflects how many people die from it in a given time, which is usually one year. So, it is:

$$MR = \frac{\text{Number of deaths due to a disorder in a given time}}{\text{Number of people at rsk}},$$

$$[10\text{-}7]$$

where the number of people at risk is the general population. However, the simplicity of this formula masks a few problems. First, if we find that the one-year mortality rate for MHE is, say, 2 per cent, is that high or low? The number by itself is difficult to interpret, and is useful only when it can be compared to mortality rates for other disorders. Second, our interest is rarely the population at large, but rather the people who have the disorder.

Case Fatality Rate

The **case fatality rate** (CFR) solves the second problem by restricting the denominator to only those who have the disorder; it is the proportion of people with MHE who die within a given time, again usually one year:

$$CFR = \frac{\text{Number of deaths due to a disorder in a given time}}{\text{Number of people with the disorder}}.$$

$$[10\text{-}8]$$

However, the first problem remains, in that we do not know if the number is high or low, except in comparison with CFRs from other disorders. We have also introduced another problem, in that we do not always know how many people there are with a given disorder. Often, we have to rely on epidemiological data, such as the CCHS 1.2 described in the Health Care in Action Box 10.1, but it did not include rare disorders such as schizophrenia (or MHE), so the denominator is often nothing more than an educated guess.

Proportional Mortality Rate

A way to avoid the problem of imperfect estimates of prevalence that we just mentioned is to look at death rates for a specific disorder in relation to deaths from all causes. One measure of this is the **proportional mortality rate** (PMR), which keeps the same numerator as in Equations 10-7 and 10-8, but uses all deaths in the denominator:

$$\text{PMR} = \frac{\text{Number of deaths due to a disorder in a given time}}{\text{Number of deaths from all disorders}}.$$

[10-9]

As with the previous indices, the number makes sense only when we compare the PMR from one disorder with those from other disorders.

Bear in mind that PMRs for a given disorder can increase over time for two different reasons. First, more people may be contracting and dying from the disorder, as may be the case with certain forms of cancer. But, a second process may also be at work: fewer people are dying from other causes. The sad fact is that, as Marcel Aymé (1956) said, "Life always comes to a bad end." Even if we jog, eat "organic" foods (is there any other type?), boost our immune system, and arrange our homes in accordance with the principles of feng shui, none of us will get out of this life alive; in the

long term, the mortality rate is 100 per cent. So, as we get better in treating heart disease, diabetes, infectious diseases, and other scourges of humanity, more people will die from something else. Over 100 years ago, William Osler, the Canadian physician who is regarded as one of the fathers of modern medicine, described pneumonia as "the old man's friend," because it was a swift, relatively painless way to die. Now that pneumonia can be successfully treated with antibiotics, its PMR is extremely low, but that for Alzheimer's disease has increased.

Standardized Mortality Rate

All of the measures we have discussed so far suffer from a similar limitation: they are meaningful only in comparison to other disorders. One index that surmounts this is the **standardized mortality rate** (SMR). It is the ratio of the number of observed deaths from a given cause in a given time to the expected number of deaths:

$$\text{SMR} = \frac{\text{Number of deaths due to a disorder in a given time}}{\text{Number of expected deaths}}.$$

[10-10]

An SMR less than one means that people with the disorder are dying at a lower than expected rate; an SMR greater than one indicates a higher than expected death rate. Most often, the expected number of deaths is derived from the general population. Saha, Chant, and McGrath (2007), for example, found that the SMR for people with schizophrenia was 2.58, meaning that they died at a rate that was slightly more than two and a half times that of the general population. Their meta-analysis analyzed the data in even more depth, looking at various **cause-specific SMRs**; that is, SMRs in a specific group due to a specific cause:

Cause-Specific SMR

$$= \frac{\text{Number of deaths for a disorder due to specific cause in a given time}}{\text{Number of expected deaths}}.$$

[10-11]

That for suicide was 12.86, reflecting the fact that those with schizophrenia kill themselves at a rate that's nearly 13 times that of the general public.

Age-standardized Mortality Rate

One remaining problem is that there are times that using the general population as the reference group may not make sense. For example, the one-year **crude mortality rate** (that is, not adjusting the MR for any other factors) in Canada is 6.70 per 1000, which is considerably higher than in Saudi Arabia, where it is only 3.56. Does that mean that they lead much healthier lives and that we should all move there? Not necessarily. One major difference between Canada and Saudi Arabia is the age structure of the population. If we look at an **age pyramid**—a graph showing age distributions—of the two regions (Figure 10.5), we see a dramatic difference. As is typical for a developed country, Canada's population has a much higher proportion of older people than is the case in a developing country like Saudi Arabia. Consequently, it is not at all surprising that the MR in Canada is also much higher; older people are more likely to die within the year than younger ones. The only way to compare the MRs fairly is to use **age-standardized mortality rates**; that is, to adjust the age distributions of the two countries so that they are the same.

This is done in Table 10.1. To keep the example simple, we've used only three broad age categories—birth to 14, 15 to 64, and 65 and older— rather than the 19 categories in Figure 10.5. If we were more interested in accuracy rather than

explanation, we would use the finer divisions, and perhaps even do the calculations separately for males and females if we thought that mortality rates differed by sex.

Column B shows the population of Canada in each of the three age categories, and Column F does the same for Saudi Arabia. Columns C and G have the number of deaths. Dividing C by B (and G and F) yields the death rate for each country for each age (Columns D and H). We are using Canada as the reference population, so Column E is simply the proportion of people in each age category. We could just as easily have used Saudi Arabia as the reference group, and we would get the same results. Often, if we were interested in comparing many countries, we would use the entire world as the standard.

Now the fun (or work) begins. We "adjust" Saudi Arabia's population so that its age structure is the same as Canada's by multiplying Saudi Arabia's total population (roughly 26 million; the last entry in Column F) by the values in Column E, which gives the numbers in Column I. So, the value for the 0–14 age group (4,072,000) is 15.69 per cent of the population of 25,958,000. Then, using the MR for that age group (Column H), we finally arrive at Column J. That tells us that, if Saudi Arabia's age structure were the same as Canada's, there should have been 7859 deaths in the age group 0 to 14, rather than the observed 14,843. The biggest difference, as we would expect, is in the oldest age group: 344,192 expected deaths instead of the actual 92,486.

Looking at the bottom row, the observed MR in Saudi Arabia is Column G (92,486) divided by Column F (25,958,000), or 3.56, which is the number we reported previously. However, the age-adjusted MR is Column J (344,192) divided by Column F, or 13.26, which is twice as high as Canada's. So, you can unpack your bags now.

The bottom line is that when we are considering any outcome that may be affected by age,

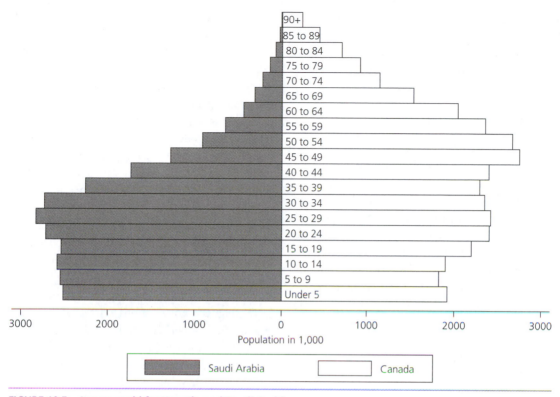

FIGURE 10.5   Age pyramid for Canada and Saudi Arabia

Source: Data from CIA World Fact Books (n.d.)

TABLE 10.1   Age-adjustment in Crude Mortality Rates for Canada and Saudi Arabia

	Canada				Saudi Arabia				
Age Group (A)	Population (x1000) (B)	No. of Deaths (C)	Death Rate (D)	Pct. of Population (E)	Population (x1000) (F)	No. of Deaths (G)	Death Rate (H)	Adjusted Population (x1000) (I)	Weighted No. of Deaths (J)
0-14	5,339	2,528	0.47	15.69	7,693	14,843	1.93	4,072	7,859
15-64	23,295	48,959	2.10	68.45	17,666	37,042	2.10	17,769	37,315
65+	5,397	176,592	37.72	15.86	599	40,601	72.63	4,117	299,018
Total	34,031	228,079	6.70	100.00	25,958	92,486	3.56	25,958	344,192

Source: Data from United Nations (n.d.).

United Nations Demographic yearbook. Retrieved from: http://unstats.un.org/unsd/demographic/products/dyb/dyb2008.htm

such as death itself or illnesses such as cancer, cardiovascular disease, or dementing disorders, we cannot compare regions that differ with regard to their age structure without adjusting for this.

Measures of Impact

Although, as we have said, life is a terminal disorder, we have set up an elaborate system of health care (or, more accurately, illness care), drug manufacturing, "wellness" spas, health food stores, and the like to delay the inevitable. The question then arises regarding how effective these are. This leads us to consider measures of the impact of our interventions, and that where we'll turn our attention to next. But first, we need to discuss the concept of *risk* and the many (and confusing) ways the term is used.

Risk, Risk Markers, Risk Determinants, and Modifiable Risk Factors

In his *Dictionary of Epidemiology*, James Last (2000) defines **risk** as:

> The probability that an event will occur, e.g., that an individual will become ill or die within a stated period of time or age. Also, a nontechnical term encompassing a variety of measures of the probability of a (generally) unfavorable outcome (p. 160).

and a **risk factor** as:

> An aspect of personal behavior or lifestyle, an environmental exposure, or an inborn or inherited characteristic which on the basis of epidemiological evidence is known to be associated with health-related condition(s) considered important to prevent (p. 160).

One important point to note in the definition of a risk factor is that it uses the term "associated with," and nowhere do we see the word "cause." Because of this, we have to differentiate

among various flavours of risk factors. A **risk determinant** is something that is causally related to an outcome. For example, workers who are exposed to asbestos have a much higher risk of developing mesothelioma, a rare form of cancer affecting primarily the lungs. It is extremely unusual for a person who was not exposed to asbestos to develop this disease. A **risk marker** is a factor that is related to a higher prevalence of an outcome, and may or may not be causally related. John Paulos (1995), who has written a number of delightful books pointing out how innumeracy can get us into trouble, cites a newspaper headline proclaiming that drinking bottled water leads to having healthier babies. Should we immediately supply bottled water to all pregnant women? We can, but it won't do anything for the neonates' birth weight. Who can afford to buy water, a commodity that's (literally) freely available, but litre for litre, costs more than gasoline when it comes with designer labels attached? Obviously, only women who have enough disposable income to do so. These women are also more likely to be able to afford prenatal care when they are pregnant and are more inclined to take care of their health in other ways. Thus, bottled water is a risk *marker* (i.e., it is correlated with birth weight), but it is not a risk *determinant*.

Finally, a **modifiable risk factor** is one that is causally related to an outcome, and whose change can affect the outcome. A modifiable risk factor is also a risk determinant, but not all risk determinants are modifiable risk factors, and confusing the two has led to many false starts. For example, blood pressure is a modifiable risk factor: a high value increases the risk of heart attack and stroke, and lowering blood pressure decreases these risks. On the other hand, a high level of plaque in the brain is associated with Alzheimer's disease, but a study that used a drug to reduce plaque levels did not slow the advance of the disease and may even have resulted in deaths among study participants (Green et al., 2009). Similarly, homocysteine levels are correlated with both cardiovascular disease and dementia, but reducing the level did not affect progression of the diseases (Stott et al., 2005); and there is growing suspicion that cholesterol levels may be risk markers rather than modifiable risk factors.

Relative Risk

With that as background, we are ready to address the issue of measuring the impact of conditions and interventions. We have said that MHE is a potentially life-threatening disorder, because these people engage in risky behaviours and their overweening egos make them prime targets for normal people's anger. But just how dangerous is it? One way to find out is to do a **cohort study**. In such a study, we assemble two cohorts of people, one of which has been exposed to the putative causal factor (in this case, the trait of MHE) and the other which has not been exposed. (In general, a **cohort** is a group that shares a common characteristic, such as year of birth or exposure to some risk factor.) We then follow them for a few years and count how many in each group have the outcome of interest; in this case, death by misadventure or homicide. Let's assume that we recruit 100 people in each group, and find the results presented in Table 10.2 after 10 years of follow-up.

Of the 100 MHE sufferers, 20 were dead by the end of 10 years. Therefore, the risk of death for them is:

$$\text{Risk}_{\text{MHE}} = \frac{A}{A+B} = \frac{20}{100} = 0.20, \qquad [10\text{-}12]$$

where the letters refer to the cells in the table. In a similar manner, the risk of death in the comparison cohort is:

$$\text{Risk}_{\text{Comparison}} = \frac{C}{C+D} = \frac{10}{100} = 0.10. \qquad [10\text{-}13]$$

The **relative risk** (RR), then, is the ratio of the risks for the two groups:

$$RR = \frac{\text{Risk}_{\text{MHE}}}{\text{Risk}_{\text{Comparison}}} = \frac{\dfrac{A}{A+B}}{\dfrac{C}{C+D}} = \frac{A\,(C+D)}{C\,(A+B)} = \frac{0.20}{0.10} = 2.00.$$

$$[10\text{-}14]$$

In other words, if you have MHE, you are two times as likely to die within 10 years than if you do not have it. An RR of 1 means that the risk is the same in both groups, and RRs less than 1 indicate a reduced risk.

In this example, we used the RR in an observational **cohort study**, in which the assignment of people to the various groups was outside of the researcher's control. However, it also finds use when we are looking at a dichotomous outcome in a **randomized controlled trial** (RCT).

TABLE 10.2 Results of a 10-year Cohort Study of MHE

		Outcome		
		Dead	Alive	Total
	MHE	20 (A)	80 (B)	100
Cohort	Comparison	10 (C)	90 (D)	100
	Total	30	170	200

An RCT is a research design where the investigator randomly assigns participants to be in either the treatment condition (often called an "arm" of the study) or in the comparison arm. Because MHE doubles the risk of dying prematurely, it is worthwhile to try to ameliorate its harmful effects by trying to teach these people a modicum of humility.

Consistent with the procedures for conducting an RCT, we will enroll 200 people who meet the criteria for it, and then randomly allocate them to one of two groups: an active therapy group or an attention-control group. This latter group will meet just as often as the therapy group but not discuss humility, in order to control for any effects of meeting and being assessed. Six months later, we will administer a diagnostic scale to all of the participants and see how many people still meet the criteria for MHE. What we find is shown in Table 10.3.

Using Equation 10-14, we can calculate the RR as:

$$RR = \frac{A(C+D)}{C(A+B)} = \frac{70+(100)}{60+(100)} = 1.17, \qquad [10\text{-}15]$$

which means people in the treatment group are 1.17 times more likely to be cured than people in the comparison condition.

Relative Risk Reduction

Another way to express these findings is to use the **relative risk reduction** (RRR), which expresses improvement (or exacerbation—it can happen) as a percentage relative to the comparison group:

$$RRR = \frac{Risk_{Treatment} - Risk_{Control}}{Risk_{Control}} \times 100$$

$$= \frac{0.70 - 0.60}{0.60} \times 100 = 16.7\% \qquad [10\text{-}16]$$

Another way to talk about these findings, then, is that there was a 16.7 per cent increase in good outcomes following therapy.

Absolute Risk Reduction

The **absolute risk reduction** (ARR) is the decrease in risk in the treatment group compared to the control or comparison group:

$$ARR = Risk_{Treatment} - Risk_{Comparison}, \qquad [10\text{-}17]$$

which in this case is 0.70 − 0.60 = 0.10. By itself, the ARR is hard to interpret; is 0.10 a lot or a little? We can't really tell, but we'll see shortly how the ARR can be used to overcome some of the problems with the RR.

Population Attributable Risk

We have seen that MHE results in premature deaths among those who have it (we are reluctant to call them "sufferers," because it's usually people around them who suffer the most). Unfortunately, though, it's not the only cause of people prematurely joining the choir invisible; people will

TABLE 10.3 Results of a Randomized Control Trail to Treat MHE

		Outcome		
		Does Not Meet MHE Criteria	Still Meets MHE Criteria	Total
	Treatment	70 (A)	30 (B)	100
Group	Control	60 (C)	40 (D)	100
	Total	130	70	200

still contract fatal illnesses, be involved in accidents that are not their fault, commit suicide, and so forth. The question that arises, especially for those involved in allocating health care resources, is how many early deaths can be prevented if we eliminate MHE. This estimate is called the **population attributable risk** (PAR)—how much the incidence of the outcome (in this case, premature death) can be reduced in the population if we were able to eliminate the risk factor (MHE).

In order to figure this out, we need two pieces of information: the difference in the risk of the outcome between exposed and unexposed people; and the proportion of exposed people in the population. We have the first from the data in Table 10.2: the risk of premature death for people with MHE is 0.20, and it is 0.10 among unexposed people, so the difference is 0.10. We don't know the second number, the proportion of people with MHE in the general population, so let's assume it's 20 per cent. We then put those numbers into the formula:

$$PAR = \text{Risk Difference} \times \text{Proportion Exposed} \qquad [10\text{-}18]$$

and we would get $0.10 \times .20 = 0.02$, or 2 per cent. So, eliminating MHE would reduce the number of early deaths by 2 per cent (and make the world a much better place, which is not quantifiable).

Problems with Relative Risk

Although the RR is perhaps the most widely used index in reporting the results of clinical trials, and especially for drug studies, it suffers from two important limitations. The first is the problem that the RR is **non-invertible**. This means that if we analyzed the data in Table 10.3 to focus on the bad outcome (still having symptoms of MHE) rather than the good outcome (cure), we would get different results. Remember that when we looked at cure, we found an RR of 1.17. Now, let's

reanalyze the data by interchanging the two columns, so that Cell A represents the number of people *not* cured by the therapy, and Cell C is the number of people not cured in the control condition. Now what we get is:

$$RR = \frac{30 \times (100)}{40 \times (100)} = 0.75, \qquad [10\text{-}19]$$

meaning that those in the treatment group are only three-quarters as likely to still have MHE after treatment as the control group. It still shows that treatment works, but the magnitude of the effect is very different. Moreover, there's no relationship between 1.17 and 0.75; one is not the reciprocal or the log or the anything else of the other. Later, we will look at another index that is invertible.

The second problem is a bit more subtle, and is based on the fact that the RR does not take into account the prevalence of the disorder. To see why this is an issue, let's repeat our RCT, but instead of having 100 people in each group, we'll have 10,000 in each. But, let's assume that the same *number* of people get better in the two conditions—70 in the treatment arm and 60 in the control group—and let's recalculate the RR. We would get:

$$RR = \frac{A(C+D)}{C(A+B)} = \frac{70 \times (10,000)}{60 \times (10,000)} = 1.17. \qquad [10\text{-}20]$$

Your eyes do not deceive you; it's exactly the same RR as we found previously, even though in the first study 10 additional people out of 100 were helped, and here only 10 more people out of 10,000 were. We might have been tempted to adopt the treatment into our practice in the first instance, but it would be a waste of time and effort based on the second study. Obviously, the RR can hide as much as it reveals, which may be one reason drug companies are so enamoured of the measure. Is there an index that can illuminate the difference between the two studies?

Number Needed to Treat and Number Needed to Harm

The answer to the above question is "Yes," and that index is the **number needed to treat** (NNT). It is the number of people who must be treated for there to be one additional positive outcome. The NNT was developed by Laupacis, Sackett, and Roberts (1998), and is the essence of simplicity:

$$NNT = \frac{1}{ARR} . \qquad [10\text{-}21]$$

If you remember, the ARR for the first study was 0.10 so the NNT = 1/0.10 = 10. For the second study, the ARR would be 0.001 and the NNT would be 1000. That means that we would have to treat 10 patients in order to have one additional cure in the first case, and we would have to treat 1000 people to help one in the second.

The question arises why the NNT was 10 rather than 1. There are two reasons. First, not everyone who receives treatment benefits from it. After all, in our (admittedly fictitious) example, 30 people in the treatment arm were not helped by the therapy. Second, and more importantly, not everyone who is untreated comes to a bad end. To use a more realistic example, not everyone who takes a statin (a drug that lowers cholesterol levels) avoids having a stroke or heart attack; and only a few people who do not take the drug have these adverse events. In fact, between 30 and 100 primary prevention patients have to take the drug for a year to prevent one event (Thompson and Temple, 2004).

The **number needed to harm** (NNH) is exactly equivalent to the NNT, but is used with adverse events: how many people must be treated to produce undesirable side-effects in one more person. In this somewhat bloodless measure, death is considered to be just another side-effect.

Odds Ratio

To repeat what we said earlier, in a cohort study, we find one group of people who have the suspected risk factor and another group that doesn't, and follow them to see how many in each group develop the outcome of interest. However, this type of design isn't feasible when the outcome is very rare; we would have to enroll a very large number of people in each group just to find the small proportion who do develop the outcome. Under these circumstances, we use a different design called a case-control study. In a case-control study, we recruit people on the basis of the outcome rather than the exposure. We then interview them or use existing records to determine if they were exposed to the putative causal factor. In our example, we would locate a group of people who suffered an untimely death (the cases) and a control group of people who are as similar as possible but who are still alive, and then determine the number in each who had symptoms of MHE. (Needless to say, we would have to rely on interviews with close friends or relatives, or use existing data bases, since interviewing people who are dead is rarely very rewarding.) Let's assume we did such as study, using 100 people in each group, and found the results in Table 10.4.

Of the 100 people who died prematurely, 20 had signs of MHE (Cell A), while of those still alive, only 10 did (Cell C). Because the table appears similar to Table 10.2, we might be tempted to calculate a RR, but it would be wrong to do so. The reason is that in a cohort study, the ratio of Cell A to Cell B and of Cell C to Cell D is determined by how strong the effect of MHE is on mortality; the more it affects the death rate, the larger A/B will be in relation to C/D. However, in a case-control study, those ratios are determined by the researcher. In this example, we decided to have an equal number of cases and controls, and the ratio of Cell A to Cell B turned out to be 2:1.

TABLE 10.4   Results of a Case-control Study of MHE

		Outcome		
		Dead	Alive	Total
	Yes	20 (A)	10 (B)	30
Exposure to MHE	No	80 (C)	90 (D)	170
	Total	100	100	200

But we could have said that we want two controls for every case or even five controls for every case in order to make our study more powerful (that is, able to detect an effect of MHE), which would change the ratio. Consequently, in case-control studies, we need some other way to determine the relationship between the exposure and the outcome. That measure is called the **odds ratio** (OR), which is sometimes called the **relative odds** (but still abbreviated as OR).

For a case, the odds that they had MHE is:

$$\text{Odds}_{\text{Case}} = \frac{A}{C} = \frac{20}{80} = 0.25. \qquad [10\text{-}22]$$

Similarly, for a control, the odds of having MHE is:

$$\text{Odds}_{\text{Control}} = \frac{B}{D} = \frac{10}{90} = 0.11. \qquad [10\text{-}23]$$

and the OR is the ratio of the two:

$$\text{OR} = \frac{\text{Odds}_{\text{Case}}}{\text{Odds}_{\text{Control}}} = \frac{\frac{A}{C}}{\frac{B}{D}} = \frac{AD}{BC} = \frac{20 \times 90}{10 \times 80} = 2.25. \qquad [10\text{-}24]$$

Figuring out an OR is easy; interpreting it is not. We *cannot* say that someone who died prematurely is 2.25 times more likely to have had MHE. Rather, it means that 2.25 people with MHE will die for every one person without MHE who dies. Not easy to wrap your head around. We can convert an OR into an RR with the formula:

$$RR = \frac{OR}{1 - \text{Risk}_{\text{Comparison}} + (\text{Risk}_{\text{Comparison}} \times OR)}. \qquad [10\text{-}25]$$

From Equation 10-13, we know that the risk in the comparison group is 0.10, so plugging the numbers into the formula, we get:

$$RR = 2.\frac{25}{1 - 0.10 + (0.10 \times 2.25)} = 2.0. \qquad [10\text{-}26]$$

Note that the OR is larger than the RR. This is always the case. The higher the prevalence of the disorder in the general population, the more the OR will exceed the RR. When the prevalence is low, though, the OR is a close approximation of the RR. To see why, let's go back to the formula for the RR:

$$RR = \frac{A(C+D)}{C(A+B)}. \qquad [10\text{-}27]$$

In low prevalence conditions, C+D is fairly close to D and A+B is nearly the same as B, so the formula reduces to AD/BC, which is the same as Equation 10-24.

We mentioned earlier that one problem with the RR is that it is non-invertible. Counterbalancing the difficulty with interpreting ORs is the fact that it is **invertible**: we get comparable results if we look at positive or negative outcomes. Using the data from Table 10.4, but using survival rather than death, we would find:

$$OR = \frac{10 \times 80}{20 \times 90} = 0.444. \qquad [10\text{-}28]$$

versus 2.25 that was found when we looked at deaths. This may not seem to help, but 0.444 = 1/2.25—that is, one is the reciprocal of the other. To make the relationship between the two even clearer, we can take the logarithm of the odds: $\log_e$ (2.25) = 0.811, and $\log_e$ (0.444) = −0.811; they are identical except for the sign. (It doesn't matter if we use $\log_e$ or $\log_{10}$; the values will change but the relationship will remain the same.)

Summary

- Part of delivering health care consists of determining the need for services, the effects of various risks factors on health, and the effectiveness of interventions (or lack thereof).

- Determining the number of people who have a disorder can be measured with indices of:

  - Prevalence—how many cases exist at any given time

  - Incidence—how many new cases are there within a time frame

- For disorders that are potentially fatal, we can determine:

  - Mortality rate—how many people die each year

  - Case fatality rate—how many people with a given disorder die yearly

  - Proportional mortality rate—how many people die yearly from a given disorder compared with deaths from all disorders

- Standardized mortality rate—comparing deaths from a specific disorder to the number of expected deaths

- Age-standardized mortality rate—which corrects for difference between regions in terms of their age structure

- When we look at the effects of risk factors or of interventions, we examine:

  - Relative risk or odds ratios—how much more (or less) people in one group have the outcome compared to a comparison group

  - Risk reduction—how much the risk is reduced because of the intervention or some protective factor

  - Number needed to treat—how many people must receive the treatment in order for one additional person to benefit

Review Questions

1. *Prevalence* is a measure of:

   a. *The impact of an intervention*

   b. *The number of new cases in a given period*

   c. *The effect of a risk factor on an outcome*

   d. *The number of existing cases in a given period*

2. *Incidence* is a measure of:

   a. *The impact of an intervention*

   b. *The number of new cases in a given period*

   c. *The effect of a risk factor on an outcome*

   d. *The number of existing cases in a given period*

3. To measure the effect of a treatment in a randomized controlled trial, we use:

   a. *The odds ratio*

   b. *The population attributable risk*

   c. *The relative risk*

   d. *The attributable risk*

4. To measure the impact of a risk factor in a case-control study, we use:

   a. *The odds ratio*

   b. *The population attributable risk*

   c. *The relative risk*

   d. *The attributable risk*

5. What is the relationship between the relative risk and the odds ratio?

   a. *The odds ratio is always higher*

   b. *The odds ratio is always lower*

   c. *It depends on the type of study*

   d. *It cannot be determined ahead of time*

Recommended Readings

Streiner, D.L., and Norman, G.R. (2009) PDQ *Epidemiology*. 3rd ed. Shelton, CT: PMPH US.

Streiner, D.L., MacPherson, D.W., and Gushulak, B.D. (2010) PDQ *Public Health*. Shelton, CT: PMPH US.

These two books provide brief, non-technical explanations to many of the concepts explained in this chapter.

Kleinbaum, D.G., Kupper, L.L., and Morgenstern, H. (1982) *Epidemiologic Research: Principles and Quantitative Methods*. New York: Wiley.

Rothman, K.J., Greenland, S., and Rothman, S.M. (1998) *Modern Epidemiology*. 2nd ed. New York: Lippincott, Williams and Wilkins.

These are much more comprehensive and mathematical looks at epidemiological research and various indices of incidence, prevalence, and impact. They are the bibles for those intending to enter into the field of epidemiology.

References

Aymé, M. (1956) *Les Oiseaux de Lune*. Paris: Gallimard.

Cairney, J., Corna, L.M., and Streiner, D.L. (2010) Mental health care use in later life: Results from a national survey of Canadians. *Canadian Journal of Psychiatry*, 55, 157–164.

Central Intelligence Agency. (n.d.). The world factbook. Retrieved from: www.cia.gov/library/publications/the-world-factbook/.

Gravel, R., and Béland, Y. (2005) The Canadian Community health Survey: Mental health and well-being. *Canadian Journal of Psychiatry*, 50, 573–9.

Green, R.C., Schneider, L.S., Amato, D.A., Beelen, A.P. Wilcock, G., Swabb, E.A., … Tarenflurbil Phase 3 Study Group. (2009) Effect of tarenflurbil on cognitive decline and activities of daily living in patients with mild Alzheimer disease. *Journal of American Medical Association*, 302, 2557–64.

Henderson, A.S., Jorm, A.F., Korten, A.E., Jacomb, P., Christensen, H., and Rodgers, B.

(1998) Symptoms of depression and anxiety during adult life: Evidence for a decline in prevalence with age. *Psychological Medicine*, *28*, 1321–8.

Kessler, R.C., Berglund, P., Demler, O., Jin, R., Merikangas, K. R., and Walters, E. E. (2005) Lifetime prevalence and age-of-onset distributions of DSM-IV disorders in the National Comorbidity Survey Replication. *Archives of General Psychiatry*, *62*, 593–602.

Last, J.M. (Ed.). (2000) *A Dictionary of Epidemiology*. 4th ed. Oxford: Oxford University Press.

Laupacis, A., Sackett, D.L., and Roberts, R. (1988) An assessment of clinically useful measures of the consequences of treatment. *New England Journal of Medicine*, *318*, 1728–33.

Norman, G.R. and Streiner, D.L. (1994) *Biostatistics: The Bare Essentials*. St. Louis: Mosby.

Patten, S., Williams, J., Lavorato, D., Bulloch, A., D'Arcy, C., and Streiner, D.L. (2012) Recall of recent and more remote depressive episodes in a prospective cohort study. *Social Psychiatry and Psychiatric Epidemiology*, *47*, 691–6.

Paulos, J. A. (1995) *A Mathematician Reads the Newspaper*. New York: Basic Books.

Public Health Agency of Canada. (n.d.). HIV and AIDS in Canada: Surveillance report to December 31st, 2010. Retrieved from www.phac-aspc.gc.ca/aids-sida/publication/survreport/2010/dec/index-eng.php.

Robins, L.N., Helzer, J.E., Weissman, M.M., Orvaschel, H., Gruenberg, E., Burke, J.D., and Regier, D.A. (1984) Lifetime prevalence of specific psychiatric disorders in three sites. *Archives of General Psychiatry*, *41*, 949–58.

Saha, S., Chant, D., and McGrath, J. (2007) A systematic review of mortality in schizophrenia: Is the differential mortality gap worsening over time? *Archives of General Psychiatry*, *64*, 1123–31.

Stott, D.J., MacIntosh, G., Lowe, G.D.O., et al. (2005) Randomized controlled trial of homocysteine-lowering vitamin treatment in elderly patients with vascular disease. *American Journal of Clinical Nutrition*, *82*, 1320–6.

Streiner, D.L., Cairney, J., and Veldhuizen, S. (2006) The epidemiology of psychological problems in the elderly. *Canadian Journal of Psychiatry*, *51*, 185–91.

Streiner, D.L. and Norman, G.R. (2009a) *PDQ Epidemiology*. 3rd ed. Shelton, CT: PMPH US.

Streiner, D.L. and Norman, G.R. (2009) Randomized controlled trials. *Community Oncology*, *6*, 83–5.

Streiner, D.L., Patten, S.B., Anthony, J.C., and Cairney, J. (2010) Has "lifetime prevalence" reached the end of its life? An examination of the concept. *International Journal of Methods in Psychiatric Research*, *18*, 221–8.

Thompson, A., and Temple, N.J. (2004) The case for statins: Has it really been made? *Journal of the Royal Society of Medicine*, *97*, 461–4.

United Nations (n.d.) Demographic yearbook. Retrieved from http://unstats.un.org/unsd/demographic/products/dyb/dyb2008.htm.

11 Quantitative Methods: Analysis

Charles H. Goldsmith

CHAPTER OUTLINE

Introduction

The basic purpose of this chapter is to prepare you to handle the data you will gather when you conduct a study in the health sciences. Without data your ideas will not be well respected; your readers or listeners will not be convinced you know that your arguments matter to health and people. Having data means that you must have defined what your concepts mean and can be turned into measurements. This is the basis of measurement and shows that the numbers have properties that reflect something about what you mean. Assignment of numbers to things is used to reflect a property of the thing, one of its essences. **Statistics** is the study of the proper use of statistical principles that allows one to understand the data in such a way as to display ideas about various properties. This chapter minimizes use of formulas and equations so you should have access to a credible statistical computing package such as **Minitab** 16. A statistical package such as Minitab has been put through extensive peer review and has had many users that have made suggestions to ensure that it uses computing formulas correctly so you do not need to remember them. Your task is to enter data correctly, choose from computer output the numbers that make sense for your study, and incorporate them in your study report.

Types of Data

Data are numbers that represent some feature of the thing you are measuring. The process of assigning numbers to the thing is called **measurement** and there are several ways this can be done. If the number represents a label for a category and the categories are **mutually exclusive** and **exhaustive**, the data are called **nominal**. Integers are generally used to label the categories, but the numbers do not make use of any other number properties. Any distinct number for each of the categories will work. One can sort the data into groups where the numbers are the same but that is all. One should not interpret the numbers to be anything other than a category label. A common example of such categories is the variable gender: Male, and Female. While the numbers could be 1 = Male and 2 = Female; however, you should not infer that Females are twice as good as Males since the categorization does not have that meaning and hence the numbers do not. Patients are often given disease labels and the numbers used to designate these labels are also nominal.

If the categories of things can be ordered in some way such as smaller to larger, before or later, or severity of a disease, then the numbers assigned to these categories should also reflect the ordering property. These numbers are called an **ordinal** scale. Numbers as labels for the categories allow one to sort by the size of the number and these then reflect the ordering property. An example of

such a scale is patient status: Dead, Moribund, or Alive. The numbers I might use are 1 = Dead, 2 = Moribund, and 3 = Alive. While these numbers are interpreted as dead being less than moribund and moribund less than alive, the number labels do not reflect any other number properties. Most humans prefer that order rather than the reverse!

If the categories of things can be put into groups that are equally spaced, and so are the numbers assigned to the categories, then the scale is called **interval**. This is because differences between the categories should have the same meaning regardless of where on the scale the difference is obtained. An example of this is the Celsius (C) temperature scale. The difference between 10 and 20 degrees C is the same as the difference between 70 and 80 degrees C.

The highest level scale with the most mathematical properties is the **ratio** scale, because ratios make sense for the numbers assigned to the categories. Ratio scales have meaningful zeros, as the zero reflects absence of the property being measured. An example of this scale is weight in kilograms. A weight of 15 relative to 5 is 3 and this means that the 15 kg object is 3 times the weight of the 5 kg object. Here zero means the object has no weight or mass.

The names of the four scales of measurement start with the letters **NOIR** and one should remember them as the word for black in French. The scale properties are summarized in Table 11.1 where the properties are columns and the scale names are rows. The table entries indicate whether the property is present for that scale.

Prior to using these scales of measurement, there may be some verbal description of concepts; however, they lack any of these scale properties so are NOT classified as measurement. The main reason why these scales of measurement matter is that they dictate the mathematical properties of the numbers assigned to the categories and so dictate which operations can be done statistically

TABLE 11.1   Scales of Measurement

Name/Property	Category Type	Order	Equal Intervals	Meaningful Ratios
Nominal	Yes	No	No	No
Ordinal	Yes	Yes	No	No
Interval	Yes	Yes	Yes	No
Ratio	Yes	Yes	Yes	Yes

with these data. I can count the objects that fall into categories with the same numerical label generated from nominal scales, and I can convert these counts into proportions and percentages, but I cannot use other operations such as sorting by order, addition, subtraction, multiplication, and division, as well as operations that depend on these properties. The counting operation can be done with all the scales. Since I add the property of order to get the ordinal scale, data from such scales and higher (interval and ratio) can be sorted from smallest to largest (or whatever concept is ordered) and so anything that needs ordering for computation can be conducted on the numbers from these scales, such as the order statistics and functions of them. Notice that this leaves out numbers that come from nominal scales, but no others. For scales that have the interval property, interval, and ratio scales, the operations of addition, subtraction, multiplication, and division can be conducted to maintain the meaning behind the numbers. This is a large number of operations done statistically so most data that are at least interval can be handled in a multitude of ways. Finally, if your data are ratio, they have the most properties and allow for more statistical operations to be computed, which include using ratios to illustrate concepts such as relative amounts of the property being measured.

One other classification for data is whether they are discrete or continuous. **Discrete** data use integers to represent the categories while numbers between the integers do not make sense. However

PRACTICAL TIP

A related discussion about the scales of measurement can be found in Chapter 7 on Measurement, The Process of Measurement Section, by D.L. Streiner. Similar words for the terms are used; however, the examples are different than those contained here.

the concept of **continuous** means that for every pair of distinct numbers used it is possible to insert another number between them and that new number makes sense for the variable being measured. For example, the coding used for the Gender example was the numbers 1 and 2. It does not make sense to have a number like 1.5 as there are exactly two genders and there is no number in between; consequently gender is a discrete variable. On the other hand two distinct weights of 5 and 6 kg could have a number such as 5.8 kg between them and this number makes sense, so weight is a continuous variable.

Data Used in This Chapter

To keep things simple, I have chosen some data collected in a study to determine if either or both isometric exercises or a sleeping neck pillow support would help patients who had chronic neck pain. You may know that neck pain is the second leading reason why people are off work in Canada.

The data were selected from one of four groups of patients who were in the study I helped to conduct. The data are listed in Appendix 1 (see page 231). and you should try to enter these data into Minitab to do the graphing and computations that are being shown in this chapter. Since the data entry is a common task that most are now familiar with because computers are so common, this task will not be discussed in detail here. I assume that you can get the documentation that comes with Minitab to get the data entered properly.

The data are taken from the group of n = 34 randomized patients who were to be in the group that was called the control group. This group did not get exercises or sleeping pillows for the study duration. More details about the study can be found in Helewa et al. (2007) (The use of n is common in statistical reporting as the size of the group data, often called the **sample size**.) The data were entered as columns in Minitab with the first column called ID for the identification of the patient with numbers that varied from 1 to 34; the second column called Sex which contains codes of 1 = Male and 2 = Female; the third column called Age was the patient's age in years at study entry recorded as two digits; and the fourth column called NPQ for the Northwick Park Neck Pain Questionnaire (NPQ) at study entry recorded as two digits. The NPQ scores came from 9 questions about neck pain that were scored from 1 to 5 and these nine scores were added to create a total score that could vary from a minimum of 9 to a maximum of 45, with higher numbers denoting more neck pain symptoms. The therapies in the study were designed to reduce the NPQ scores in patients. For these variables, Sex was nominal and discrete, Age was ratio and continuous while NPQ was interval and discrete. Notice that NPQ does not have a 0 on the scale and so one should not read into the data that patients with a total score of 9 have absence of any pain and the ratios of total scores make sense.

Graph Your Data

The first step in understanding your data is to **graph** them with some common tools that allow you to see data patterns. Humans can see patterns easily even if they are not present in the data, and so you need to learn how to decide whether a pattern is worth paying attention to during the revelation of the story your data have to tell. (Notice that data is a plural word; datum, from Latin, is singular.) You need to learn what patterns to look for in your data and then how they can be used to tell if this matters to your study. Graphs called **Pareto charts**, **stem and leaf plots** (SLP), **box plots,** and **scatter plots** will be used to display your data and help you find patterns in your data. To create these graphs, you will need to learn how to enter your data into Minitab and then have Minitab plot the graph for you. Once your data are plotted you should concentrate on finding the relevant patterns in the plot.

The first graph to be shown is a Pareto chart. With data from the Sex variable, I clicked on Quality Tools and then Pareto Chart in Minitab and put the Sex variable in the location to get it plotted. The resulting graph is shown as Figure 11.1.

Notice that the Sex code at the bottom (on the **x axis**) put the group labelled with 2 before the group coded as 1 because the Count was larger. The Pareto chart plots the groups in the data from largest to smallest counts from left to right. There were 19 females (56 per cent) and 15 males (44 per cent). The left **y axis** shows the counts and the right y axis shows the cumulative percentages. In the plot, the left bar is drawn to the height of 19 (using the left hand y axis) and the right bar is drawn to height of 15 (also using the left hand y axis). The dot at the top of the left hand bar starts at about 55 per cent (using the right hand y axis) and ends at 100 per cent above the right bar (also using the right y axis). The Pareto chart can be extended to more than two categories of a nominal scale.

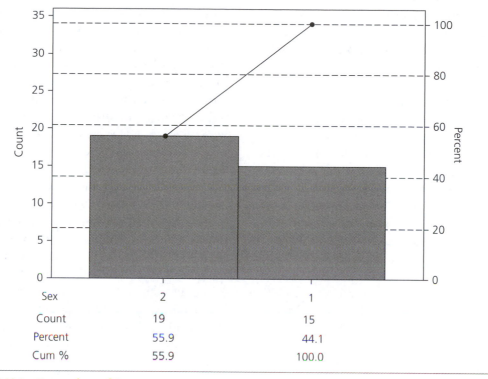

FIGURE 11.1   Pareto chart of Sex

The Pareto chart is particularly useful for nominal data as it does not pay attention to the numerical coding and uses the counts of the codes to create the plot.

The second graph is a stem and leaf plot (SLP). SLP can be used whenever the scale of measurement is at least ordinal (including interval and ratio) as the chart sorts the data from the smallest to the largest to create the order statistics, and then creates the graph out of the ordered data. I will use the Age variable in Minitab to create this plot. In Minitab, click on Stat and then **Exploratory Data Analysis** (EDA) and choose Stem and Leaf plot. This produces output in the Session window that is displayed next.

Stem-and-Leaf Display: Age

Stem-and-leaf of Age N = 34

Leaf Unit = 1.0

1	3	4
5	3	7999
10	4	13344
11	4	9
16	5	11444
(2)	5	79
16	6	012223344
7	6	5677899

The interpretation of the SLP is as follows: the variable plotted is named as Age with a sample size of 34; however, Minitab prints it as a capital N. If you want your output to have the lower case n, you need to edit it in your report. On the next row of output is the leaf unit, which means in this case it is in the units position of a two-digit number.

Depths in the first column reading downward are the **cumulative frequencies**: 1 in the first row, 5 in the second row, down to the 2 in round brackets. Similarly from the bottom of the first column, the last row is 7 and the second last row is 16 until the 2 in round brackets is encountered. One can check that the entire sample size has all been plotted by adding the numbers on either side of the number or numbers in the round brackets as well as the numbers in the rounded brackets to get 16+2+16 = 34, the sample size. These depths are handy for reading off the order statistics if you want to use them. The second column shows the stems. Notice that they are repeats of the numbers 3 to 6. The first three place holds for leaves that are between 0 and 4 while the second three place holds for leaves between 5 and 9. In this case there is one leaf next to the first three, indicating that the age of 34 years is the youngest person in this sample. This also accounts for the 1 in the first column to the left of the first three. The reason there is a 5 in the first column of the second row is because 1 + 4 = 5; there are four leaves in the second row that indicate there was one patient who was 37 and three who were 39 years for Age.

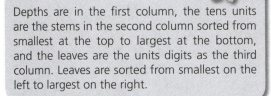

PRACTICAL TIP

Depths are in the first column, the tens units are the stems in the second column sorted from smallest at the top to largest at the bottom, and the leaves are the units digits as the third column. Leaves are sorted from smallest on the left to largest on the right.

This plot is akin to asking for age groups of length five years. Minitab lets you pick lengths of 1, 2, 5, or 10 to create a graph the shape you find most appealing for your data display. Once printed the SLP can be rotated 90 degrees counter clockwise to show a **distribution** of the data. At the bottom of the SLP you notice that there are seven leaves, one each of 5, 6, and 8 and two for each of 7 and 9. As well, the largest Age comes from the largest leaf 9 in the last stem of 6 to make a patient of Age 69 years in the data set. By inspecting the leaves carefully you can see that there are three locations where there are three leaves together, one at each of 39, 54, and 62. Also the general shape of the overall plot is like a wedge that starts small at the bottom end of the data and grows to be large at the top end of the ages. This is called a **skewed left** distribution. If the shape was flat or in the shape of a bell it would be called **symmetric**, and if the wedge started at the top and went to the bottom it would be called **skewed right**.

Stem and leaf plots can be used for two or more data sets that you want to compare using the same stems, and appear in Minitab output below each other for the different data sets. This will be left as an exercise for those who are interested in seeing how this feature works.

The third graph is a box plot. A box plot is created from the ordered data as was the SLP; however, it highlights some important indicators that take some additional computation with the SLP. It can also be done with more than one group, which will be shown later. I will use the NPQ data to illustrate the box plot and its interpretation. In Minitab, click on the Stat and then EDA (Exploratory Data Analysis) and choose Box plot. This produces the graphical output that is displayed next in Figure 11.2.

Notice the box is plotted vertically. It can be plotted horizontally if required. In Figure 11.2 the bottom of the box is the **lower quartile** while the top is the **upper quartile**. The line in

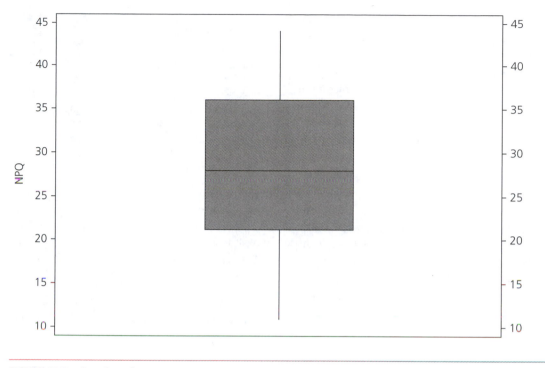

FIGURE 11.2   Boxplot of NPQ

the middle of the box is the **median**. A median cuts the ordered data into two equally frequent parts while the quartiles cut the ordered data into four equally frequent parts. (The median is the second quartile.) The length of the box is called the **interquartile range** (IQR) and is computed as the difference between the upper quartile and the lower quartile. It is important to note that this is a single number, not what is often found in many health journals, which list the lower and upper quartiles separated with a dash (–) but call them the IQR. The lines that extend from the top and bottom of the box are called **whiskers** (think cat). They are plotted from the quartiles outward until the end of the data on that end as long as the data points are not outliers. If the end of the data set contains outliers they will be displayed

as * values on the plot. If one sees them, then they should be examined carefully as they may be **errors** or data points that might be **set aside** (but reported) as they could be from groups other than the group being plotted. In this case the graph shows no outliers, so there are none in the NPQ data for this group. This boxplot also shows that the NPQ data are relatively symmetric, although it might be more obvious if I created a SLP for these data. (This will be left as an exercise for those interested.)

The fourth graph is a scatterplot with a **straight line** superimposed on it. A scatterplot is designed to show the graphical relationship between two **variables** that are both at least ordinal, ideally at least interval. If it is clear that one variable is a **response variable** and the other is an **input variable**, then the response variable should be plotted on the y axis while the input variable is plotted on the x axis.

In Minitab, click on Graph and then Scatterplot with a fitted straight line. This produces the graphical output that is displayed next in Figure 11.3.

Notice that the plot seems to have a relatively even vertical scatter as your eye moves from left to right as Age increases. The straight line seems to have a slight dip as Age increases; however, it looks to be very small. Later I will see if this is supported by a more detailed analysis. If this is correct, then it appears to be that NPQ is not related to Age. If you were still in Minitab before plotting the Figure 11.3 here in this text, you could click on the line to see the magnitude of the **intercept** and **slope**. (This will be shown in

PRACTICAL TIP

Sometimes response variables are called dependent variables and input variables are called independent variables; however, this notation causes problems with new learners when they encounter the concepts of independence and dependence as statistical terms; so this chapter does not use them. In epidemiology usage, the input variables may be called exposure variables and the response variables called disease variables. However, this is not true in this chapter; nor is it generally used that way in statistical texts.

As an example I show a scatterplot of the two variables NPQ and Age from the data set. Since Age cannot be a response to NPQ I have chosen to plot NPQ on the y axis and Age on the x axis. If you would like to see the plot with the axes reversed, that is left as an exercise.

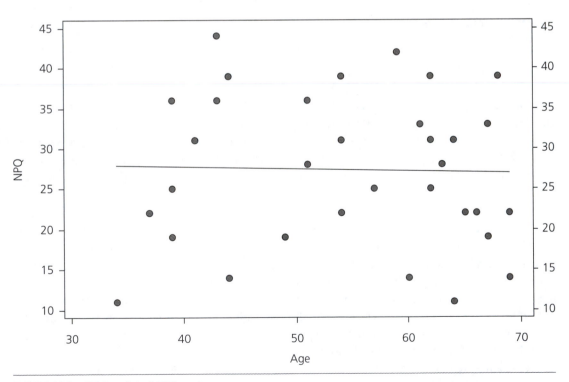

FIGURE 11.3   Scatterplot of NPQ vs Age

a later section when I discuss confidence intervals and hypothesis tests.)

Describe Your Data Numerically

To describe your data you must compute a small set of numbers that communicate the essence of the patterns in your data to reflect the data properties you consider to matter for your study. Usually the numbers are called **descriptive statistics** because they happen to describe properties of the data and their distribution. Some of these properties are the extremes, the location, the variation and the shape the data plot has using symmetry, and tail direction. Sometimes one set of data is compared to another set of data and the properties of the two data sets are compared. This is particularly true when you have two groups in your study. Each group can be described by itself and then the two groups can be compared. You will see how to relate one variable to another using a measure of the **straight line relationship** between them and this is called a **correlation coefficient**. If the straight line is a good summary of the relationship between the variables the slope and intercept are used to describe the equation of the straight line that links the output variable to the input variable. Sometimes these ideas are extended to more than two groups; however, I will use no more than two groups in this chapter.

One Group of Data

If the data you want to describe consists of **one group** you might want to find a set of summary statistics that properly reflect what is important for the set of data. Common measures include the lowest data extreme that is called the **minimum** for the smallest number in the set. To find

and report this number you must make sure that the data are at least ordinal otherwise there is no point of stating that it is a minimum; likewise for the largest observation or **maximum**. Both extremes are at the edges of the SLP as seen in the example for Age where the minimum was 34 and the maximum was 69 years. Sometimes it is useful to compute the difference between the extremes as the maximum minus the minimum; this difference is called the **range** and is a single number. The range is a **measure of variation**. For the Age variable the range is 35 years. The range, as well as many other measures, can be computed by Minitab and printed simultaneously as part of the output. This will be shown later. (Also note that this definition of the range is not always properly shown in health science publications. Like the IQR some journals show the extremes separated with a dash as minimum – maximum but call the two numbers the range.)

Besides the extremes, other locations are often chosen to summarize the data, the most common being near the centre of the data. If the data are at least ordinal then the **median** can be computed as the number that bisects the ordered data into two equally frequent parts. Recall that the median is plotted as the centre line on the boxplot. The median is 28 for the NPQ data while it is 58 years for the Age data. Other commonly used location measures are the other two quartiles. Along with the median partition, the data are ordered into four equally frequent parts. The first and third quartiles define the bottom and top edges of the box in the boxplot. Once the quartiles are known the difference between them is the IQR and is the length of the **middle 50 per cent** of the ordered data. Like range, the IQR is a single number and is also a measure of variation. For the Age data the lower (first) quartile is 43.75, the upper (third) quartile is 64, and the IQR is 20.25 years. The most common measure of location if your data are at least interval is the **mean**, which is also computed in Minitab. It is like the fulcrum of the data if each observation had a weight distributed on a teeter totter with the mean at the balance point or middle. For these data the mean for Age is 54.8 years (rounded to one **decimal place** (dp) even though it may be computed to more) and for NPQ is 27.4. Another common measure of variation is the **standard deviation**, computed by Minitab and is a measure of how much each observation varies from the mean. For the Age data the standard deviation is 10.9 years (also rounded to one dp) and the NPQ is 9.2. Notice that the measuring units are expressed with the summary measures if the units are known.

Sometimes you may want to use more than one measure at a time in your description of the data. Almost always you should report the sample size. It is common to include a central measure of location as well as measure of variation. If the data distribution is symmetric or bell-shaped it is common to include the sample size, mean, and standard deviation with units for the latter two if appropriate. Because the NPQ data looked fairly symmetric the sample size was 34 while the mean was 27.3, and the standard deviation was 9.2. However, because the Age data were not quite symmetric it would be better to use the median and IQR as measures of the location and variation. So a **three number report** would be: a sample size of 34 with a median of 28 and an IQR of 20.25 years. You could also report the IQR 20.2 in the report to one dp to be consistent with other reporting. (A note of caution: some health science journals use a plus/minus (±) between the mean and standard deviation. I and many other biostatisticians think one should not suggest mathematical operations without conducting them for the reader. I have also found that few humans are good doing these computations in their heads, so I recommend against doing so.)

The final summary measure I shall discuss in this chapter is the measure of symmetry called skewness. Minitab computes a skewness measure as part of the descriptive statistics. The skewness measure can vary most commonly between −1 and 1. Values around 0, say between −0.1 and 0.1, usually mean the distribution is close to symmetric while values less than −0.3 indicate that the distribution is **skewed** to the **left** or has a tail that is longer on the left than it is on the right. On the other hand values above 0.3 generally indicate that the distribution of the data is **skewed right** or has a longer tail on the right than on the left. Examples of left skewed data are lifetimes of people and electronic devices such as computers while right skewed data come from the length of stay of patients in a hospital. The skewness measure for the Age data is −0.43, which is less than the criterion of −0.3, and so suggests that the data are left skewed. However, the NPQ data have a skewness measure of −0.08 which is between −0.1 and 0.1 suggesting that the distribution is close to symmetric. One can get these two measures by clicking on the skewness measure in the descriptive statistics section of Minitab for these two variables.

If you want more numbers in your summary then a **five-number summary** would add the extremes to the sample size, mean and standard deviation or to the sample size, median, and IQR. Even others would use the extremes added to the three quartiles without computing the IQR. Note again that the median is the second quartile. Of course it is possible to include either the SLP or boxplot as a graph for your summary. Once you have made your choice as to the form of your summary, describe it in the Methods section of your report (see later) and report the numbers in a table if there is more than one variable. If there is only one variable include it in a sentence without losing space to a table. An example of the extremes, sample size, mean, and standard deviation is: for the Age measured in years, the sample size was 34, the minimum 34, mean 54.8, standard deviation 10.9, and maximum 69. As a form using medians and quartiles because the data were not symmetric: for the Age variable, the sample size was 34, the minimum 34, lower quartile 43.75, median 58, upper quartile 64, and maximum 69 years. One could also round the lower quartile to 43.8 to one dp like the other location measures. Notice that this form has six numbers and some books and journals would drop the sample size to make the summary into five measured numbers. Be sure to check with the journal where you plan to publish your report to see if they have a preference for one of these formats.

Two Groups of Data

If one wanted to describe **two groups** of data the same descriptive statistics can be used with Minitab. All it takes is to have the data you want as output in a single column such as what was already done for the Age and NPQ data; however, I need another column such as the Sex column with two levels to create the two groups of interest for either the Age or NPQ data. Minitab is a column oriented statistical package and as such you can create descriptive statistics for each group separately with the software. The commands are similar except the subset variable (Sex) is used to create the two groups. They are Stat>Descriptive Statistics using Age for the Variable, Sex for the By variable, and clicking Statistics for the sample size, mean, standard deviation, minimum, maximum, and median. From these you can create the number summaries for Males and Females as follows:

Descriptive Statistics: Age

Variable	Sex	N	Mean	StDev	Minimum	Median	Maximum
Age	1	15	54.80	9.24	39.00	54.00	67.00
	2	19	54.84	12.30	34.00	61.00	69.00

From this output you can see the minimum for males (coded 1) is 39 while for the females (coded 2) it is 34; similarly the maximum is 67 for males and 69 for females. So the females have more spread in their data than the males. Notice also that the male median of 54 is seven years younger than the female median at 61; yet the means are close to each other. The female standard deviation is slightly larger at 12.3 than for the males at 9.2. Some of these features can be also seen in the boxplot computed for each group in the same plot shown next. The Minitab commands for this are Graph>Boxplots>With Groups and choosing the Graph variable as Age and the Categories variables as Sex.

Notice that the middle line (median) of the box for the females (coded 2) is higher than for the males (coded 1) and length of the box is larger for the females than the males indicating slightly more variation. This plot supports what was seen with the grouped descriptive statistics.

Correlation

One reason why someone might conduct such a study is to see whether one variable is related to another variable. A measure of the straight line relationship between two variables is called a **correlation coefficient**. The word starts with letters "co" to indicate it is a relationship of two measures at a time. The correlation coefficient comes in many forms, the most common being the product moment correlation coefficient. (I will not discuss the other types of correlation

PRACTICAL TIP

The use of > between the different parts of the pull down menus means that you need to click on each heading to get the procedure you want to use.

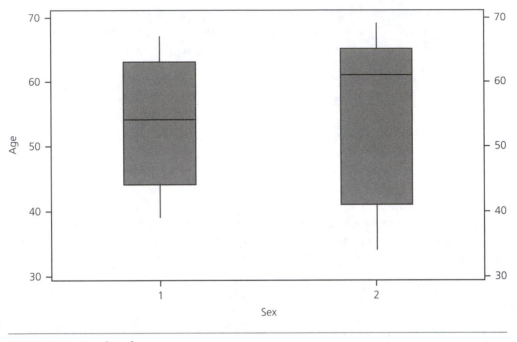

FIGURE 11.4   Boxplot of age

coefficients in this chapter.) When I mention correlation in this chapter, I mean the product moment correlation coefficient. The two variables should be each measured on scales that are at least ordinal, and ideally at least interval to make the correlation coefficient easy to interpret. Minitab computes the correlation coefficient when you specify the two variables. Correlation is written as a numerical value between −1 and 1. When values are close to 0, say between −0.2 and 0.2, it is likely that there is no straight line relationship between the two variables; however, the relationship can be more complicated and still have a correlation value close to 0. Positive values above 0.2 generally show that the straight line is going up to the right when you investigate a scatterplot of the two variables. Values between 0.2 and 0.5 are called moderate, values between

0.5 and 0.7 are large and those above 0.7 to 1 are considered to be very large. Negative values have a similar interpretation; however, the straight line goes down to the right when looking at the scatterplot.

To compute the correlation from the data we have in this chapter using Minitab, click on Stat>Basic Statistics>Correlation and then select NPQ and Age to produce the output:

Correlations: NPQ, Age

Pearson correlation of NPQ and Age = −0.032

Notice that the numerical value is −0.032 and since this is between −0.2 and 0.2 we conclude that the plot of NPQ versus Age is not a straight line pattern; even though we will indeed fit a straight line to these data as a regression equation next.

The Regression Equation

Recall that Figure 11.3 plotted using a scatterplot for the NPQ values against Age and there was a straight line in the plot as well. If you want to see the equation of that straight line, it can be obtained in Minitab by using the commands Stat>Regression>Regression and choosing NPQ as the Response variable and Age as the Predictor variable. The output is:

The **regression equation** is
NPQ = 28.9 – 0.028 Age

Predictor	Coef	SE Coef	T	P
Constant	28.863	8.369	3.45	0.002
Age	–0.0275	0.1498	–0.18	0.855

From this output I can see that the intercept of the straight line is 28.9 and the slope of the straight line is –0.028. I will look at the rest of the output later in the sections on confidence intervals and hypothesis testing. (Indeed the large p value of 0.855 suggests that the straight line in age does not predict NPQ well.)

Create Confidence Intervals for Your Data

As well as descriptive data for point estimates, you may wish to have a way to express your conclusion as an interval on the same scale as the original data that you collected. A **confidence interval** (CI) is such a statement, usually computed at the confidence coefficient of 95 per cent. This means that 95 per cent of the time the true value in the population will be contained in the interval if the study were to be repeated many times. Usually a study is conducted once where the interval bounds are created from the one study; however, one still expresses confidence with an interval that should contain the truth. A CI is described by two numbers: a **lower bound** and an **upper bound**, and

is called a **two-sided confidence interval**. (One-sided confidence intervals will not be discussed here.) Minitab computes these bounds for you when you select the proper type of parameter you want to use for the creation of the CI. A **parameter** is a characteristic of a distribution of a variable in a population that was used to generate the sample.

Ideally your sample should be **selected at random** or created as part of a **randomized controlled trial** to ensure the groups represent the population. Without this random feature your sample might be biased and hence your CI may not reflect what is happening in the population. Another assumption that one often uses is that your data are an **independent sample** from the population. Generally if the observations in your sample are selected from distinct objects being measured, independence is satisfied. (This does not have the same meaning as an independent variable and so the latter is avoided in this chapter.)

For some CIs the data themselves need to be **normally distributed** for the CI to cover the parameter with the interval. If all three of these assumptions are satisfied, one says assuming the sample is RIN for random, independent, and normally distributed. (There are more advanced statistical procedures for checking these assumptions; however, they will not be covered in this chapter.)

Finally a CI is a statement about a characteristic in a population that was used to generate the sample and as such is called a **statistical inference**, rather than a descriptive statistic that was used to describe the sample of data selected from the population. The value 95 per cent is called the 95 per cent **confidence coefficient**, and could be chosen with other high numbers such a 90 per cent or 99 per cent; however, 95 per cent is commonly used. If you read newspapers or listen to TV news, you might hear about surveys of the population that report findings are precise to within some stated percentage points 19 times out of 20; well 19/20 = 0.95 and this expression of a proportion is scaled up by 100 to a percentage when discussing CIs.

For the first example of a CI, suppose I was interested in the population interval from which the sample of females and males were drawn as I wanted to estimate the proportion of females. I know from Figure 11.1 and the Pareto chart that there were 19 females in the sample size of 34. Going to Minitab in Stat>Descriptive Statistics>1 Proportion>Summarized, I note from the data that 19 is entered as the numerator and 34 as the denominator. The output gives the sample proportion as 0.558824 and the 95 per cent CI as (0.378858, 0.728150). I can recognize that the proportion (shown as a percentage) from the Pareto output, which was 55.9 per cent, is also the proportion as seen in the CI output. However, for a report it would be fine to record this as 0.56 with a 95 per cent CI as (0.38, 0.73). Notice that the interval is expressed with round brackets and there is a comma between the two boundaries. (Some health science journals like to use a dash rather than a comma; however, this is not a good practice since it may be confused with a negative sign.) So in the population I should expect that the percentage of females to be between 38 and 73 per cent. Notice that this interval also contains the value of 50 per cent, which would be the value for an equal distribution of both males and females. The **assumptions** needed for this CI are R and I, which I have used since this group came from a randomized trial and the 34 patients were separate individuals so they are independent. (I did not need to assume normality for this CI as the computations do not depend on this assumption.) Suppose you want to report a 95 per cent CI for the mean of the population from which the 34 patients were selected for the NPQ values. Assuming this is a random sample from independent patients and that the NPQ values are normally distributed, the 95 per cent CI can

be computed from the 1 sample t-test in Minitab as Stat>Basic Statistics>1 Sample t and clicking on the column where the NPQ data are stored to get n = 34, mean = 27.35, 95 per cent CI (24.13, 30.58) which can be rounded for a report to mean = 27.4, 95 per cent CI (24.1, 30.6) years. I do not compute a 95 per cent CI for the Age data as they are skewed and hence likely do not satisfy the assumption of normality, even though they would satisfy R and I. Minitab does not compute a CI for the median, so I will not use Minitab to get one. A book by Hubbard (2011) shows how to do it if you need to create one. Confidence intervals can be computed for any parameter one wants in a population; however, you might have to search in different software packages to get them computed as easily as they are done in Minitab.

From the regression output when I plotted NPQ versus Age, the output showed that the slope was -0.0275 with **standard error** (SE) of 0.1498. If I assume a Student's t **criterion value** of t (0.975, df = 32) = 2.037 (I can get this in Minitab; however it will not be shown how here.) I can compute the 95 per cent CI bounds for the slope as: lower bound = −0.0275 − (2.037)(0.1498) = −0.0275 −0.3051 = −0.3326 or rounded to −0.33; likewise the upper bound is −0.0275 + (2.037)(0.1498) = −0.0275 + 0.3051 = 0.2776 or rounded to 0.28. So in summary the slope is −0.03 with a 95 per cent CI of (−0.33, 0.28). Notice that this CI contains 0 so it supports the fact the slope could be 0 in the population from which these data were selected. In other words NPQ has no straight line relationship with Age.

(Version 16 of Minitab does not compute this CI. If one is interested in an **approximate CI** for the slope and the sample size is at least 30 then one could use the value 2 instead of the t criterion value of 2.037. This would result in the CI bounds being lower bound = −0.0275 − (2)(0.1498) = −0.0275 − 0.2996 = −0.3271, or rounded to −0.33; likewise the upper bound is −0.0275 + (2)(0.1498) = -0.0275 + 0.2996 = 0.2721 or rounded to 0.27.

So in summary the slope is –0.03 with a 95 per cent CI of (–0.33, 0.27). Notice that this is very close to the exact calculation shown earlier.)

It is also possible to compute a confidence interval for the **difference between the means** of the males and females as two groups with some additional assumptions. Within each group the RIN assumptions should be met and the groups should also be independent of each other. This usually means that the two groups contain different subjects or units being measured. The Minitab commands to generate the confidence output are Stat>Basic Statistics>2 Sample t and for Samples in One Column insert Age for Samples and Sex for Subscripts; also checking the box for **equal variances**. The output gives a 95 per cent CI for the difference between males and females as (–7.83, 7.74) which may be rounded to (–7.8, 7.7). Notice that 0 is contained in this interval, so the male and female ages are likely not different in the population from which these samples were selected.

Test Your Hypothesis

Hypothesis testing is another way to draw an inference about the population from which the sample of data was collected. Testing will be done in a series of steps. Step 1 is to compute a test statistic (that Minitab will do). Step 2 is to compute a p value from the test statistic from a suitable **referent distribution** (that Minitab will also do). Step 3 is to compare the p value to a **criterion standard** called α, alpha, the first letter of the Greek alphabet. The value of α is set by you the experimenter; however, the choice of 0.05 is very common in the health sciences literature. Here I will use two-sided p values that are the standard printed by Minitab. Step 4 is the interpretation where if the p value is less than the alpha value the hypothesis is rejected in the population and said to be **statistically significant**. If the p value

is larger than alpha, then the hypothesis cannot be rejected in the population. (Drawing a conclusion for the population when the p value is larger than alpha depends on the power of the test and the sample size for the study. These issues will not be discussed in this chapter.) Generally one creates a **null hypothesis** that one expects to be rejected. This null hypothesis is a parameter statement that is specific to the needs of the analysis and is usually a single number for the parameter in the population. It is compared to the **alternative hypothesis**, which generally contains all the rest of the values that the parameter could take on in the population. The p value computed from the referent distribution is usually done as two-sided, or what is called a **two-tailed test**, because both larger as well as smaller values of the test statistic can lead to rejection of the null hypothesis.

For example, suppose I wanted to test that the proportion of females in the population was 0.5 and I wanted to use the data from Figure 11.1, where the sample contained 34 patients, of which 19 were female and 14 were male. Suppose I chose alpha as 0.05 and the sample was RI; random and independent. To do the test in Minitab, click Stat>Basic Statistics>1 Proportion and then enter 19 as the Number of Events, 34 as the Number of Trials and check the box for Perform Hypothesis Test and enter 0.5. The output is:

Test and CI for One Proportion

Test of p = 0.5 vs p not = 0.5

Sample	X	N	Exact p-value	95% CI	p value
1	19	34	0.558824	0.378858, 0.728150	0.608

Notice that the output claims the test p = 0.5 vs. p not = 0.5. The latter includes all values between 0 and 1 except the value 0.5 and is the alternative, while the former is the null. Notice that the estimated proportion is printed along with the 95 per cent CI and the p value of 0.608. Since 0.608 is > 0.05, the value of alpha, I cannot reject the null hypothesis. So I conclude that the population could be 50 per cent female. Notice that the p value is said to be exact, because it is computed from a **binomial distribution** exactly and not an approximation as the binomial is the exact referent distribution. (Sometimes the p value is computed from a referent distribution that is an approximation to the exact distribution when the exact distribution is unknown or when it is difficult to compute.)

This time I consider hypothesis testing for the mean. Suppose I thought that the population had patients with NPQ scores with a mean of 35 that I set as the null hypothesis. Again I can use Minitab with Stat>Basic Statistics>1 Sample t, clicking on the box for Hypothesis testing and entering 35 into the box. The output is:

One-Sample t: NPQ

Test of $\mu = 35$ vs not $= 35$

Variable	N	Mean	StDev	SE Mean	95% CI	t	p
NPQ	34	27.35	9.24	1.58	(24.13, 30. 58)	−4.83	0.000

This time the output suggests that the test of the null hypothesis is $\mu = 35$ vs not $= 35$ as the alternative. Here μ is the Greek letter for mean. The output also consists of showing the test statistic as −4.83 and the p value is 0.000. This p value is impossible for a report so the convention is to express it as $p < 0.001$ with a 1 in the last dp of the output. Since this is less than 0.05, the null hypothesis is rejected and the conclusion is that the population mean is NOT 35. The assumptions needed for this test are RIN, and they seem to be satisfied.

Suppose I want to see if the ages by gender are the same in the population by testing that the population means for males and females are the same as

the null hypothesis and that they are different as the alternative. The Minitab commands to generate the p value output are Stat>Basic Statistics>2 Sample t and for Samples in One Column insert Age for Samples and Sex for Subscripts; also checking the box for **equal variances**. The output is:

Two-Sample t-Test and CI: Age, Sex

Two-sample t for Age

Sex	N	Mean	StDev	SE Mean
1	15	54.80	9.24	2.4
2	19	54.84	12.3	2.8

Difference $= \mu(1) - \mu(2)$

Estimate for difference: −0.04

95 per cent CI for difference: (−7.83, 7.74)

t-test of difference $= 0$ (vs not $=$): t value $= -0.01$, p value $= 0.991$, DF $= 32$

Both use pooled StDev $= 11.0636$

The null hypothesis of no difference between the male and female population means is set to 0 and the alternative is not $= 0$. Notice that the test statistic is −0.01 and the p value is 0.991 with 32 df. While it does not say so the reason for the value of df $= 32$ is that the referent distribution needs this value to compute the correct p value. Because the equal variance box was checked the pooled standard deviation was used to create this test statistic. Since the p value of 0.991 > 0.05, the null hypothesis cannot be rejected. It is reasonable to conclude that the population means are similar.

To test the null hypothesis that the correlation coefficient is 0, one can use Minitab to get the output for correlations as I did to get the summary statistic: click on Stat>Basic Statistics>Correlation and then select NPQ and Age to produce the output and it is printed as a p value along with the summary statistic. Since 0.855 > 0.05, we are unable to reject the null hypothesis that the population correlation is zero.

Pearson correlation of NPQ and Age = −0.032

p value = 0.855

The regression example can be used to test the null hypothesis that the slope of the line is 0 vs not = 0. The same output is reproduced that was used to create the 95 per cent CI for the slope as:

The regression equation is

NPQ = 28.9 − 0.028 Age

Predictor	Coef	SE Coef	t	p
Constant	28.863	8.369	3.45	0.002
Age	−0.0275	0.1498	−0.18	0.855

Now the test statistic for the slope is −0.18 with a p value of 0.855. Since 0.855 > 0.05 I am unable to reject the null hypothesis that the slope is 0. So I conclude the slope could be zero in the population.

Some health science journals like confidence intervals and some like p values, some allow either or both to be used. You should be comfortable creating both so as not to restrict where you publish your report findings. Similar conclusions should be obtained from the two ways of dealing with samples from populations as long as the alpha value used is the compliment of the confidence coefficient, 0.95 on the probability scale vs 95 per cent on the percentage scale. The assumptions needed for each are essentially the same. I like to use both confidence intervals and p values to accommodate the readers who prefer one over the other.

Be careful when your data come from samples that are not from randomized trials or are not randomly selected from a known population as the samples may be biased for the things you want to say about the population. A safe rule of thumb for your studies is when there is choice, randomize or randomly sample. Otherwise some form of selection bias may be the thing that is being measured and not differences between the groups you think are there. (I will not discuss how to randomize in this chapter; however, the strategy can be found in many basic biostatistics books.)

Write Your Report

Once you have completed your graphing and analyses you should be in a position to write a **report** on your findings so your results will be available to others who may be interested. If you have funding to conduct your study, there is a moral obligation to make your findings available to others who may have provided the funding, and to the general public if your research support came from public taxes. Ideally you should try to publish your findings in some medium that is open to the public such as journals, websites, professional meetings, and talks you may give about your study.

If you are writing a report that may see its way into a journal you should look at the format that the journal requires for papers that appear in it. A common format is: **Introduction**, **Methods**, **Results**, and **Discussion**, or the phrase **IMRaD**, created from the first letters of the headings. In the Introduction you might state why you did the study and what was known about the topic area or research question before your study was designed. This might include a summary of the literature that you read over about the ideas relevant to your study. It could include a research question such as **PICOST**, where P is for **Patients** (or subjects), I is for the **Intervention**, C is for the **Comparison**, O is for the **Outcome**, S is for the **Study** design, and T is for the **Time** the outcome was measured. This section helps to put your study into the context of the world literature. You should be able to read your research question out loud in a single breath. It could serve as your elevator talk when telling others about your study.

In the Methods section you would state all the things that are relevant to allow an intelligent reader who knows the research area to assess what you did and answer the questions Who, What, Why, When, Where, and How, the W^5H. Any measurement instruments should be described and referenced as to their relevant measurement properties: **reliability**, **validity**, and **responsiveness**. Any statistical methods and software used to handle the data and analyses should be documented. Some health science journals require these details for the statistical reviewer, and then do not make them available to the typical reader; however, I think they should do so. It is useful to document the computer used as it sometimes plays a role in the veracity of the findings. A subsection on Statistical Methods might be appropriate if your analyses are unusual and need to be documented using the statistical literature to make them transparent to readers.

The Results section is where the detailed findings of your study should be reported. Things like a **CONSORT** (Schultz et al., 2010) flow chart and check sheet should be included along with any relevant tables and graphs to understand the study results (Schulz, K.F, et al). This is where your descriptive statistics, confidence intervals, hypothesis tests, and graphs are reported. You might want to use the graphs you created to show the key study findings and leave the other graphs to a presentation. Tables are often better in written reports than graphs as graphs often need more explanation of the details.

The Discussion section is where you attempt to interpret your findings. This should include a brief summary of your findings in less detail than the results section; how your findings relate to what was known before in the literature, which you summarized in the Introduction; the strengths and weaknesses of your study; and your findings as well as the impact on future research and the health of people if that is why you did your study.

The final paragraph could be a summary of what your study adds to the world literature.

Some journals require a format other than IMRaD, so you should check the journal requirements before you write your report by looking at the journal's **website** and **Instructions to Authors**. This can prevent much grief when it comes to writing your report. Before you submit your report, ask a friendly colleague to read over your report to see that it makes sense and meets the requirements for the journal where you would like to see it submitted.

Software

While I have used Minitab 16 to do the computations for the examples in this chapter, there are many other highly developed statistical packages that will do the same things. Another very good package is JMP 8 from the SAS Corporation. Both Minitab and JMP require you to get a paid copy for your own computer; however, many university computer laboratories have such packages available free for students registered in suitable courses that use these packages. If you do not have the resources to buy or rent your own copy of Minitab or JMP, you might consider an open source package called R. R is a little more complicated to use than either Minitab or JMP; however, it is used by statisticians throughout the world to do their research and eventually every useful statistical technique appears on it to do the computations you may need. You may want to Google R to see how to download your own copy.

Extensions and More Complicated Analyses

There are sometimes other things that constitute a statistical analysis because the data collected may not be handled by the methods I have used in this chapter. This could be because the outcome variables are not handled by the methods I have described, there are more than two groups, or the data may need a more complicated model than the simple straight line function I showed in this chapter. For these, there are references to more advanced books, which have been shown to be helpful for handling more complicated data and multiple variable models of more complexity.

Books such Altman (1991) and Kleinbaum et al. (1998) cover more methods for handling these as well as other types of quantitative statistical techniques, many of which can be conducted with Minitab.

Summary

- This chapter describes scales of measurement and how when they are used to collect data in the health sciences a reader might use a statistical package such as Minitab to compute descriptive statistics, create graphs and reports on one or two variables collected in a health sciences study.
- Descriptive statistics include extremes, quartiles, mean, median, mode, standard deviation, skewness, confidence intervals, simple hypothesis tests, and graphical techniques to display single and two group data such as stem leaf plots and scatterplots.
- Simple straight line regression and the product moment correlation are described to graph and model two variables.

Review Questions

1. What scale of measurement is the set of scales of measurement in Table 11.1?

2. What scale of measurement is time at a location? What scale of measurement is a time interval, such as how long a task took to complete?

3. Create a SLP for the NPQ data. What do you see in the plot? Try to change the number of leaves per stem and decide on what plot you like best and why.

4. Discuss whether you think that using random digit dialling with a telephone selects a random sample from the population of Canadians.

5. Do you think that two measurements conducted on the same patient are independent of each other?

6. What is the impact on the two-sample 95 per cent CI if you had coded Females as 1 and Males as 2 instead of what was used?

7. Create a two-group SLP by using the By command as Sex in Minitab with the Age data.

8. Create a SLP for the NPQ data. Try varying the number of leaves per stem with 1, 2, 5, and 10, and choose the plot you like the best. Why did you like the one you chose?

9. Create a scatterplot of Age versus NPQ with a straight line superimposed. Compare this plot with Figure 11.3. What if anything did you learn from this plot and its comparison with Figure 11.3?

10. What is meant by a 90 per cent CI for a parameter?

11. What word would you use to describe a correlation coefficient of size −0.6?

12. For the regression output from the straight line fit of NPQ on Age, test the null hypothesis that the intercept is zero vs. the alternative that it is not zero. Use alpha of 10 per cent.

13. Compute a 95 per cent CI and get a p value to see if there is no difference between male and female NPQ scores in the population from which these data were selected. What assumptions did you make?

14. Discuss the difference between a p value and the alpha level.

15. Find the reporting format for a health sciences journal you regularly read and compare it to IMRaD.

References

Altman, D.G. (1991) *Practical Statistics for Medical Research*. London, UK: Chapman and Hall.

Helewa, A., Goldsmith, C.H., Smythe, H.A., Lee, P., Obright, K., Stitt, L.W. (2007) Effect of therapeutic exercise and sleeping neck support on patients with chronic neck pain. A randomized clinical trial. *Journal of Rheumatology*, 34(1):151–158.

Hubbard, D.W. (2011) *How to Measure Anything. Finding the Value of Intangibles in Business*. Toronto, ON: Wiley.

Kleinbaum, D.G., Kupper, L.L., Muller, K.E., and Nizam, A. (1998) *Applied Regression Analysis and Other Multivariable Methods*. Pacific Grove CA: Duxbury Press.

Schulz, K.F., Altman, D.G., Moher, D., for the CONSORT Group (2010) CONSORT 2010 Statement: Updated guidelines for reporting parallel group randomised trials. *BMC Medicine*, 8, 18.

Appendix 1

Raw data for examples used in this chapter

Row	ID	Sex	Age	NPQ
1	1	2	62	25
2	2	2	37	22
3	3	1	39	19
4	4	2	41	31
5	5	2	51	36
6	6	2	49	19
7	7	2	61	33
8	8	1	43	44
9	9	1	43	36
10	10	2	39	36
11	11	1	44	39
12	12	1	63	28
13	13	2	66	22
14	14	2	59	42
15	15	1	64	11
16	16	2	65	22
17	17	1	54	31
18	18	2	34	11
19	19	1	67	33
20	20	1	54	22
21	21	1	60	14
24	24	1	54	39
25	25	1	62	31
26	26	2	69	22
27	27	2	63	28
28	28	2	64	31
29	29	1	51	28
30	30	2	39	25
31	31	1	57	25
32	32	2	69	14
33	33	2	62	39
34	34	2	68	39

12 Reporting Health Research

Donald C. Cole

CHAPTER OUTLINE

Introduction

Reporting is an essential part of conducting health research. We have a responsibility to share our findings to inform, to guide, to persuade, or to challenge ourselves and others to improve the health of individuals and populations. We may communicate verbally and visually through other forms of knowledge translation and exchange, but we often start with written abstracts or summaries of our research, which we elaborate into longer papers or reports. The process of writing up our research helps us clarify our ideas, gain perspective, deepen our interpretation in relation to practice and relevant literatures, delineate our argument, and focus our key message(s) (Booth et al., 1995).

Given your extensive education to date, you are already writers, though with different approaches to writing, varied voices, and distinct styles. The following sections invite you to consider the *structure* of a research report, to delve into the *craft* of writing, to reflect upon the *purpose* of your research, to adopt different *approaches* depending upon your methodology, and to speak clearly to your *audience*(s). You may find one section more compelling than another; in which case start with that one, as the sections are not necessarily sequential.

The *Structure* of a Research Report

Similar to the way we consult online maps as guides to where we are going, having a clear idea of potential structures can provide a mental map of the placement of various components of a research report. The Practical Tip box on the adjacent page provides an outline of these components, in a common sequence.

Different research traditions and placements or venues for research reports, can require adaptations to this structure. For example, social science journals may place substantial emphasis on theories, while these may barely be mentioned in the introduction of pragmatic clinical research reports. Social and psychological sciences often require an extended literature review, which many clinical journals will not have space for (hence the +/– in the Practical Tip box). Some research reports combine results and discussion, accompanying the exposition of key themes or exemplary quotations or tables with interpretative comments and refer-

ence to relevant literature. Abstracts of research reports may leave the structure implicit, or make it explicit as exemplified in the Health Research in Action boxes 12.1–12.3. However, most abstracts do not describe the weaknesses or limitations of the research, as these are seldom part of the key messages that those reporting the research want to convey to the reader. Nevertheless, the outline in box 12.1 can give you, as early health researchers, somewhere to start.

The *Craft* of Writing

For many of us, getting down to writing is hard, even with a magnificent looking outline. It takes sufficient forward planning to start, to make time for writing the first complete draft, and to leave enough grace time for re-writing as needed (Booth et al., 1995). For example, most academic terms are pretty short to squeeze in health research and the grace period available to most professors or research supervisors who must submit marks shortly after the end of term or a research internship is very short!

Choosing a Voice

An important initial choice is the voice and person in which you are going to write. Unlike much traditional "scientific" writing, an increasing number of writers and editors prefer active voice for its parsimony in words and greater clarity on who says or does what. So, in this chapter, I use primarily active voice. Although historically most researchers encouraged their students to write in a more disembodied third person, critics of positivism have argued that all research is affected in its conception and execution by the researcher, so trying to create an aura of "objectivity" is inappropriate. Hence, many editors now accept, and, in some qualitative research traditions, demand first

PRACTICAL TIP

A Structure for Reporting Health Research*

Title and authors

Abstract + keywords

Introduction/Background

- Statement of the problem or issue
- Relevant literature on the research problem or issue
- Gaps in previous studies (theory, coverage, methods and implementation rigour)
- Purpose statement

Research questions or objectives

+/− Broader literature review

Methods

- Type of research design +/− definition
- Visual diagram of study flow
- Sample recruitment-selection
- Data collection +/− measures
- Data analysis

If mixed methods or multiple components these may be grouped for ease of understanding

Results (or Findings)

- Sample description (in epidemiological, clinical and some program evaluation traditions)
- Descriptive results or initial themes
- Modeling or more synthetic results

Discussion

- Summarize key findings in relation to existing literature
- Note weaknesses and strengths
- Indicate potential research directions
- Provide guidance to practice or policy, as appropriate

+/− Conclusion or Key Message box

References +/− Appendices or other Supplemental Material

---

*   Structure may be adapted, depending on the nature of the research, the type of report, and course, funder, or journal requirements.

12.1   Health Research in Action

The Meaning of Health in Rural Children: A Mixed Methods Approach (Bilinski et al., 2010)

Background: Gaining an understanding of the meaning of health in children may provide insight into factors that contribute to effective programs aimed at preventing diseases such as childhood obesity.

Objective: To explore the meaning of health of rural pre-adolescent Saskatchewan children.

Methods: A mixed methods, explanatory, sequential design. The Health Behaviour in School Aged Children (HBSC) Survey questionnaire (WHO, 2007) was administered and height and weight collected from 51 children in grades four to six of one school. A focused ethnographic approach was used to explore the meaning of health in a subset of children (nine to 12 years old), with at least two brief audiotaped interviews. Transcribed interviews underwent four stages of analysis. Contextual data was collected through a windshield survey of physical surroundings and activity patterns in the community.

Results: Using the international standards for childhood obesity, 10 children were classified by their body mass index score (BMI) as a healthy weight and nine as having an unhealthy weight (overweight or obese). Healthy weight children were more likely to be female, exercise more than four hours/week, eat fruit at least once/day and eat french fries less than once/week.

Regardless of BMI, children described their meaning of health as Knowing Stuff, Having a Working Body, and Feeling Happy. They suggested that Feeling Happy was most meaningful. The rural environment appeared to provide a sense of safety, security, and freedom.

Conclusion: The research team discovered factors associated with healthy weight and the value rural children placed on psychosocial aspects of health.

12.2   Health Research in Action

Regions, Hospitals and Health Outcomes Over Time: A Multi-level Analysis of Repeat Prevalence Among a Cohort of Health-care Workers (Cole et al., 2009a)

Background: The relative importance of region, workplace, and individual determinants of health burden is debated.

Objective: To model the contribution of hospital characteristics to employee mental and musculoskeletal disorders.

Methods: We linked employment records of nurses and support services' staff with health records, neighbourhood census, and hospital administrative data. We conducted multi-level logistic regression analyses with three levels: year (I), employee characteristics (II), and hospital characteristics (III).

Results: Northern region hospitals experienced lower disorder prevalences (odds ratios (OR) 0.58, 95 per cent confidence intervals (0.40, 0.82) for mental and 0.56 (0.44, 0.73) for musculoskeletal disorders). Hospitals with yearly workloads of the highest versus lowest quintiles of inpatient days/1000 employee hours (> 86.0 vs. < 42.6) and surgical cases/1000 employee hours (>10.5 vs. < 3.9) had greater odds of mental (1.29 (1.05, 1.57); 1.22 (1.05, 1.42)) and musculoskeletal (1.38 (1.21, 1.58); 1.21 (1.09, 1.34)) disorders.

Conclusion: Opportunities exist for reduction in burden with hospital workload reduction. Further exploration of regional effects is needed.

12.3   Health Research in Action

The Role of Nursing Best Practice Champions in Diffusing Practice Guidelines: A Mixed Methods Study (Ploeg et al., 2010)

Background: While the importance of nursing best practice champions has been widely promoted in the diffusion of evidence-based practice, there has been little research about their role.

Objective: The researchers aimed to determine how nursing best practice champions influence the diffusion of Best Practice Guideline recommendations.

Methods: a mixed method sequential triangulation design with two phases: (1) QUAL - key informant interviews with 23 champions and (2) QUAN - a survey of champions ($N = 191$) and administrators ($N = 41$). Qualitative findings (QUAL) informed the development of surveys and were used in interpreting quantitative information (QUAN).

Findings: Qualitative and quantitative findings suggested that champions influence the use of Best Practice Guideline recommendations most readily through: (1) dissemination of information about clinical practice guidelines, specifically through education and mentoring; (2) being persuasive practice leaders at interdisciplinary committees; and (3) tailoring the guideline implementation strategies to the organizational context.

Conclusion: Understanding best practice champions' multi-dimensional role can help service organizations and the nursing profession more fully capitalize on their potential to influence and implement evidence-based practices in order to advance positive patient, organizational, and system outcomes.

---

person writing. I write here in all three persons i.e., including myself as a health researcher (first) (e.g., I/we), speaking directly to you as student health researchers (second) (e.g., you), and citing others' experience, approaches or guidance (third) (e.g., he/she/it/they).

Deciding on Language

As Canadians, we must struggle with our own particular mid-Atlantic version of spelling. For this Canadian book, I can use the *Gage Canadian Dictionary* as a resource but for US journals, I have to switch my word processing program to US English, and for UK journals, UK English. I recently had a paper returned from an international journal asking me to make up my mind with regards to spelling and stick with it, so clearly I am not always successful!

Related is the effort to eliminate unnecessary jargon or language pertinent to only a small group of researchers. A good trick is to try out words with your potential audience verbally, e.g., at a student research day. If your student colleagues ask what a word or concept means, or for a fuller explanation, then you likely need to both describe more in the text and construct a glossary of key terms. Similarly, one must clearly explain acronyms and abbreviations early on in one's research report, and often include them in a list up front or at the end. For example, colleagues with whom I have done research use many phrases and acronyms to describe work-related musculoskeletal disorders (MSDs), or health problems in the muscles, tendons, and other soft tissues that can be caused or aggravated by work. Because of the variety of terms used, we have to explain our usage in most of our research reports and journal articles.

In addition, out of respect for our participants, our colleagues, our readers, and the wider public, we must avoid the use of sexist, racist, paternalist, or disablist language. Sometimes our perception of such language is different from that of the person who may feel slighted by its use. Think of your own identity and social location, and pass it by a person who might be aggrieved by your language. For example, as a man, I have asked women colleagues to read research papers that I have written about gender, as they sometimes ask me to read their papers.

Assessing Contributions

Even as novice health researchers, you may be making an intellectual contribution which deserves recognition. Most universities have clear policies around intellectual "property," particularly at the graduate student level. In research teams and with collaborators from other organizations, we must explicitly work through the delicate process of recognizing contributions to a manuscript. At the Institute for Work and Health (Toronto, Ontario), we developed a guide with scores (0 nothing to 3 large) for each item of contribution to a manuscript. We grouped the items into categories, with different weights applied to all items in that category, depending on its importance. Category A, the most important and hence weighted 4, includes items on conception, theory development, design, analysis and interpretation. So an author who made a large contribution on each of these could receive (five items)*(score of 3)*(weight of 4) = 60 for this category alone. Category B includes two items on drafting the manuscript or making critical revisions to the text, each weighted 3. Category C items (weighted 2) include project coordination, running literature searches, interviewing, coding data, standard data analysis, and other more routine research tasks.

Category D (weighted 1) includes administrative, technical, or material support and different kinds of advice around searching, reviewing, statistics, or editing i.e., more distant involvement. We put together a spreadsheet to facilitate calculation of scores for each contributor, with a threshold of 20 for authorship. Those below 20 can be acknowledged. With strong encouragement to discuss contributorship early in the process, we have found that it has facilitated frank discussions, and made the process of sorting through authorship more harmonious.

Referencing Others

Good guides to nailing down details abound, e.g. Maloy's (2001) "Guidelines for Writing a Scientific Paper." Some details may seem interminable, e.g. citing all your sources in the precise form required for a particular journal, including the URLs of websites and date of access. Of particular importance is going back to original publications behind a source. For example, if you think one of the references in this chapter seems particularly good, retrieve it and read it directly before you cite it. Related is the task of distinguishing between the first place some new research was reported (the primary source) and subsequent descriptions, often summaries, of the research findings (secondary sources). Textbooks and websites are common secondary sources, while original books and journal articles are often primary sources.

I have taken up the practice of developing my reference list and listing abbreviations as I write, while others input all their references into reference manager software (a better option!). On the positive side, we recognize how we learn from the work of others; an advantage in going to primary sources. At the same time, we are showing basic respect for their intellectual contributions to our own research. On the negative side, we must avoid even a semblance of plagiarism, something universities and journals are become appropriately strict about.

Different *Purposes* of Research Require Different Write-ups

Reporting Reviews

Often health research students start writing up through some type of literature review for a course paper or a summer internship. As you have encountered in Chapter 4, reporting of scoping and systematic reviews have their own requirements including: clear sections on the search strategy (for reviews and primary studies), the assessment of relevance at the title and abstract and full study stage, classification of the kinds of studies encountered and criteria for selection, description of the nature +/− assessment of the quality of included studies, and synthesis method chosen to produce inferences or recommendations (see the Canada's National Collaborating Centre for Methods and Tools website for a guide). Researchers adapt these components to their purpose(s). For example, the meta-narrative review of environmental health and vulnerable populations in Canada led by a health geographer (Masuda et al., 2008) includes a strong emphasis on research and policy gaps. The review of divergence between qualitative and quantitative results in mixed methods studies (see explanation below) by a Montreal team (Pluye et al., 2009) includes multiple search strategies, classification of ways of dealing with divergence, a report of divergence in a pilot study on handheld computer use as an electronic knowledge resource in a family medicine clinic, and discussion of these results in a health research course with novice researchers—a full exposition for us as readers!

Describing Findings

When the purpose is description of a population's health status and/or experience, a relatively straightforward exposition of quantitative results and qualitative findings is adequate. The Health Research in Action box 12.1 describes rural Saskatchewan children's weight status and key behaviours associated with it quantitatively (Bilinski et al., 2010). The researchers then explored these pre-adolescents' understandings of health, uncovering a rich description of their experience.

Conveying Analyses of Relationships

When analyzing relationships among predictors and health outcomes, complex modelling often requires more extensive quantitative analysis sections and staged presentation. For example, our interest in the effects of health care workplace characteristics on employee health led us to use several sources of data at different hierarchical levels (Table 1 from paper highlighted in Health Research in Action box 12.2). With Ministry of Health administrative data on acute care hospitals we could calculate workload per year as the number of inpatient days and surgical cases per hours worked (Table 2). On the employees, we had information from their health benefits provider on their job type (nurse or support staff), their years of experience, and their neighbourhood of residence (for socioeconomic status) which we could link with the occurrence of a mental health or musculoskeletal disorder in each of five years, derived from multiple British Columbia linked health databases (Table 3). To bring this all together, we had to use multi-level models to show prediction of outcomes by factors from each level (Tables 4 and 5). A complex story, but one which was powerful, because we could fairly confidently assert that employees in hospitals with yearly workload in the top quintile had a 20–30 per cent greater odds of experiencing an adverse health outcome compared to those working in hospitals at the lowest quintile of workload. The paper took a long time to write, reanalyze according to methods which reviewers suggested (see the section "Writing for Different *Audiences*" about responding to reviewers), and revise through several iterations. Perhaps all that work meant that health service stakeholders found it useful!

Evaluating Programs

Program evaluation brings its own requirements, including a detailed description of the program and its implementation (Spratt et al., 2004). For example, we evaluated a program of participatory ergonomics interventions in Ontario workplaces using a mixed methods, multiple case study approach (Cole et al., 2009b). Writing the paper was a way for us to draw upon the strengths of a multidisciplinary research team and reflect upon why we didn't find the expected improvements in pain among workers, despite the changes which the workplace teams implemented—an example of analyzing and constructing an argument through writing (as per section on "*Approaches* with Different Methodologies and Designs" below).

Influencing Health Policy

For policy research, Erica Bell (2010: 147) describes "techniques for writing the report in a way that delivers the policy story, from understanding the nature of political reasoning in policy-making contexts to special issues in data presentation for policy makers. [Her chapter 7] emphasizes that delivering findings in this genre is not just about research rigour—it is about particular strategic written communication skills." Such writing is highly relevant to achieving knowledge translation (see Chapter 13).

Approaches with Different Methodologies and Designs

As Chapter 2 noted, different research paradigms (qualitative, quantitative, mixed methods) have implications for different study designs and, in the case here, different research reports.

Qualitative Research

In studies using qualitative methods (Chapter 9), you may already have been writing considerable amounts of text as part of your analysis, describing the themes which emerged, or weaving together your results into a coherent conceptual framework which captures the relationships among different themes. The process of "writing as analysis" has been well described by Harry Woolcott (2009) in his book devoted entirely to writing up qualitative research, a must-read for those of you reporting a qualitative study. Two organizational researchers (Golden-Biddle and Locke, 1997) described this process as "composing qualitative research," with allusions to literary writing. They focus on generating and developing a "storyline" to convey your argument (Booth et al., 1995), leading the reader to discover your findings with you. Setting forth a clear narrative or argument which leads logically from one point to the next in a cascading, imaginative yet concise fashion is one of your key challenges as a writer.

Quantitative Research

For studies using quantitative methods (Chapters 10–11), you likely wrote during the design phase, but may not have been writing as much during the analysis phase until you feel the set of tables and/or figures is "right." Nevertheless, a back and forth process between analyzing and writing up results will likely help your interpretation and may stimulate further analyses. In the natural sciences, colleagues have set out a helpful algorithm for writing up a research paper, starting with the tables and figures (O'Connor and Holmquist, 2009). Consultation with reporting guidelines for different kinds of primary health research can be very helpful. For example, expert groups have developed detailed guidelines to strengthen the reporting of observational studies in epidemiology (STROBE) and to make more transparent the reporting of evaluations with non-randomized designs (TREND). These not only provide a specific structure for a research article, but they have helped me several times realize gaps in my research article drafts!

Mixed Methods Research

You may not have explicitly encountered mixed methods research so far. Mixed methods researchers believe that "the use of qualitative and quantitative approaches in combination provides a better understanding of research problems than either approach alone" (Plano Clark and Creswell, 2010: 5). Mixed methods studies may appeal to a wider audience, as stories are more convincing for some and numbers for others. Canadian researchers have surveyed the use of mixed methods in their particular health disciplines. For example, Mortenson and Oliffe (2009) examined the substantial use of mixed methods research in occupational therapy (14 per cent of research articles published between 2000 and 2005). Increasingly, resources are available to guide design and implementation (Griffiths and team in "Readings and Websites" section below), and writing up (O'Cathain, 2009) of mixed methods health research. Writing up mixed methods research builds upon the different chapters in the book or different steps in research design, which are re-visited when writing up research. Although somewhat more complicated in mixed methods research, it is feasible to describe the methods

for each component, lay out the research implementation sequence, indicate the joint analysis, and present merged results succinctly, as Health Research in Action box 12.3 demonstrates.

Critical Appraisal of Your Own Report

As you approach the end of your writing up phase, you can appraise your own study as you did other studies in your literature review (Chapter 4). For example, the UK Critical Appraisal Skills Programme (in "Readings and Websites" below) has tools for different kinds of primary studies: clinical (diagnostic test studies, randomized controlled trials); epidemiological (case-control, cohort); and other designs (economic evaluation, qualitative). Carrying out a critical appraisal of your own research can inform the weaknesses and strengths section of your discussion, generate ideas for further research, and sometimes temper your enthusiasm for practice and policy suggestions!

Writing for Different Audiences

When writing up our health research, we must focus not only on what we want to communicate but also to whom. In each of these writing tasks, you need to consider a distinct readership.

Fellow Students and Professors

Your first set of readers may be your fellow students for peer review of an assignment or in a poster at a student conference. A second would be your professor for a project proposal or a term paper or, if you are doing an honours thesis or capstone project, your supervisor. For each of these readers, you may want to share something about why your research project is important to you or your group, about your challenges in implementing the research, and your learning from your findings i.e. highlighting yourself as the "storyteller," as is common in qualitative traditions (Golden-Biddle and Locke, 1997).

Research Ethics Board Members

During a summer internship or practicum, a year-long research assistantship, or a master's project, you may help write a research ethics board (REB) application. These are good examples of tailoring one's writing to a particular format. In addition to the justification and research design, you will need to pay attention to the REB's stringent requirements for protecting research participants, informing them, and justifying the societal benefits which your research team hopes to generate. Similarly, each year one has to report on the implementation of one's research, including recruitment of participants and any variances from a study protocol. Chapter 5 provides more details on ethics in health research.

Participants, Stakeholders, Funders, and Policy Makers

During a research project, there are a host of research report writing tasks. During an internship, you may be asked to record minutes of research team meetings, in which decisions are made about recruitment or analysis or of stakeholder advisory committees about how to interpret the findings. You may then need to draft feedback of preliminary group results to present to participants, often via a newsletter. If you are close to an annual or final report being due to a funder, you may play a role in producing a research report according to the funder's specified format. More excitingly, you may be asked to produce summaries of the research to inform change (Kirby and McKenna, 1989) and

convince policy makers (see Bell [2010] in section on "Influencing Health Policy" above).

Peers

Finally, you may have the opportunity to draft a chapter for a book or a paper for a peer-reviewed journal. In the latter case, you may ask: what results and methods can we publish for what likely audience, in which journal, at what length, and, to a journal with open source availability, for how much money? Your supervisor may also be concerned about the journal's impact factor, a measure which reflects the average number of citations to recent articles published in that journal. I ask students whom I supervise to put together a spreadsheet of journal options, with the information on each journal laid out in rows and some examples of articles that are on related topics or use similar methods. That way we can jointly decide which journal to start with, and which journals are back-ups when we get rejected by our first choice!

Reviewers

Most important is learning to respond constructively to critical feedback from your peers, supervisor, mentor or reviewers. The latter can be particularly challenging, as you may feel that a piece of writing is already pretty good but the reviewer has all kinds of questions, comments on gaps, and critiques of deficiencies. I generally take some deep breaths before reading reviews, let them percolate through my thinking over a few days, and discuss them with colleagues. When we have roughly worked out what to do, including modifications, additions, or deletions, then we set about addressing reviewers' comments, point by point. We end up improving our paper or report for the very readers we want to reach and convince about the value of our research.

PRACTICAL TIP

Putting Yourself in Your Readers' Shoes—Questions to Ask Yourself when Reviewing Your Write-up

Overall

- Are you clear on whom you are writing to or for?
- Do you have clear signposts in the course of your written work, so that readers are clear about what to expect next and why it is there?
- Does your written work meet the word or character count limitations imposed by your course, institution, funder, journal, or publisher?

Literature and research questions

- Is your discussion of the literature critical (positively and negatively) yet succinct?
- Have you indicated how your research questions relate to the literature you have read and/or to practice or policy?

Methods

- Have you clearly outlined:
  - Why you chose a particular design? And method(s)?
  - How you selected participants? Data sets? Or studies?
  - Steps you took to ensure that your research was ethically responsible?
  - Why you collected data in a particular way?
  - Why and how you analyzed your data?

Results

- Have you presented your data in a manner that respects your methodology(ies)? How do your data relate to your research questions? Does it comply with any explicit requirements for results presentation?

Discussion

- Have you explained the limitations of your study?
- Do your conclusions make clear the answers to your research questions? And their implications?

References and supporting material

- Have you fully acknowledged the work of others, so that you cannot be accused of plagiarism? Have you checked that your list of references includes all items referred to in your text? And no additional ones?
- Does your referencing method follow precisely the style which your course, institution, funder, journal, or publisher requires?
- Have you included appendices or supplemental material that you might need to or be able to provide, e.g., interview schedules, letters requesting access, ethical approvals, detailed analyses?

Mentoring and Reflection

Essential to all of the above is mentorship by a more senior researcher, i.e., it could be a senior study coordinator or doctoral student working in the same research group. Building in a personal reflection capacity is also important, aided by sets of questions like those in the Practical Tip box on the previous page.

Hopefully, this chapter will also help you make writing choices which enable you to think creatively, communicate clearly, respond constructively, and be successful research writers.

Summary

- Writing up research is a responsibility and a complex challenge, yet it can bring great satisfaction to you, the researcher, and to others who learn from your research.
- You must consider your reader and the kind of research report you are producing, the rationale behind your question or purpose of your research, the research design you used, the kind of research results you produced, your interpretation of your results in light of the literature, and the storyline or argument which runs through them all.
- The nuts and bolts of writing up are not trivial, so be diligent, take time, and recognize others who work with you!

Review Questions

1. What are key sections of a research report?
2. What constitutes a primary source for citation?
3. How can criteria for authorship and/or contributorship be useful?
4. How can different purposes of research influence your write-up?
5. How does writing up differ for primarily qualitative, quantitative, or mixed methods research?
6. In what ways might a report on the results of your research be different if you are writing for a fellow student, a researcher in your field, a health practitioner, or a policy maker?

Recommended Readings and Websites

Booth, W. C. Colomb, G. G., and Williams, J. M. (1995) *The Craft of Research*. Chicago, USA: The University of Chicago Press.

The best overall guide to writing up research, finding your voice, crafting arguments, drafting approaches, and revising iteratively.

Bryman, A. and Bell E. (2007) *Business Research Methods* 3e. Oxford University Press Online Resource Centres. http://global.oup.com/uk/orc/busecon/business/brymanbrm3e/ and 3e Research Project Guide http://global.oup.com/uk/orc/busecon/business/brymanbrm3e/01student/project_guide/

A very accessible, point form with elaborations, step-by-step approach to writing up.

Canada's National Collaborating Centre for Methods and Tools. www.nccmt.ca/registry/view/eng/87.html

This site has guides for particular designs from a range of sources such as the UK National Health Service Public Health Resources Unit Appraisal Tools. Immensely helpful to critique one's own study in relation to what is needed and essential for systematic reviews. Wide range of clinical (diagnostic test studies, randomized controlled trials), epidemiological (case-control, cohort) and other designs (economic evaluation, qualitative).

Frances Griffiths and team have mounted a great website on Mixed Methods for Health Research at www2.warwick.ac.uk/fac/med/research/hsri/primary_care/research_/centrepatexp/complexityhealth/mixedmethods/. These pages

are for health professionals who want to design and conduct a research project using mixed methods in a health related field.

Maloy, S. Guidelines for writing a scientific paper. October 2001. Retrieved 20 Aug 2012 from www.sci.sdsu.edu/~smaloy/MicrobialGenetics/topics/scientific-writing.pdf

Strengthening the Reporting of Observational Studies in Epidemiology (STROBE) at www.strobe-statement.org and Transparent Reporting of Evaluations with Nonrandomized Designs (TREND) www.trend-statement.org provide reporting guidelines for these kinds of primary studies.

UK Critical Appraisal Skills Programme www.casp-uk.net has useful critical appraisal tools against which to check your research report.

References

Bell, E. (2010) Telling the health policy story. In *Research for Health Policy* (147–80). Oxford, UK: Oxford University Press.

Bilinski, H.N., Duggleby, W., and Rennie, D. (2010) The meaning of health in rural children: a mixed methods approach. *Western Journal of Nursing Research, 32*(7), 949–66.

Cole, D.C., Koehoorn, M., Ibrahim, S., Hertzman, C., Ostry, A., Xu, F. (2009a) Factors associated with mental and musculoskeletal health outcomes in a cohort of health-care workers—a multi-level analysis. *Journal of Health & Place, 15,* 1046–57.

Cole, D.C., Theberge, N., Dixon, S.M., Rivilis, I., Neumann, W.P., Wells, R.P. (2009b) Reflecting on a program of participatory ergonomics interventions: A multiple case study. *Work, 34*(2),161–78.

Golden-Biddle, K. and Locke, K.D. (1997) *Composing Qualitative Research*. Thousand Oaks, USA: Sage.

Kirby, S. and McKenna, K. (1989) Presenting the analysis. In *Experience, Research, Social Change—Methods from the Margins* (155–68). Toronto, ON: Garamond Press.

Masuda, J., Poland, B., Yupanski, T., and Cole, D.C. (2008) Environmental health equity in Canada: mapping the landscape of research. *Canadian Geographer, 52*(4), 427–50.

Mortenson, W.B. and Oliffe, J. L. (2009) Mixed methods research in occupational therapy: a survey and critique. *OTJR: Occupation, Participation and Health, 29*(1), 14–23.

O'Cathain, A. (2009) Reporting mixed methods projects. In Andrew, S., Elizabeth J. Halcomb (eds). *Mixed Methods Research for Nursing and the Health Sciences* (135–58). Chichester, UK: John Wiley & Sons, Blackwell Publishing.

O'Connor, T.R. and Holmquist, G.P. (2009) Algorithm for Writing a Scientific Manuscript. *Biochemistry and Molecular Biology Education*, *37*(6), 344–8.

Plano Clark V.L. and Creswell, J.W. (2010) Writing and evaluating mixed methods research. In *Designing and Conducting Mixed Methods Research* (151–66). Thousand Oaks, CA, USA; Sage.

Ploeg, J., Skelly, J., Rowan, M., Edwards, N., Davies, B., Grinspun, D., Bajnok, I., and Downey, A. (2010) The role of nursing best practice champions in diffusing practice guidelines: a mixed methods study. In *Worldviews on Evidence-Based Nursing, Fourth Quarter* (238–51).

Pluye, P., Grad, R.M., Levine, A., and Nicolau, B. (2009) Understanding divergence of quantitative and qualitative data (or results) in mixed methods studies. *International Journal of Multiple Research Approaches*, *3*, 58–72.

Spratt, C., Walker, R., and Robinson, B. Critical reviewers: Terry Allsop, Richard Freeman and Bernadette Robinson. Module A5: Mixed research methods in PREST (*Practitioner Research and Evaluation Skills Training in Open and Distance Learning*). Unit 4 on program evaluation and writing evaluation reports. © 2004 Commonwealth of Learning. Retrieved 3 Jan 2013 from www .col.org/SiteCollectionDocuments/A5.pdf.

Woolcott, H.F. (2009) *Writing up Qualitative Research*. 3rd ed. Thousand Oaks, USA: Sage 2009.

13 Knowledge Translation

Elliot M. Goldner

CHAPTER OUTLINE

Introduction

Amongst health researchers, there has been a rapid growth of interest in methods of **knowledge translation** (KT). This growth has been sparked by the realization that practitioners, patients, and decision makers do not pick up many potentially beneficial research findings, i.e., the new *knowledge* does not get *translated* into action. Moreover, new knowledge that does get translated into action does so only after a lengthy lag time (Institute of Medicine, 2001). Many promising discoveries and health interventions fail to achieve their maximum potential and/or reach those most in need (Panisset et al., 2012).

Naturally, researchers are dissatisfied with the prospect of their findings collecting dust on a shelf and want to see effective KT methods used to optimize uptake and application of new knowledge. Many research funding agencies and governments who invest in research also emphasize the essential role of KT methods (e.g., Lomas, 2000; Graham and Tetroe, 2009). Most funding organizations now require a well-developed KT plan as a component of every grant application. Consequently, familiarity with KT has become essential fare for virtually all health researchers.

In the past, researchers were likely to consider their work complete once their findings were published in a scientific journal. Although scientific journals remain an important means of diffusing research knowledge, they have a limited audience. Readers of scientific journals are primarily research scientists (and possibly a few proud mothers of authors!). In order to move new findings beyond the relatively small audience of researchers who seek out articles on specific topics, additional KT efforts are needed in most circumstances.

In certain areas of health research, policy, and practice, the need for intensified KT activity is particularly prominent, for example, when there is a strong rationale to bring about a widespread change of practice by health care providers, such as when a new intervention has been found to have benefits over existing practices (e.g., better outcomes, lower costs or improved safety). Similarly, when it is important to influence policy or decision makers or achieve changes in patient behaviour, KT methods are of crucial importance.

This chapter provides a theoretical foundation to understand KT, offers practical examples of the application of KT methods relevant to health research, describes prominent findings that have been made, and discusses research approaches that are likely to advance the field of KT.

Defining Knowledge Translation

Sometimes described as "closing the gap between what we know and what we do" (Graham and Tetroe, 2009), KT is nevertheless difficult to define. A plethora of related terms exists and the distinctions amongst terms such as knowledge transfer, knowledge exchange, knowledge mobilization, research utilization, dissemination, and implementation are often used in varying ways by different groups. In a study of health research funding agencies, Tetroe and colleagues (2008) identified 29 different terms used to signify KT, often without definition (see Table 13.1).

Graham and colleagues (2006) note the incoherent and ambiguous terminology that has characterized the field in their paper entitled "Lost in translation: Time for a map?" and offer an antidote through provision of a conceptual map of the Knowledge to Action process (described later in this chapter).

The following definition of KT advanced by the Canadian Institutes of Health Research (2010) has been widely adopted in the field of health care:

TABLE 13.1 Terms Used for Knowledge Translation by Participating Funding Agencies (As Reported in Semi-Structured Interviews)

Applied health research	Knowledge translation
Capacity building	Linkage and exchange
Competing, cooperation, co-optation	Popularization of research
Diffusion	Research into practice
Dissemination	Research mediation
Exploitation	Research transfer
Getting knowledge into practice	Research translation
Impact implementation	Science communication
Knowledge communication	Teaching
Knowledge cycle	The "third" mission
Knowledge exchange	Translation
Knowledge management	Translational research transmission
Knowledge mobilization	Utilization
Knowledge transfer	

Many overlapping and ill-defined terms related to KT were found to be in use within a group of international research funding organizations. This appears to reflect widespread ambiguity in terminology within the field of KT. (From Tetroe, Graham, Foy et al. 2008)

Source: Tetroe, J.M., Graham, I.D., Foy, R. et al. (2008). Health Research Funding Agencies' Support and Promotion of Knowledge Translation: An International Study. *The Milbank Quarterly*. 86(1): 125–55.

[A] dynamic and iterative process that includes synthesis, dissemination, exchange and ethically-sound application of knowledge to improve the health of Canadians, provide more effective health services and products and strengthen the health care system. This process takes place within a complex system of interactions between researchers and knowledge users. . .

In this definition, KT constitutes a broad concept. According to Tetroe (2007): "It encompasses all steps between the creation of new knowledge and its application to yield beneficial outcomes for society." The concept of KT is thus an umbrella term that includes many activities such as technology transfer, knowledge management, knowledge utilization, continuing education, consensus guideline development, and translational research.

Interestingly, the KT process often brings knowledge that has been developed through *scientific research* into contact with knowledge developed through other means. Other forms of knowledge

can be gained through the experience people have accumulated by living with a certain health problem, through experience gained being a close family member or friend of someone with a health problem, through providing treatment as a health care provider to various people with the health problem or by being involved with cultural, policy, educational, or political processes that address health care issues. Two forms of knowledge, i.e., **explicit knowledge** and **tacit knowledge** are often distinguished, however, they can be viewed as co-existing across a continuum (Kothari et al., 2012). Explicit knowledge follows logic, can be codified, written down, and effectively communicated to others. Tacit knowledge is developed from direct experience and action, is highly pragmatic and situation-specific, and is often understood and applied subconsciously and is thus difficult to articulate or codify, but is usually shared through interactive conversation and shared experience.

Naturally, scientists are keen to apply explicit knowledge acquired through scientific methods, including systematic observation, data collection, hypothesis development or testing, etc., and are generally uncomfortable accepting other forms of knowledge unless they have been put through scientific filters. Conversely, non-scientists often feel that their tacit knowledge, often gained through years of experience, should be recognized without the impediment of detailed scientific study. These conflicting perspectives may cause tensions within the KT process, however this can be a *creative* tension; it is often through the interplay amongst these perspectives that highly valuable knowledge is created and moved into action. Figure 13.1 illustrates the complex interactions that occur amongst multiple stakeholders in KT addressing health care issues. We will return to a discussion of the interactive nature of KT later in the chapter.

Background and Development of KT Science

Interest in KT is not confined to the field of health care and is deemed important amongst many disciplines and enterprises including: agriculture, education, marketing, engineering, economics, information technology, community development and various business enterprises. In the field of health care, Canadian contributors have often been at the forefront of developments in KT research, theory and practice (e.g., Barwick et al., 2009; Dobbins et al., 2009; Dreidger et al., 2010; Gagnon, 2011; Estabrooks, Thompson, and Lovely, 2006; Jacobson, Butterill, and Goering, 2003; Lavis, Wilson, and Grimshaw, 2011; Lomas, 1993; Mitton et al., 2007; Straus, Tetroe, and Graham, 2009).

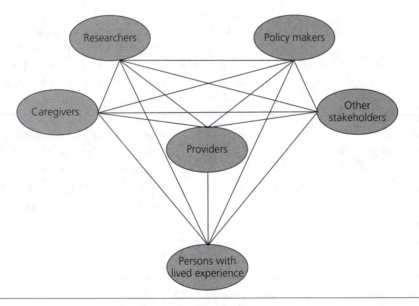

FIGURE 13.1   The Activated Knowledge Exchange "Diamond"

The Activated Knowledge Exchange "diamond" (Mental Health Commission of Canada 2011) illustrates the complex interactions that occur amongst multiple stakeholders in KT relevant to health care. Researchers play an important role through applying scientific methods to build and shape knowledge and influence KT. However, interactions amongst various stakeholders are critical to the KT process. The term "Persons with lived experience" refers to individuals directly affected by health conditions whereas "Caregivers" denotes family members, friends, or others who provide physical, emotional, and financial supports. "Providers" refers here to service providers, such as physicians, nurses, and other health care workers, but also to those who provide administrative oversight, or offer other necessary services and supports related to health care. "Other stakeholders" that often play important roles in KT include journalists and others working in media and communications, educators, employers, and people involved in the justice system.

Source: Mental Health Commission of Canada (2011). Activated Knowledge Exchange Framework. https://kec.mentalhealthcommission.ca/about_kec/keframework. Retrieved February 11, 2013.

A key figure who has played an instrumental role in the development and recognition of KT within health care is Jonathan Lomas, cofounder of the centre for health economics and Policy Analysis at McMaster University and the inaugural chief executive officer of the Canadian Health Services Research Foundation, a nationally endowed organization founded in 1997 to improve the relevance and use of health services research in health system **decision making**. Dr Lomas has been prescient in his recognition of the importance of understanding and advancing the role and impact of research evidence in health systems decision-making and is often viewed as the "godfather of knowledge translation." In recognition of Dr Lomas' eminent contributions to the field, the Canadian Institutes of Health Research have instituted a special award in his name, the Jonathan Lomas KT Doctoral Research Award Supplement (Canadian Institutes of Health Research, 2012).

The roots of KT science have grown from many different sources, including such fields as: communications, education, network theory, psychological studies of individual and organizational behaviour change, studies of policy decision-making, and economics, particularly in relation to financial incentives to behaviour change. Consequently, it is not surprising that a number of different "pockets" or thematic areas can be found in the scientific literature in relation to KT.

An important subset of KT science is known as **implementation science**, and this field is supported by a high quality scientific journal bearing the same name. Implementation science focuses on the use of strategies to adopt and integrate evidence-based health interventions and change practice patterns within specific settings. Initially, this area of study tended to focus on the implementation of evidence-based findings into practice through interventions geared toward clinical practitioners. However, more recent developments have expanded the focus of implementation

science to address multiple levels of health care delivery: i.e., the patient level, the provider team or group level, and the organizational level, or the market/policy level (Damschroder et al., 2009).

A number of other pockets of literature and scholarship are highly relevant to KT science. These include the fields of **community-based and participatory-action research** and **shared decision-making** studies. These areas of study emphasize efforts to bring together researchers and knowledge users in order to achieve meaningful refinement, uptake, and application of scientific knowledge in order to optimize successful outcomes. When hoping to influence the uptake and utilization of knowledge by patients and the general public, the field of **health literacy** seeks to improve the degree to which individuals have the capacity to obtain, process, and understand health information and services needed to make appropriate health decisions. The full range of literature relevant to KT is scattered across a variety of disparate research themes that are not often assembled or considered together.

The potential value of KT in achieving improvements in health care delivery and health outcomes has generated substantial enthusiasm and KT has become a prominent element within Canadian health research funding organizations (e.g., Lomas, 2000; Graham and Tetroe, 2009). Evidence for the effectiveness of KT remains limited (Mitton et al., 2007) but is accumulating gradually through work in various research centres and by groups such as the Cochrane Public Health Group (CPHG, 2012), a review group of the Cochrane Collaboration.

Effective KT Strategies

Evidence about the effectiveness of various KT strategies in addressing health related issues is now accumulating. In general, passive forms of knowledge translation (e.g., information campaigns, posting information on websites) appear to be relatively ineffective in comparison to more active approaches (e.g., use of opinion leaders, or use of reminders and feedback) (Bero et al., 1998; Boaz, Baeza, and Fraser, 2011; Grimshaw, Thomas, and McLennan, 2001). In general, multifaceted interventions (in which two or more interventions are combined in the KT approach) are more effective than single interventions (Boaz, Baeza, and Fraser, 2011); however, there are circumstances in which simple, single interventions can be optimal (Grimshaw and Eccles, 2004). An example of a multi-faceted intervention is one that combines incentive payments, education of health care professionals, and provision of self-management tools for patients.

In the following sections, information is summarized about evidence for the effectiveness of KT strategies that aim to influence the behaviour of each of the following three important groups: health care providers, the general public and patients, and policy decision makers. Factors that influence the effectiveness of KT strategies are also described.

KT Strategies That Aim to Influence Health Care Providers

A number of high-quality studies, including systematic reviews and overviews of systematic reviews, have been conducted to examine the effectiveness of KT strategies that aim to influence health care providers (e.g., Bero et al., 1998; Boaz, Baeza, and Fraser, 2011; Francke et al., 2008; Grimshaw et al., 2001; Jamtvedt et al., 2006; Locock et al., 2001; O'Brien et al., 1999; 2007).

The following specific KT interventions have been identified to be effective in changing the behaviour of health care providers, producing small to moderate improvements in the delivery of health care services and patient outcomes:

Educational outreach visits

Also known as "academic detailing," **educational outreach visits** refer to a personal visit by a trained, credible person to health professionals in their own settings in which evidence-based, tailored information is provided for the purposes of influencing specific practice behaviours.

Audit and feedback

Audit and feedback refers to the provision of information to health care providers about their own clinical performance, allowing comparison of their performance with that of their peers. Often, such information is collected through clinical databases and fed back through individualized reports and summaries.

Use of opinion leaders

Defined as influential members of a community or field of practice, **opinion leaders** are individuals whom other health care providers often turn to for advice, opinions and clinical direction. Although there is evidence that the use of opinion leaders can be effective in promoting changes in health care providers' behaviour, the mechanisms through which such influences operate are not well understood (O'Brien et al., 1999).

Reminders and prompts (either manual or computerized)

These include various formats (e.g., paper reminders in patient charts, computerized decision support, algorithms) that help clinicians optimize evidence-based protocols and practices at the point of care. Increasingly, computerized prompts are being developed, utilized, and integrated as an application of electronic health care records.

Interactive educational meetings

Continuing education, such as courses, workshops, and seminars can improve professional practice and the achievement of treatment goals by patients, when delivered alone or in combination with other KT interventions. However, the effect on professional practice tends to be small (Forsetlund et al., 2009; O'Brien et al., 2001). It has also been found that interactive formats have more beneficial effects than didactic educational approaches. Educational strategies found to be most effective applied multiple interventions, two-way communications, printed and graphic materials in person, and locally respected health personnel as educators (Cauffman et al., 2002). Grimshaw and colleagues (2001) reported that the distribution of educational materials and provision of didactic educational sessions had little or no effect on influencing health care providers' behaviour.

Further study is needed to examine the effectiveness of financial incentives in changing health care providers' behaviour. A systematic review by Scott and colleagues (2011) found insufficient evidence to determine whether or not financial incentives are effective in improving health care services delivered by primary care physicians.

Another approach requiring further study is the use of **communities of practice** (also known as communities of interest), i.e., self-organized networks of peers with skills and experience in an area of practice or profession. Such groups provide health care providers with opportunities to share information, enhance their skill and capacity to adopt evidence-based knowledge, and foster continuous learning. Barwick and colleagues (2009) found that health care practitioners randomized to participate in communities of practice did not report their practices to have changed any more than their colleagues in the "practice as usual" group. However, they suggest

that communities of practice are worthy of further study as a means of supporting the implementation of evidence-based practice.

KT Strategies That Aim to Influence the General Public and Patient Behaviour

There is an extensive history of efforts to mobilize knowledge to foster improved health outcomes amongst the general population and within subgroups who are at high risk or who have particular health conditions. For example, efforts to decrease tobacco use, increase levels of physical exercise, influence dietary behaviour and alcohol use, diminish behaviours that risk the transmission of infectious disease, and increase adherence to screening protocols and evidence-based treatment protocols, have been addressed using various strategies. Despite limitations in research examining the effectiveness of such strategies, there is ample evidence that many of these interventions are effective in achieving behavioural change (Jepson et al., 2011). It may be artificial to consider individual strategies in isolation, since multiple strategies are often underway concurrently and these tend to multiply, expanding awareness, reinforcing consistent messages over time and eventually resulting in changes to social values and behaviour within the population (Murphy, 2005). The following strategies have been found to be effective under certain circumstances.

Mass media campaigns

These are determined efforts used to promote health behaviour through television, radio, the Internet and print or other media. **Mass media campaigns** can effectively produce positive changes in health behaviour across large populations; however, positive outcomes may be difficult to achieve (Wakefield, Loken, and Hornik, 2010).

Since the media environment is increasingly cluttered with messages and entertainment that compete with efforts to capture attention of the public, considerable challenges exist in the use of mass media campaigns to effectively influence health behaviour. Wakefield and colleagues (2010) also point out that mass media campaigns are more effective when the target behaviour is one-off or episodic in nature (e.g., screening, vaccination, children's aspirin use) rather than routine or ongoing (e.g., food choices, sun exposure, physical activity).

Social marketing approaches

These strategies apply commercial marketing technologies and techniques to initiatives that seek to improve the welfare of individuals and society. Features of **social marketing** approaches include the use of consumer research to understand consumer values and needs, and subsequent use of segmentation variables to tailor interventions for use with specific segments of the population. Consideration is given to the so-called eight "P's" of social marketing: Product, Price, Place, Promotion, Publics, Partnership, Policy, and Purse Strings (Weinreich, 2011). Studies indicate that social marketing approaches can be effective in achieving health behaviour change in target populations (Gordon et al., 2006). Depending on the target population, approaches might utilize a range of approaches, relaying messages through traditional media communications, digital electronic or communication channels, social media, printed materials, educational programs and marketing initiatives delivered in schools, workplaces, health care environments, or other locations.

Community mobilization

Community mobilization refers to community-wide efforts to address a health or social issue and may bring together local, provincial, and federal governments, professional groups, religious groups, businesses, and individual community members. The process includes mobilizing necessary resources, disseminating information, generating support, and fostering cooperation across public and private sectors in the community in order to bring about changes in relevant health behaviours (Roussos and Fawcett, 2006).

Laws and regulations

These have been applied by governments in order to achieve substantial public health accomplishments (Moulton et al., 2009). Widely-implemented examples are tobacco control laws that have reduced rates of many chronic illnesses, laws addressing the operation of motor vehicles while under the influence of alcohol that have reduced accident-related fatalities and injuries, regulations regarding the addition of iodine to table salt (in order to prevent thyroid disorders commonly caused by iodine deficiency), and school immunization laws that have helped reduce rates of infectious disease. The effectiveness of legal tools to address some health-related behaviours, such as substance misuse, is a complex area and must take into careful account the relative harms that may be created through inappropriate criminalization of individuals in society (Babor et al., 2009).

Financial incentives and disincentives

The use of excise taxes and pricing has been found effective to change health-related behaviours, such as reduction of tobacco and alcohol use, amongst members of the general public; however, such strategies have a greater effect on the behaviour of people with less disposable income (Chaloupka, Straif, and Leon, 2011). The effects of positive financial incentives, such as payments provided to individuals for using prevention services or completing educational programs (known as conditional cash transfers), are unclear (Marteau, Ashcroft, and Oliver, 2009).

Self-management

This is a KT approach to enhance an individual's ability to manage the symptoms, treatment, physical and psychological consequences, and life style changes associated with a health condition. **Self-management** approaches recognize the important contributions that individuals can make themselves in achieving good outcomes and are also considered to support movement toward collaborative models of care in which expertise is shared between patient and professional (Du and Yuan, 2010). Self-management may be undertaken when individuals obtain tools, resources, or guidebooks through their own initiative, from websites, or in various print, video, or interactive computer-based formats. In addition, health care providers or organizations may provide patients with self-management tools and support, either as an initial step in a stepped-care approach or as an integral component of a multi-faceted treatment approach. Self-management has been demonstrated to be effective for various health conditions (Lorig and Holman, 2003), but research is needed to examine long term outcomes, cost effectiveness, and comparative outcomes of different self-management strategies (Coulter and Ellins, 2007).

Supported self-management (also known as "guided self-management") signifies the involvement of a health care provider in translating knowledge to patients for the purpose of self-management, or coaching patients to support their efforts at self-management, either in individual or group formats. Self-management approaches limited to the provision of information are mostly unsuccessful, but educational and self-help programs that are actively supported by clinicians have been found to improve health outcomes for patients with depression, eating disorders, asthma, diabetes, and hypertension (Barlow et al., 2002). Self-management may also be supported by lay educators or peers (rather than health professionals). A systematic review of such approaches found modest, short-term improvements in patients' confidence to manage their condition and perceptions of their own health; however, they did not produce clinically significant reductions in pain or other symptoms, improve quality of life, or reduce health care utilization (Foster et al., 2009).

KT Strategies That Aim to Influence Health Policy Decision Makers

There is little evidence available regarding the effectiveness of KT strategies aimed to influence health policy decision makers. Orton and colleagues (2011) undertook a systematic review to synthesize empirical evidence on the use of research evidence by public health decision makers in settings with universal health care systems (including European countries, Canada, Australia, and New Zealand). They concluded that although decision makers access a wide range of research evidence, the extent to which it is used remains unknown. Use of research evidence is often indirect and operates alongside many other influences on decision making, including "organizational, political and strategic factors; financial and resource constraints; personal experience; common sense; expert opinion; stakeholder and public pressure; community views and local competition" (p. 8). In addition to these competing influences, the authors identified the existence of substantial barriers to the use of research evidence. These include the "gulf" between researchers and decision makers (including some decision makers' negative perceptions of research evidence and its usefulness); the culture in which decision makers function; and practical constraints.

In their review, Orton and colleagues (2011) found a dearth of evidence regarding the effectiveness of strategies to improve uptake of research evidence by decision makers. They compiled a list of requirements identified by decision makers to improve uptake of research evidence, reproduced here in Table 13.2. Although largely untested, the following were identified to have potential to improve KT amongst researchers and decision makers: creating a means for sustained dialogue between researchers and decision makers, building capacity to increase researchers' abilities to create and disseminate evidence geared to decision makers' needs and improve decision makers' abilities to appraise and interpret research, and changing the culture within which policy makers work to increase the value placed on the use of research evidence.

Governments and research funding organizations in some jurisdictions have initiated programs to increase the capacity of decision makers to utilize research evidence, such as the Executive Training for Research Application (EXTRA) Program developed by the Canadian Health Services Research Foundation. An initial evaluation of the EXTRA program indicated that participants reported significant improvements in their research knowledge, skills in assessing the quality of evidence, knowledge of change management, and ability to improve their own organization's context for informed decision making (Anderson and Lavoie-Tremblay, 2008).

A unique study by Dobbins and colleagues (2009) stands as a unique investigation that has directly evaluated the effectiveness of KT interventions on health policy decision makers. This study and its findings are summarized in Health Research in Action box 13.1.

Factors Influencing the Effectiveness of KT

Various factors have been found to influence the effectiveness of KT interventions. KT is more effective when addressing topics that are perceived by knowledge users to be relatively simple

---

TABLE 13.2   Public Health Decision Makers' Requirements of Research

Researchers should clearly summarize their main findings.

Research approaches should show effectiveness (through study design and/or statistical presentation) and consensus.

Researchers should align evidence with current and future policy environments.

Evidence must identify relevant indicators for health targets.

Research should make suggestions for implementation.

Research evidence must be designed so it is easily incorporated with colloquial/experiential/common sense knowledge.

Evidence is required at a local, micro level.

Evidence should arise from sources which are seen as unbiased (such as peer-reviewed research), authoritative, and credible; and provide methodological details so rigor can be assessed.

Funding should be provided for longer term and longitudinal research.

Research evidence should be made more widely available to decision makers through the use of email bulletins, public health professional organizations or clearinghouses.

Source: Orton et al. (2011).

13.1   Health Research in Action

Maureen Dobbins, a Professor at McMaster University's School of Nursing, and her colleagues studied the effectiveness of KT interventions in a national sample of 108 Canadian public health departments (Dobbins et al., 2009). The researchers selected a specific policy issue, i.e., applying available research evidence to plan and implement effective healthy body weight promotion programs and services for children to prevent obesity and associated chronic disease.

They undertook a randomized trial to study three KT interventions that are widely used to promote evidence-based decision making: access to an online registry of research evidence (providing summaries of research evidence on various topics); tailored, targeted messaging (that was individualized and matched relevant research evidence to specific decision makers' needs); and use of **knowledge brokers** (each of whom were trained to work on a one-to-one basis with decision makers to facilitate evidence-informed decision making). The study hypothesis was that health departments randomized to the targeted, tailored messages and knowledge broker groups would report greater evidence-informed decisions than departments in the group randomized to simple access to the registry of research evidence. Furthermore, it was hypothesized that organizations that highly valued the use of research evidence in decision making would have more improvement in evidence-informed decisions than those who placed a low value on research evidence.

No significant effect was observed for the primary outcome, i.e., the extent to which a specific area of research evidence was used in a recent program decision by health departments. However, a significant effect of the intervention was observed for the secondary outcome, i.e., the number of policies or programs being delivered at health departments that incorporated the specific area of research evidence. This effect was observed only for tailored, targeted messages and no significant effects were associated with an online registry of research evidence or use of knowledge brokers. The effect was moderated by organizational research culture, i.e., departments that placed a higher value on use of research evidence were found to show a greater improvement in the number of evidence-based policies or programs delivered than departments that attributed less value to research evidence.

The study findings support the notion that passive KT strategies, such as access to highly synthesized evidence, are insufficient to facilitate evidence-based decision making, whereas the more active intervention of targeted, tailored messaging is effective in having decision makers incorporate the evidence into program decisions. However, it is surprising that the study found that health departments randomized to the knowledge broker group did not show a significant effect. Knowledge brokers are trained to assist in the assessment, interpretation, and adaptation of evidence to local contexts. In the study, knowledge brokers were prepared at the Master's level, had extensive knowledge and expertise in public health decision making, and possessed knowledge of the research process. They sought to ensure relevant research evidence was transferred to decision makers in ways that were most constructive and relevant to local practice, and aimed to assist decisions makers to develop skill and capacity for evidence-informed decision making. As the most resource-intensive and interactive of the three interventions tested in the study, one might have anticipated that health departments randomized to receive the support of a knowledge broker would have demonstrated an effect in primary or secondary outcomes. The study has raised a series of questions as to how to best interpret its findings and has sparked novel research approaches to pursue intriguing areas of enquiry.

and when tools (e.g., guidebooks and decision aids) are in place to support the intended behaviour changes (Titler, 2008). Factors associated with better uptake of evidence-based innovations by organizations include larger size, decentralized decision making, greater resourcing, and closer proximity to urban centres; however, these account for a relatively small degree of variance (Greenhalgh et al., 2005).

A "learning organizational culture" promotes absorptive capacity and facilitates the identification, capture, sharing, reorientation and implementation of evidence-based knowledge (Titler, 2008). Organizational characteristics that contribute to good capacity include clear vision and strong leadership, workforce and skills development, ability to access research (library services), fiscal investments, acquisition and development of technological resources, a knowledge management strategy, effective communication, a receptive organizational culture, and a focus on change management (Peirson et al., 2012).

KT Frameworks and Guides

Various theoretical frameworks to conceptualize and approach KT within the field of health care have been produced (e.g., Bowen and Zwi, 2005; Graham et al., 2006; Hogan and Logan, 2004; Kitson, Harvey, and McCormack, 1998; Lavis et al., 2003; Stetler, Damschroder, and Helfrichm, 2011). A number of frameworks have been compiled, summarized and reviewed by the National Collaborating Centre for Methods and Tools (NCCMT)—you will find information about the NCCMT website at the end of this chapter in the section entitled Recommended Readings and Websites. A few frameworks are described briefly here.

The Knowledge to Action Cycle

The *Knowledge to Action Cycle* (Graham et al., 2006) is a framework that has been adopted and promoted by the Canadian Institutes of Health Research (see Figure 13.2). This framework conceptualizes two components: (i) a *knowledge creation funnel* where new knowledge is generated, surrounded by (ii) a series of action steps that are needed to bring knowledge to action. The latter may occur either in sequence or simultaneously. The authors of the framework consider the process to be complex and dynamic, without boundaries between the two components or among the various phases they have described.

In the circle at the centre of Figure 13.2, the process of *knowledge creation* is shown to move through a series of phases leading gradually to refined, clearer and more actionable findings and knowledge products. The initial phase (knowledge inquiry) often involves various research studies that first signify beneficial, new findings whereas the subsequent steps (knowledge synthesis and production of knowledge tools and products) bring together results from various sources and produce knowledge that is ready for action. This is represented in Figure 13.2 by a broader base of knowledge inquiry that gradually narrows, toward the point of the triangle, signifying more refined and actionable knowledge.

The Knowledge to Action cycle describes a series of action steps involved in mobilizing new knowledge (in Figure 13.2, these are illustrated as surrounding the knowledge creation efforts). The framework authors describe this cycle as a dynamic process in which all phases in the cycle can influence one another. The following action steps are described:

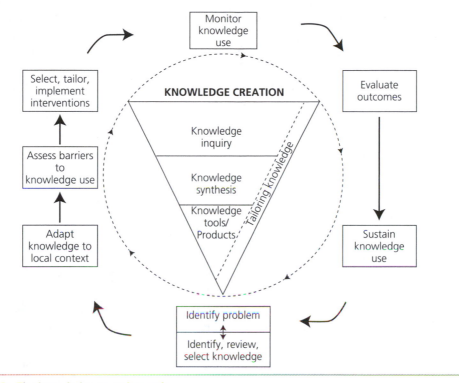

FIGURE 13.2   The knowledge to action cycle

Source: From the *Journal of Continuing Education in the Health Professions*, Vol. 26, No. 1, Graham, I. D. et al., Lost in knowledge translation: Time for a map, pp. 13–24, copyright © 2006, John Wiley & Sons, Inc.

- Identify and understand a problem; identify, review and select the knowledge or research relevant to the problem;
- Adapt the identified knowledge or research to the local context;
- Assess barriers to using the knowledge;
- Select, tailor and implement interventions to promote the use of knowledge (i.e. implement the change);
- Monitor knowledge use;
- Evaluate the outcomes of using the knowledge; and
- Sustain ongoing knowledge use.

The Promoting Action on Research Implementation in Health Services (PARiHS) Framework

Originally developed by Kitson and colleagues (1998), the PARiHS model has subsequently been revised by members of the original research team and by other authors who have also developed a companion guide to apply the framework (Stetler, Damschroder, and Helfrichm, 2011). The framework describes three core elements that affect implementation of research into practice, i.e., evidence, context, and facilitation (see

Table 13.3), and can be expressed as the formula: $SI = f(E, C, F)$, where SI = successful implementation, E = evidence, C = context, F = facilitation, and f = function.

The PARiHS framework provides descriptions of each of the core elements and allows one to assess whether they are strong or weak, thereby helping to identify opportunities to strengthen elements that could improve implementation outcomes.

ments to meet the following requirements: to demonstrate effectiveness (i.e., "it works"), show the need for policy action (i.e., "it solves a problem"), guide effective implementation (i.e., "it can be done"), and demonstrate cost-effectiveness (i.e., "it is affordable and may even save money"). The framework also emphasizes the need for systems to have capacity in place to "adopt, adapt, and act" in order to achieve effective and sustained successful public health action.

The Evidence-Informed Policy and Practice Pathway

Developed by Bowen and Zwi (2005), this framework is geared to KT efforts within policy decision making environments. It purposely uses the term "evidence-informed" (instead of evidence-based) to signify that policy environments are influenced by various factors in addition to research evidence.

As illustrated in Figure 13.3, there are three stages in the pathway: (1) sourcing the evidence, (2) using the evidence, and (3) implementing the evidence. Evidence is sought in policy environ-

The Innovation to Implementation (I2I) Guide

Keeping in mind the caveat attributed to Friedrich Engels, a German economist: "An ounce of action is worth a ton of theory," a useful guide for working through individual KT plans entitled "Innovation to Implementation (I2I)" has been developed through the Mental Health Commission of Canada's Knowledge Exchange Centre (Bilsker, Petermann, and Goldner, 2012) and is available for download at the Mental Health Commission of Canada website. Built upon Lavis et al.'s (2003) framework, which expressed

---

Table 13.3   The Promoting Action on Research Implementation in Health Services (PARiHS)

Goals	To provide a map that explains the complexities of implementation and provides the elements that must be attended to in order to achieve successful implementation of research into practice
Elements	Implementation is a function of three elements:
	Evidence (E): codified and non-codified sources of knowledge Context (C): characteristics of the environment or setting Facilitation (F): support to help people change their attitudes, habits, skills, and ways of thinking and working
Overview	The PARiHS framework identifies key elements that determine the likelihood of success of implementation efforts. Assessment of the strength or weakness of various elements allows for opportunities to identify elements that could be strengthened in order to increase the success of implementation efforts.

Source: Adapted from Stetler, Damschroder, and Helfrichm (2011).

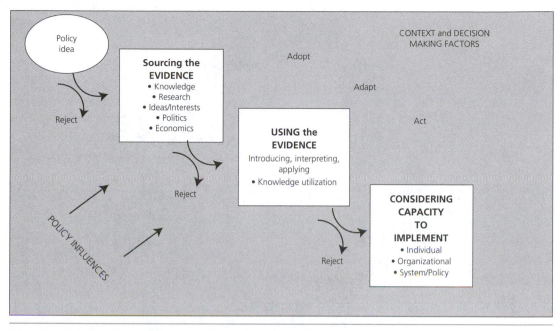

FIGURE 13.3 **The evidence-informed policy and practice pathway**

Source: Developed by Bowen and Zwi (2005)

basic questions to guide KT activities, the I2I is a practical, step-by-step guide to achieving successful KT. It highlights the importance of bringing a wide range of participants to the table, stresses the importance of incorporating various knowledge perspectives and lays out seven practical steps (see Figure 13.4).

Additional KT Concepts

"Push" and "Pull"

The **push** of KT refers to efforts to enhance the movement of knowledge from those who generate knowledge outward to those who may be able to benefit from its utilization. It involves gathering, synthesizing, and funnelling high quality information. In marketing (the field in which the terms "push" and "pull" originate), a push strategy is used when there has been a development or improvement of a new product that is unknown to the consumer. As there is no demand in the product launch, the product and the information are pushed to the consumer by distribution and promotion. In health care, push strategies may involve scientific publications, reports, systematic reviews, guidelines, online materials, conference presentations, courses, webinars, educational outreach, prompts, social marketing efforts, financial incentives, and media campaigns.

In marketing, **pull** refers to movement instigated by consumer requests in which the product is pulled through the delivery channel. In health care,

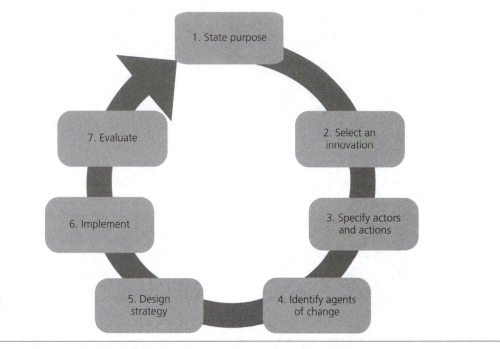

FIGURE 13.4   Steps for effective KT from "Implementation to Innovation (I2I)"

Source: Developed by the Mental Health Commission of Canada Knowledge Exchange Centre (Bilsker, Petermann & Goldner (2012)

Bilsker, D., Petermann, L., Goldner E.M. (2012). Innovation to implementation (I2I): A practical guide to knowledge translation in healthcare. Mental Health Commission of Canada. https://kec.mentalhealthcommission.ca/documents/knowledgeexchangeframework/i2i-innovation-to-implementation-workbookpdf.

knowledge is "pulled" when health care providers, policy makers or patients seek out the knowledge that is needed to guide their actions. Such efforts can be facilitated by effective search tools that can locate high quality information, access to knowledge syntheses and databases, training in the identification and application of research findings in decision making, critical appraisal skill development, and creation of rapid response units and government-university liaisons.

Some authors have suggested that there has been a progressive movement away from the use of pull mechanisms in health care over recent decades with a shift of responsibility now resting upon researchers to push scientific evidence into decision processes (Brousselle, Contandriopoulos, and Lemire, 2009; Mitton et al., 2007).

Integrated Knowledge Translation

Integrated Knowledge Translation signifies that potential knowledge users have been meaningfully engaged in the entire research process, involved from the outset and instrumental in shaping, refining and optimizing research development and implementation. There is an emphasis on researchers and knowledge users working closely together to design the research process, refine and undertake data collection processes, interpret findings, and communicate and implement knowledge that is produced. Research approaches in which such efforts are prominent are also described as *participatory action research* or *collaborative research* and they emphasize the importance of *co-production of knowledge*.

PRACTICAL TIP

By following each of the seven steps shown in Figure 13.4 and applying the tools provided in the I2I guide, one can assemble an approach to KT that is likely to be most effective. For example, if a program of research produced substantial evidence of improved detection rates, safety and cost-effectiveness of a new approach to prostate cancer screening, and you wished to undertake a KT plan, then the first step, "State the purpose of your KT plan," would be straightforward: i.e., the purpose would be to improve prostate cancer screening. The second step. "Select the innovation around which your KT plan will be built," would also be clear: i.e., a new prostate cancer screening procedure Y is more effective and safer, and should replace screening procedure X, which is currently used widely in Canada. The third step, "Specify the actors and actions: who needs to do what differently?," might be formulated to include health care providers across the country (who would need to shift from using screening procedure X to Y), local administrators (who would need to facilitate the cessation of procedure X and adopt the less expensive procedure Y), individuals likely to be at risk (i.e., adult and older adult males, who would need to be aware that they should be prescribed the more effective procedure Y), and government policy makers involved in funding and implementing prostate cancer screening (who would need to foster movement from procedure X to Y). To address the fourth step, "Identify the best agents of change: who should be delivering knowledge about this Innovation?," one must consider who is likely to be most effective in carrying the message to the target audience. Individuals and agencies with high credibility (such as well-respected prostate cancer specialists who are local opinion leaders) cancer agencies, and professional associations might be identified to be the best messengers to reach health care providers and administrators, whereas lobby groups, patient representatives, and economic policy researchers (who can demonstrate the economic savings) may be optimal messengers in addressing government policy makers and others.

In order to address the fifth step, "Design your KT plan," it is necessary to utilize best evidence about effective means of influencing the target audience and achieving change. Where they exist, the findings of implementation research studies relevant to the desired change (or a very similar initiative) should be applied. In this case, for example, educational outreach (academic detailing) would constitute an evidence-based KT method to influence practice by health care providers. Educational outreach is a KT method modeled upon successful interventions by pharmaceutical companies in which a detailer (i.e., a trained person) meets with health care providers in their practice setting to provide information with the intent of changing the provider's performance, e.g., by holding a lunch meeting in a group practice setting to review evidence on managing a particular condition. In designing the KT plan, one will also need to take into account the resources that are available to promote desired outcomes. In the next step, "Implement the plan," you might choose to implement your KT plan all at once or in a gradual manner. Where there is low readiness to adopt the Innovation, it may prove best to use a phased approach to implementation where the Innovation is gradually introduced to different parts of the system and community. Also, as you implement your plan, it is useful to get feedback about its perceived relevance, acceptability and feasibility, and this will allow you to tailor your KT plan accordingly. The final step in the cycle, "Evaluate your success," is crucial whether or not any formal evaluation of impact is planned. The entire KT initiative should be guided by the impact or outcome that one hopes to achieve. In this example, we hope to see the replacement of a commonly used screening procedure with a more effective and more economical approach. Ideally, this could be demonstrated through changes in practice, costs, detection rates, and patient outcomes.

Knowledge that is co-produced may result in scientific information being enhanced by knowledge gained through experiences of patients, family members, clinical providers, and others. Moreover, stakeholder groups that have contributed to knowledge production will have a greater "stake" in the uptake and utilization of knowledge. Collaborative efforts in KT allow stakeholder groups to undertake different and complementary efforts that could not be accomplished by any one group (e.g., patient groups may be able to successfully lobby for changes in policy or practice that would be impractical or unfeasible for researchers to achieve).

Integrated KT efforts may be considered particularly important in research addressing vulnerable populations, ethno-cultural minority groups, and people who are subjected to stigma and discrimination. In such circumstances, concerted efforts may be necessary to prevent dominant cultural values and beliefs from oppressing the creation and translation of relevant knowledge. Cargo and Mercer (2008) have developed a framework for participatory research that includes attention to integrated KT.

Diffusion, Dissemination, and Implementation

According to Lomas' (1993) taxonomy, **diffusion**, **dissemination**, and **implementation** are progressively more active steps in the process of moving research into action.

Diffusion refers to relatively passive and horizontal (i.e., amongst peers) activities, such as publishing findings in journals, presenting papers at academic meetings, or posting information on websites. Despite their limitations as means of effective KT, diffusion activities remain important and form a foundation for the development of more action-oriented KT efforts and opportunities exist to improve the likelihood that dif-

fused knowledge will reach relevant users. For example, although scientific journal publications are, for the most part, read by researchers (Pless, 2005), certain journals have readerships that consist of specific health professional groups or policy decision makers. Researchers can improve the likelihood that their work will reach a relevant audience by submitting papers to a journal selected with careful attention to the journal's readership. Other factors that are important in selecting journals include the journal's accessibility (e.g., whether it is widely available in library databases, is available online, and has "open access") and its "impact factor" rating (calculated on the basis of the numbers of citations of recent articles and considered a proxy measure for the relative importance of a journal within its field).

Dissemination delivers messages that are tailored to the target audience and uses effective delivery channels. Such efforts include the development and distribution of materials formatted to match the needs of particular stakeholder groups. Similarly, dissemination efforts may involve briefings, educational sessions, media communications, and other activities that are designed for specific target audiences.

Implementation is described by Lomas (1993) as the most active process in KT and one that is undertaken primarily at a local level, where barriers to the use of new knowledge can be effectively addressed and overcome. In general, effective implementation requires persistent and multi-faceted efforts that may be directed through various routes and means.

Linkage and Exchange

The gulf between researchers and decision makers, described previously by Feldman (1999) as "strangers in the night dimly aware of each other's presence," may be bridged through efforts to link these groups together in order to exchange knowledge

PRACTICAL TIP

The Canadian Health Services Research Foundation (CHSRF) has developed an approach to creating research summaries that are targeted for policy decision-makers using the "1:3:25" format.

One Page of Main Messages: These main messages are the lessons decision makers can take from the research and should articulate what implications the findings have for policy decision-makers.

Three Pages of Executive Summary: The executive summary is not an academic abstract but should be written like a newspaper story with the most prominent findings and key implications written first, followed by the background and context and less important information further down. The essence of the research findings should be communicated succinctly.

The (up to) 25 Page Report: CHSRF allots up to 25 pages for the complete report (double-spaced with 12-point type and 2.5 cm margins). They warn the researcher to refrain from lapsing into academic style to ensure that the writing suits the busy decision-maker, i.e. "intelligent and interested, but not an academic."

more effectively. Health research funding organizations have sought to foster such **linkage and exchange** by various means. They have provided innovative funding mechanisms that build linkage networks, released funding opportunities for groups that bridge research and practice environments, and have facilitated engagement between researchers and decision makers through specific requirements for active collaboration in grant applications. Various university programs have developed units that focus their activities on KT efforts addressing specific health care issues and these often work closely with community agencies, health care providers, governments, patients, and families. Some government ministries have provided funding to support university research programs that liaise closely with decision makers through an active linkage and exchange process.

KT Research Methods and Designs

A wide range of research designs is applicable to the study of KT and researchers have often applied mixed methods. The use of multiple, integrated methods may be particularly useful in the evaluation of the effects of complex health interventions such as those relevant to KT. However, Lewin and colleagues (2009) found that it was uncommon for qualitative studies to be undertaken alongside randomized trials, even where relatively complex KT interventions were being evaluated. Quantitative research designs applied to KT may involve randomization, such as cluster randomized controlled trials, randomized controlled trials, and quasi-experimental studies, as well as non-randomized designs, such as controlled before and after studies, interrupted time series designs, cohort studies, case-control designs, and cross-sectional studies. Randomized designs are more likely to provide unbiased information than are non-randomized designs in examining the differential effects of alternative KT interventions. However, there are instances in which KT interventions cannot be randomized or are unlikely to be studied in randomized trials whereas non-randomized designs may be feasible and provide meaningful information. Qualitative approaches applied to KT utilize grounded theory, phenomenological approaches, case studies, participant observation, and other ethnographic methods and apply various means of coding and content analysis, including computerized methods of data analysis (see Health Research in Action box 13.2).

Researchers studying KT have utilized systematic review methods frequently, including various reviews published through the Cochrane

13.2   Health Research in Action

A qualitative, participatory action-research study was undertaken to explore Indigenous approaches to KT by Dr Janet Smylie of the University of Toronto, Dr Nili Kaplan-Myrth of the University of Melbourne, Dr Kelly McShane of St Michael's Hospital in Toronto, and members of the Métis Nation of Ontario, the Pikwakanagan First Nation and the Tungasuvvingat Inuit Family Resource Center (Smylie et al., 2009). The investigators explored local Indigenous processes of knowledge creation, dissemination, and utilization in three Indigenous communities in Canada and applied these understandings to health-related KT activities. Local Indigenous community leaders, primary health care providers, traditional healers, youth counsellors, Elders, adults, and youth representatives of an urban Inuit, an urban Métis, and a semi-rural First Nations community collaborated with a multidisciplinary group of academics that included physicians, epidemiologists, anthropologists, lawyers, and psychologists, in order to design, facilitate, analyze, and evaluate the project.

The team recruited a purposive sample of diverse community members including health directors, frontline health workers, traditional knowledge experts, local Indigenous political leaders, youth, adults, and Elders to participate. Data collection included a combination of focus groups and key informant interviews in which participants were asked questions such as how they obtain information about physical, mental, emotional, or spiritual health issues, how they appraise the quality of such information, and how they would seek to spread such information in their community. An iterative process that involved repeated community corroboration was applied to data analysis.

Although the study found some commonalities amongst the Indigenous approaches to KT, they identified distinctive differences and unique features characteristic of each of the Inuit, Métis, and First Nations communities participating in the study.

One theme common to all three communities was the value of experiential knowledge, i.e., that medicines, health care providers, programs and services are evaluated based on the personal experiences of community members. Another theme common to the three communities was the use of family and community networks to disseminate health information.

In each of the three communities, themes that were considered specific to the community were identified and a few examples are provided here. The study identified that face-to-face interactions are important to the Inuit and that Inuit-specific health services have the most cultural relevance whereas other services, including those for First Nations, are perceived as non-Inuit and therefore less relevant. The study found that the First Nations participants identified concerns about privacy and stigma within their own community and indicated a preference for individual, rather than group-based, services in the context of a small community. The study found that Métis described the absence of a cohesive community information network as the result of increasingly disrupted community structures.

The authors concluded that KT activities are likely to be ineffective in the three participant communities without the local and specific understandings generated by community participants.

collaboration. As a new and emerging field of research, some novel research approaches to study KT have been developed and applied. For example, Valente (2010) has applied Social Network Analysis, Brousselle and colleagues (2009) have used Logic Analysis, and Ebener and colleagues (2006) have applied Knowledge Mapping as a technique to study KT.

TABLE 13.4 Studies That Provide Instruments Considered Promising for Evaluation of KT Impact and Implementation

Study	Instrument(s)
Ammendolia et al. (2004) Implementing evidence-based guidelines for radiography in acute low back pain: A pilot study in a chiropractic community.	(Name of instrument not given) A brief mailed survey to assess use of radiography for acute low back pain.
Dufault and Willey-Lessne (1999) Using a collaborative research utilization model to develop and test the effects of clinical pathways for pain management.	(1) Use of innovations questionnaire (2) Pain assessment audit instrument (3) Competency in research utilization (4) Attitudes towards research utilization scales
Neitzel et al. (1999) Improving pain management after total joint replacement surgery.	The knowledge and attitude survey regarding pain The survey measures knowledge and attitudes and consists of 39 questions in true/false, multiple choice, and case history formats.
Shirazi et al. (2008) Effects on readiness to change of an educational intervention on depressive disorders for general physicians in primary care based on a modified Prochaska model—a randomized controlled study.	Modified Prochaska questionnaire Used to assess readiness for change in a research transfer program, and consists of 11 statements answered by "yes" or "no" corresponding to the attitude stage, intention stage, and action stage.
Sung, Chang, and Abbey (2008) An implementation programme to improve nursing home staff's knowledge of and adherence to an individualized music protocol.	(1) Music knowledge questionnaire Modified from nursing staff's knowledge assessment tool of individualized music consisted of 18 true–false items. (2) Audit checklist A 10-item, self-report audit checklist to assess nursing staff's adherence to the music protocol containing yes–no items on implementation of the music protocol.
Titler et al. (2009) Translating research into practice intervention improves management of acute pain in older hip fracture patients.	(1) The perceived stage of adoption instrument Measures nurses' and physicians' adoption of practices that have a research base. (2) Medical record abstract form A 19-page abstract instrument used to determine nurse and physician conformance to a clinical guideline in acute pain management practices. (3) Summative index (SI) of quality care pain management Eighteen variables selected by consensus representing aspects of evidence-based pain management, scored 1 or 0, summed to yield SI score. (4) Barriers to optimal pain management tool Addresses the extent that system and practice issues are perceived by nurses and physicians as barriers to pain management. (5) Use of research findings in practice scale A nine-point scale that asks respondents to select one statement that best reflects use of research-based acute pain management practices in the organization.

Source: Adapted from Van Eerd et al. (2008)

Various measures have been utilized to examine KT outcomes ranging from citation indices and other bibliometric measures, self-reported measures of knowledge, behaviour or practice, ratings made through semi-structured audits of clinical records or program outputs, and specific instruments developed for the purpose of measuring KT impact. Van Eerd and colleagues (2011) undertook a systematic review of the quality and types of instruments used to assess KT implementation and impact. They found few well-developed instruments in which reliability or validity was

adequately assessed, and that most studies did not clearly report instrument measurement properties and did not utilize context-specific instruments. Table 13.4 lists the studies that contained instruments that they considered to be promising for the evaluation of KT implementation and impact, and Table 13.5 shows the studies of the instrument development they considered to be of good quality. It is likely that the field of KT will see further development of reliable and valid measures and the application of strong research designs in the future.

TABLE 13.5   Studies of Instrument Development Considered Promising for Evaluation of KT Impact and Implementation

Study	Instrument
Bahtsevani et al. (2008) Developing an instrument for evaluating implementation of clinical practice guidelines: a test-retest study.	(Name of instrument not given) A 23-item instrument for evaluating implementation of clinical practice guidelines. Includes questions on respondent characteristics and on use, implementation and evaluation of the clinical practice guideline. Some items include visual analogue scales constructed using statements drawn from the PARiHS framework and related to patients' experiences.
Grad et al. (2008) Impact of research-based synopses delivered as daily e-mail: a prospective observational study.	Cognitive impact assessment scale A 10-item pop-up questionnaire to examine the global construct of cognitive impact of health information by email alert called Info POEM.
Shiffman et al. (2005) The GuideLine Implementability Appraisal (GLIA): development of an instrument to identify obstacles to guideline implementation.	GuideLine Implementability Appraisal Consists of 31 items, arranged into 10 dimensions. Decidability and Executability are critical dimensions. Other dimensions are Global, Presentation and Formatting, Measurable Outcomes, Apparent Validity, Flexibility, Effect on Process of Care, Novelty/Innovation, and Computability. Questions from nine of the 10 dimensions are applied individually to each recommendation of the guideline.

Source: From Van Eerd et al. (2008).

Summary

- KT is defined to be a broad concept that encompasses all steps from the creation of new knowledge to its application in the production of beneficial outcomes.

- Passive forms of knowledge translation appear to be relatively ineffective in comparison to more active approaches.
- KT strategies effective in influencing health care providers include educational outreach,

audit, and feedback; use of opinion leaders, reminders, and prompts; and interactive educational meetings.

- KT strategies effective in influencing the general public and patient behaviour include mass media campaigns, social marketing approaches, community mobilization, laws and regulations, financial incentives and disincentives, and self-management.
- A KT strategy that is effective in influencing policy decision makers is targeted, tailored messaging.
- Factors that influence the effectiveness of KT strategies include the simplicity of KT mes-

sages and various organizational characteristics related to absorptive capacity.

- Various frameworks and guides have been developed to assist KT activities.
- Concepts that underlie KT theory and practice include push and pull, integrated KT, diffusion, dissemination, implementation, and linkage and exchange.
- A wide variety of quantitative and qualitative study designs have been applied in KT research.
- Although various measures have been developed to study KT, few of these have been shown to have adequate reliability or validity.

Review Questions

1. How would you define the concept of KT?

2. Which KT strategies are effective in influencing health care providers, the general public and patients and policy decision makers?

3. What factors influence the effectiveness of KT strategies?

4. Describe a framework or guide that has been proposed for KT.

5. Compare and contrast: diffusion, dissemination, and implementation.

6. Describe a research design that has been used to study KT and explain its strengths and limitations.

Recommended Readings and Websites

Institute for Work and Health. From research to practice: A knowledge transfer planning guide. Retrieved from www.iwh.on.ca/system/files/at-work/kte_planning_guide_2006b.pdf.

A practical guide to the creation of a KT plan.

Sudsawad P. Knowledge translation: Introduction to models, strategies, and measures. The National Center for the Dissemination of Disability Research, The University of Wisconsin–Madison. Retrieved from www.ncddr.org/kt/products/ktintro/.

A review of KT that includes descriptions of frameworks and research measures that have been utilized.

National Collaborating Centre for Methods and Tools website: Knowledge translation methods and tools for public health. Retrieved from www.nccmt.ca/methods_and_tools-eng.html

Provides summaries and reviews of tools and frameworks that have been developed to addresss KT.

Canadian Health Services Research Foundation. Resources for Researchers. Retrieved from www.chsrf.ca/PublicationsAndResources/ResourcesForResearchers.aspx.

Provides a series of tools and tips designed to help researchers in undertaking KT activities.

Bilsker, D., Petermann, L., and Goldner E.M. (2012) Innovation to Implementation (I2I): A practical guide to knowledge translation in health care. Mental Health Commission of Canada. Retrieved from https://kec.mentalhealthcommission.ca/documents/knowledgeexchangeframework/i2i-innovation-to-implementation-workbookpdf.

References

Ammendolia, C., Hogg-Johnson, S., Pennick, V. et al. (2004) Implementing evidence-based guidelines for radiography in acute low back pain: a pilot study in a chiropractic community. *Journal of Manipulative and Physiological Therapeutics, 27*(3), 170–9.

Anderson, M. and Lavoie-Tremblay, M. (2008) Evaluation of the Executive Training for Research Application (EXTRA) Program: Design and early findings. *Health Care Policy, 4*(2): e136–e48.

Babor, T.F., Caulkins, J.P., Edwards, G. et al. (2009) *Drug Policy and the Public Good.* Oxford: University Press.

Bahtsevani C, Willman A, Khalaf A, et al. (2008) Developing an instrument for evaluating implementation of clinical practice guidelines: A test-retest study. *Journal of Evaluation in Clinical Practice. 14*(5), 839–46.

Barlow, J., Wright, C., Sheasby, J. et al. (2002) Self-management approaches for people with chronic conditions: A review. *Patient Education and Counseling, 48*(2), 177–87.

Barwick, M., Peters, J. and Boydell, K. (2009) Getting to uptake: Do communities of practice support the implementation of evidence-based practice? *Journal of the Canadian Academy of Child and Adolescent Psychiatry, 18*(1), 16–29.

Bero, L.A., Grilli, R., Grimshaw, J.M. et al. (1998) Closing the gap between research and practice: An overview of systematic reviews of interventions to promote the implementation of research findings. *British Medical Journal, 317*, 465–8.

Boaz, A., Baeza, J., Fraser, A. (2011) Effective implementation of research into practice: An overview of systematic reviews of the health literature. *BioMed Central Research Notes. 4*:212.

Bowen, S. and Zwi, A.B. (2005) Pathways to "evidence-informed" policy and practice: A framework for action. *PLoS Medicine, 2*(7), e166.

Brousselle, A., Contandriopoulos, D., and Lemire, M. (2009) Using logic analysis to evaluate knowledge transfer initiatives: The case of the research collective on the organization of primary care services. *Evaluation, 15*(2), 165–83.

Canadian Institutes of Health Research. (2012) The Jonathan Lomas KT Doctoral Research Award Supplement. Retrieved Feb 27, 2012 from www.cihr-irsc.gc.ca/e/36548.html.

Cargo, M. and Mercer, S.L. (2008) The value and challenges of participatory research: Strengthening its practice. *Annual Review of Public Health, 29*, 325–50.

Cauffman, J.G., Forsyth, R.A., Clark, V.A. et al. (2002). Randomized controlled trials of continuing medical education: What makes them most effective? *Journal of Continuing Education in the Health Professions, 22*(4), 214–21.

Chaloupka FJ, Straif K, Leon ME. (2011). Effectiveness of tax and price policies in tobacco control. *Tobacco Control, 20*(3), 235–8.

Cochrane Public Health Group (CPHG). (2012) Retrieved March 1, 2012 from http://ph.cochrane.org/.

Colquhoun, H.L., Letts, L.J., Law, M.C., et al. (2010) A scoping review of the use of theory in studies of knowledge translation. *Canadian Journal of Occupational Therapy, 77*(5): 270–9.

Coulter, A., Ellins, J. (2007) Effectiveness of strategies for informing, educating, and involving patients. *British Medical Journal, 335*, 24-7.

Damschroder, L.J., Aron, D.C., Keith, R.E. et al. (2009) Fostering implementation of health services research findings into practice: A consolidated framework for advancing implementation science. *Implementation Science, 4*(50), 1–15.

Dobbins, M., Hanna, S.E., Ciliska, D., Manske, S., Cameron, R., Mercer, S.L. et al. (2009) A randomized controlled trial evaluating the impact of knowledge translation and exchange activities. *Implementation Science, 4*(61), 23.

Driedger, S.M., Kothari, A., Graham, I.D. et al. (2010) If you build it, they still may not come: Outcomes and process of implementing a community-based integrated knowledge translation mapping innovation. *Implementation Science, 16*(5), 47.

Du, S. and Yuan, C. (2010) Evaluation of patient self-management outcomes in health care: A systematic review. *International Nursing Review, 57*(2), 159–67.

Dufault, M.A. and Willey-Lessne, C. (1999) Using a collaborative research utilization model to develop and test the effects of clinical pathways for pain management. *Journal of Nursing Care Quality. 13*(4), 19–33.

Estabrooks, C.A., Thompson, D.S., Lovely, J.J.E. et al. (2006). A guide to knowledge translation theory. *The Journal of Continuing Education in the Health Professions, 26*, 25–36.

Feldman, S. (1999) Strangers in the night: Research and managed mental health care, *Health Affairs, 18*(5), 48–51.

Forsetlund, L., Bjørndal, A., Rashidian, A. et al. (2009) Continuing education meetings and workshops: effects on professional practice and health care outcomes. *Cochrane Database of Systematic Reviews*, (2), CD003030.

Foster, G., Taylor, S.J.C., Eldridge, S.E. et al. (2007) Self-management education programmes by lay leaders for people with chronic conditions. *Cochrane Database of Systematic Reviews*, (4), CD005108.

Francke, A.L., Smit, M.C., de Veer, A.J., Mistiaen, P. (2008) Factors influencing the implementation of clinical guidelines for health care professionals: a systematic meta-review. *BMC Medical Informatics and Decision Making, 8*(1), 38.

Gagnon, M.L. (2011) Moving knowledge to action through dissemination and exchange. *Journal of Clinical Epidemiology, 64*(1), 25–31.

Gordon, R., McDermott, L., Stead, M. et al. (2006). The effectiveness of social marketing interventions for health improvement: What's the evidence? *Public Health, 120*(12), 1133–9.

Grad, R.M., Pluye, P., Mercer, J. et al. (2008) Impact of research-based synopses delivered as daily e-mail: A prospective observational study. *Journal of the American Medical Informatics Association. 15*(2), 240–5.

Graham, I.D., Logan, J., Harrison, M. et al. (2006) Lost in translation: Time for a map? *Journal of Continuing Education in the Health Professions, 26,* 13–24.

Graham, I.D. and Tetroe, J.M. (2009) Getting evidence into policy and practice: Perspective of a health research funder. *Journal of the Canadian Academy of Child and Adolescent Psychiatry, 218*(1), 46–50.

Grimshaw, J.M., Shirran, L., Wensing, M., Dijkstra, R., Donaldson, C., Thomas, R.E. et al. (2004) Effectiveness and efficiency of guideline dissemination and implementation strategies. *Health Technology Assessment, 8*(6), 1.

Greenhalgh, T., Robert, G., Bate, P. et al. (2005) *Diffusion of innovations in health service organisations: A systematic literature review.* Malden, MA: Blackwell.

Grimshaw, J. and Eccles, M. (2004) Is evidence-based implementation of evidence-based care possible? *Medical Journal of Australia, 180,* S50–S1.

Grimshaw, J.M., Shirran, L., Thomas, R. et al. (2001) Changing provider behavior: An overview of systematic reviews of interventions. *Medical Care, 39*(8 Suppl 2), II2–45.

Grimshaw, J.M., Thomas, R.E., MacLennan, G. et al. (2004) Effectiveness and efficiency of guideline dissemination and implementation strategies. *Health Technology Assessment, 8*(6), iii–iv, 1–72.

Hogan, D.L. and Logan, J. (2004) The Ottawa model of research use: A guide to clinical innovation in the NICU. *Clinical Nurse Specialist, 18,* 255–61.

Institute of Medicine. (2001) *Crossing the Quality Chasm: A New Health System for the 21st Century.* Washington, D.C.: National Academy Press.

Jacobson, N., Butterill, D., and Goering, P (2003) Development of a framework for knowledge translation: Understanding user context. *Journal of Health Services Research and Policy, 8,* 94–9.

Jamtvedt, G., Young, J.M., Kristoffersen, D.T. et al. (2006) Audit and feedback: effects on professional practice and health care outcomes. *Cochrane Database of Systematic Reviews,* (2), CD000259.

Jepson, R.G., Harris, F.M., and Platt, S. (2010) The effectiveness of interventions to change six health behaviours: A review of reviews. *BMC Public Health, 8,* 10, 538.

Kitson, A., Harvey, G., and McCormack, B. (1998) Enabling the implementation of evidence based practice: A conceptual framework. *Quality in Health Care, 7*(3), 149–58.

Kothari, A., Rudman, D., Dobbins, M. et al. (2012) The use of tacit and explicit knowledge in public health: A qualitative study. *Implementation Science, 20*(7), 20.

Lavis, J. N., Robertson, D., Woodside, J. M. et al. (2003). How can research organizations more effectively transfer research knowledge to decision makers? *The Milbank Quarterly, 81*(2), 221–48.

Lavis, J.N., Wilson, M.G., Grimshaw, J.M. (2011) Effects of an evidence service on health system policymakers' use of research evidence: A protocol for a randomized controlled trial. *Implementation Science, 6*(1): 51.

Lewin, S., Glenton, C., and Oxman, A.D. (2009) Use of qualitative methods alongside randomised controlled trials of complex health care interventions: Methodological study. *British Medical Journal, 339,* b3496.

Locock, L., Dopson, S., Chambers, D. et al. (2001) Understanding the role of opinion leaders in improving clinical effectiveness. *Social Science and Medicine, 53:* 745–57.

Lomas, J. (1993) Diffusion, dissemination and implementation: Who should do what? *Annals of the New York Academy of Sciences, 703,* 226-35.

Lorig, K.R. and Holman, H. (2003) Self-management education: History, definition, outcomes, and mechanisms. *Annals of Behavioral Medicine*, 26(1), 1–7.

Mitton, C., Adair, C.E., McKenzie, E.,et al. (2007) Knowledge transfer and exchange: Review and synthesis of the literature. *Milbank Quarterly*, 85, 729–68.

Marteau, T.M., Ashcroft, R.E., and Oliver, A. (2009) Using financial incentives to achieve healthy behaviour. *British Medical Journal*, 338, 983–985.

Mental Health Commission of Canada (2011) Activated knowledge exchange framework. Retrieved February 11, 2013 from https://kec.mentalhealthcommission.ca/about_kec/keframework.

Moulton, A.D., Mercer, S.L., Popovic, T. et al. (2009) The scientific basis for law as a public health tool. *American Journal of Public Health*, 99(1), 17–24.

Murphy, E.M. (2005) *Promoting Healthy Behavior, Health Bulletin 2*. Washington, DC: Population Reference Bureau.

Neitzel, J.J., Miller, E.H., Shepherd, M.F., and Belgrade, M. (1999) Improving pain management after total joint replacement surgery. *Orthopaedic Nursing*, 18(4), 37-45.

O'Brien, M.A., Freemantle, N., Oxman, A.D. et al. (2001) Continuing education meetings and workshops: effects on professional practice and health care outcomes. *The Cochrane Database of Systematic Reviews*, (1), CD003030.

O'Brien, M.A., Oxman, A.D., Haynes, R.B. et al. (1999) Local opinion leaders: effects on professional practice and health care outcomes. *The Cochrane Database of Systematic Reviews*, (1), CD000125.

O'Brien, M.A., Rogers, S., Jamtvedt, G. et al. (2007) Educational outreach visits: effects on professional practice and health care outcomes. *The Cochrane Database of Systematic Reviews*, (4), CD000409.

Orton, L., Lloyd-Williams, F., Taylor-Robinson, D. et al. (2011) The use of research evidence in public health decision making processes: Systematic review. *PLoS ONE*, 6(7): e21704. doi:10.1371/journal.pone.0021704.

Panisset, U., Koehlmoos, T.P., Alkhatib, A.H. et al. (2012) Implementation research evidence uptake and use for policy-making. *Health Research Policy and Systems*, 10, 20.

Peirson, L., Ciliska, D., Dobbins, M., et al. (2012) Building capacity for evidence informed decision making in public health: A case study of organizational change. BMC *Public Health*, 12, 137.

Pless, I.B. (2005) Do scientific publications change anything? *Injury Prevention*, 11, 193–4.

Roussos, S.T. and Fawcett S.B. (2000) A review of collaborative partnerships as a strategy for improving community health. Annual Review of Public Health, 21, 369–402.

Rycroft-Malone, J. (2004) The PARiHS framework: A framework for guiding the implementation of evidence-based practice. *Journal of Nursing Care Quality*, 19, 297–304.

Scott, A., Sivey, P., Ait Ouakrim, D. et al. (2011) The effect of financial incentives on the quality of health care provided by primary care physicians. *The Cochrane Database of Systematic Reviews*, (9), CD008451.

Shiffman, R.N., Dixon, J., Brandt, C. et al. (2005) The GuideLine Implementability Appraisal (GLIA): Development of an instrument to identify obstacles to guideline implementation. *BMC Medical Informatics and Decision Making*, 5, 23.

Shirazi, M., Zeinaloo, A.A., Parikh, S.V. et al. (2008) Effects on readiness to change of an educational intervention on depressive disorders for general physicians in primary care based on a modified Prochaska model—A randomized controlled study. *Family Practice*, 25(2), 98–104.

Smylie, J., Kaplan-Myrth, N., McShane, K. et al. (2009) Indigenous knowledge translation: Baseline findings in a qualitative study of the pathways of health knowledge in three indigenous communities in Canada. *Health Promotion Practice*, *10*(3), 436–46.

Stetler, C.B., Damschroder, L.J., Helfrich, C.D. et al. (2011) A guide for applying a revised version of the PARiHS framework for implementation. *Implementation Science*, 6, 99.

Straus, S., Tetroe J., and Graham, I.D. (Eds.) (2009) *Knowledge Translation in Health Care: Moving from Evidence to Practice*. Oxford, U.K.: Wiley-Blackwell.

Sung, H., Chang, A.M., and Abbey, J. (2008) An implementation programme to improve nursing home staff's knowledge of and adherence to an individualized music protocol. *Journal of Clinical Nursing*. *17*(19), 2573–9.

Tenopir, C. and King, D.W. (2001) The use and value of scientific journals: Past, present and future. *Serials: The Journal for the Serials Community*, *14*(2), 113–20.

Tetroe, J.M., Graham, I.D., Foy, R. et al. (2008) Health research funding agencies' support and promotion of knowledge translation: An international study. *The Milbank Quarterly*, *86*(1), 125–55.

Titler, M.G. (2008) The evidence for evidence-based practice implementation. In Hughes, R.G. (Ed.), *Patient Safety and Quality: An Evidence-Based Handbook for Nurses*. AHRQ Publication No. 08-0043. Rockville, MD: Agency for Health care Research and Quality.

Titler, M.G., Herr, K., Brooks, J.M. et al. (2009) Translating research into practice intervention improves management of acute pain in older hip fracture patients. *Health Services Research*, *44*(1), 264–87.

Valente, T.W. (2010) *Social Networks and Health: Models, Methods, and Applications*. New York: Oxford University Press, 2010.

Van Eerd, D., Cole, D., Keown, K., Irvin, E. et al. (2011) *Report on knowledge transfer and exchange practices: A systematic review of the quality and types of instruments used to assess KTE implementation and impact*. Toronto: Institute for Work and Health.

Wakefield, M.A., Loken, B., and Hornik, R.C. (2010) Use of mass media campaigns to change health behaviour. *The Lancet*, *376*(9748), 1261–71.

Weinreich, N.K. (2011) *Hands-On Social Marketing: A Step-by-Step Guide to Designing Change for Good*, 2nd ed. Thousand Oaks, California: Sage Publications.

Xu, X. and Chaloupka, F.J. (2011) The effects of prices on alcohol use and its consequences. *Alcohol Research and Health*, *34*(2), 236–45.

Glossary

absolute risk reduction the difference in risk when comparing the treatment group with the comparison group

acquiescence bias a tendency to agree with items on a scale, irrespective of their content (also called *yea-saying bias*); a tendency for participants to respond in a manner that makes the participant look good in the eye of the interviewer

activities of daily living (ADL) daily self-care activities, such as bathing, dressing, grooming, work, housekeeping, and so forth

adjectival scale an item response format consisting of adjectives that convey a gradation in the attribute of interest (e.g., None/A Little/Somewhat/A Lot)

age pyramid a type of graph that depicts the age distribution of various groups in a population of interest

age-standardized mortality rate the proportion of people who die in a given population during a particular time period, controlling for age differences during the reference period

alternative hypothesis an explicit statement of some relationship between the exposure of interest and the disease or outcome of interest; typically a rival statement to the null hypothesis

anonymous data information about a person that can never be associated with or linked to that person

assent an agreement or willingness to participate in research from those with at least a minimal level of understanding

assumptions conditions that allow for valid conclusions to be drawn from a test statistic

audit and feedback the provision of information to health care providers about their own clinical performance, allowing comparison of their performance with that of their peers

autoethnography a qualitative research method that seeks to describe and systematically analyze self-narratives and personal experiences in order to link them to cultural experiences and practices.

bias a distortion; any procedural or systematic error that distorts how the collected data can speak of the population and lead to conclusions that differ from the truth; sources of bias are numerous, and include selection bias, acquiescence bias, and non-response bias

bimodal distribution a continuous data distribution with two nearly equal peaks or *modes*

binomial distribution a discrete data distribution that summarizes the likelihood of one of two outcomes under a given set of assumptions.

bipolar scale an item response format where the scores are extreme at either end and neutral in the middle (contrast with *unipolar scale)*

blind (assignment) allocation of a participant to a treatment or control group where the participant is not told which group they are being allocated to; a method of exposure allocation used in an effort to reduce bias

bound the extreme values of an interval such as a confidence interval

> **lower** the smallest number for the parameter of interest

> **upper** the largest number for the parameter of interest

box plot a graphical display that summarizes key descriptive characteristics of the data collected

case-control (study) a study design in which individuals with the disease or outcome of interest (cases) and without (controls) are selected for participation based on their disease status and compared with respect to the exposure of interest

case fatality rate the proportion of individuals with a disease or health problem of interest who die within a given time frame

categorical judgement a family of response options consisting of discrete categories (e.g., *Likert scale*, adjectival scale, *Harter scale*)

cause-specific standardized mortality ratio the ratio of the number of observed deaths from a given cause to the expected number of deaths over a given time period

central tendency an index showing where most of the data cluster (see *mean*, *median*, and *mode*)

classical test theory a psychometric theory that assumes a test score is composed of a *true score* plus *random error*

clinical epidemiology a field concerned with applying the principles of epidemiology in a clinical setting; the critical evaluation of diagnostic and therapeutic practices used in health care

cluster sampling a probability based method of selecting individuals or units from a population for study participation that is used when the population is divided into groups, or clusters, where groups are randomly selected rather than individuals or units

Cochrane Handbook of Systematic Reviews of Interventions the official document that describes in detail the process of preparing and maintaining Cochrane systematic reviews on the effects of health care interventions

cognitive interviewing various techniques of questioning individuals to determine if they understand the wording and intent of an item; used to evaluate the quality of the response or to help determine whether the item is generating the information intended

cohort a group of people who share a common factor (e.g. year of birth, exposure to a suspected risk factor)

cohort study a research design in which individuals are recruited to participate on the basis of their exposure status. Participants are followed over time and disease status outcomes are compared by exposure status.

communities of practice (also known as "communities of interest") self-organized, networks of peers with skills and experience in an area of practice or profession

community-based and participatory action research research in which there is a strong emphasis on partnership between the researchers and the community of interest, ensuring that members of the community under study have meaningful roles in the planning, design and implementation of the research

community mapping a qualitative technique where community members pool their knowledge and experiences of their community, represented in a graphic form or map

community mobilization community-wide efforts to address a health or social issue; may bring together local, provincial, and federal governments, professional groups, religious groups, businesses, and individual community members

comparison an alternative intervention often used as the reference intervention when contrasted with an intervention of interest

compositional factors variables or attributes that describe the characteristics or parts of some whole (e.g. attributes that describe characteristics of individual cases within a population)

concealment of allocation a procedure used to ensure that the researcher who assigns participants to a treatment group does not know whether participants will be assigned to the intervention group or the control group; a procedure intended to prevent selection bias

conceptual definition the process where a notion or idea is translated or defined as a measurable variable; provides the specific meaning of the concept

conference proceedings in academia, proceedings are the collection of papers published in the context of an academic conference

confidence coefficient a number expressed as a percentage that indicates how likely the population parameter is to be included in a confidence interval; usually 95 per cent

confidence interval an estimated range of values (interval) in which the population parameter is likely to fall within; the estimated range is supported by the sample data and is usually stated in the original units of measurement

two-sided an interval with both a lower and an upper bound for the values of the parameter in the population

95 per cent confidence interval the range of values in which the estimated parameter is likely to fall 95 per cent of the time; alternatively, 95 times out of 100, the true population value lies within a particular range

confidentiality refers to the researchers' obligation to safeguard and protect private information that participants provide during data collection

conflict of interest (CoI) a situation where there are two or more actual or potential contradictory interests that are held by a person or organization in a decision-making position

consequentialism the theory that an action, rule or decision is morally right because it produces certain outcomes (e.g., maximizes benefit or pleasure)

CONSORT an acronym for Consolidated Standards for Reporting Trials; see www.CONSORT-statement.org

constant comparison a method that is used to compare and analyze qualitative data; serves as the foundation for developing grounded theory

construct validity the extent to which a scale, or the operationalization of a concept, performs as the theory predicts it will

constructionism a philosophy of knowledge creation that posits that scientific knowledge is constructed by scientists through measurements and models of the world; opposes the philosophy of objectivism

content coverage the degree to which a scale measures all aspects of a construct (see content validation)

content irrelevance a judgment surrounding whether a scale contains any items that are not pertinent to the construct (see content validation)

content validation the degree to which a scale measures all aspects of a construct and does not contain any irrelevant content (see *content coverage*, *content irrelevance*, and *content validity ratio*)

content validity ratio a number between −1 and +1 that measures the degree to which raters or experts feel the items of a scale are relevant to the construct being measured (see content validation)

contextual factors variables or attributes that describe the characteristics of an environment

continuous a statement about a set of numbers that continue uninterrupted in sequence; allows for sensible numbers to be inserted between any two distinct numbers where the inserted number makes sense, such as mass in kilograms where 2 and 5 would permit any number such 3.6 to be within these two numbers and it makes sense as a mass

continuous judgement a response format in which the respondent places a mark along a continuum (e.g., a visual analogue scale)

control group the comparison group in a research study that receives standard treatment, placebo treatment, or no treatment rather than being exposed to the experimental treatment of interest

control variable a variable that does not change or is held constant in data analysis in order to assess the relationship between the exposure and outcome of interest without interference

constructionism an ontological position that emphasizes the social construction of meaning

correlation coefficient a measure of the straight line relationship between two variables; values range between –1 and 1; values below 0 indicate a negative relationship where one variable is increasing as the other variable is decreasing and values above 0 indicate a positive relationship where both variables are increasing

criterion standard another name for the level of significance represented by the first Greek letter alpha, α

criterion value a value of the referent distribution that separates statistical significance from non-significance

critical appraisal the use of explicit, transparent methods to assess published research evidence surrounding factors such as internal validity, relevance, adherence to reporting standards, conclusions, and generalizability

critical race theory a set of practices and theories that recognizes that racism is engrained in the fabric, system, and structure of society and aims to redress the existing power structures and social inequalities

critical realism an epistemological position that emphasizes the structural underpinnings of observable phenomena

critical theory a broad theoretical approach that tends to rely on reflective dialogue through assessment and critique in order to question or challenge the natural order; is often concerned with power and how power produces structural inequalities in society

Cronbach's alpha a measure of the degree to which items in a scale are correlated with one another; reflects the *internal consistency* of a scale

cross-sectional study/survey a study design that measures exposure and disease status at the same point in time

crude mortality rate the number of people who die during a given time period (usually one year) divided by the average population size (usually 100,000); not adjusted for any other factors

cumulative frequency used to determine the number of observations that lie above or below a particular value in the data; expressed as a percentage

data a collection of information that represents features of a measured unit; often used as a basis for reasoning

decimal place the number of digits to the right of the decimal point; e.g., 1.234 would be said to have three decimal places

decision making refers to the day-to-day work undertaken by politicians, government bureaucrats and/or administrators in making decisions regarding policy, financing, practices or programs that may have a substantial impact on patients, health care providers and others

deduction a form of reasoning in research that typically begins with a theoretical position where hypotheses are derived and tested, leading to specific conclusions and the generation of new knowledge

deontology an ethical theory that focuses on the nature of actions and motives, with less overt attention to consequences

dependent variable the outcome or disease factor of interest in a study; the factor that is effected in an experiment

depth the number of observations seen from the lower or upper end of the distribution data presented in a *stem and leaf plot*

descriptive statistics quantitative measures used to describe the main features of a set of data; usually includes measures of *central tendency* and of *dispersion*

diffusion efforts to communicate knowledge that are considered relatively passive and horizontal (i.e., amongst peers) in nature, such as publishing findings in journals, presenting papers at academic meetings or posting information on websites

discourse analysis an analytic framework that examines how language both shapes and reflects dynamic cultural, social, and political practices, where the researcher aims to understand how people use language to create and enact identities and activities

discrete a statement about a set of numbers that cannot have values between them; separate and distinct numbers that make sense, for example 2 and 4 make sense, however, 3.7 does not make sense; usually expressed as whole integers

discussion the part of a written report that puts the findings of a study into context as they relate to the existing literature; this section of the written report also documents the strengths and limitations of the study

dissemination efforts to communicate knowledge that are tailored to the target audience

dispersion a statistical term reflecting the degree of variability or spread in a measure

distribution a numerical or graphical display of frequency data

document study a qualitative research study in which documents are interpreted by the researcher to give voice and meaning around a topic of interest; documents can include: public records, personal records, or artifacts

double-barrelled question an item that, overtly or covertly, asks two questions simultaneously

double-blind assignment approach allocation of participants to the treatment or control groups where neither the participants nor the researchers know which group the participant has been allocated to; a method of exposure allocation used in an effort to reduce bias

drop-outs the number of participants who start a study and do not complete it

ecological study a study in which the exposure and/or disease data are measured at the group level as opposed to the individual level

EDA the acronym for exploratory data analysis

educational outreach visits (also known as "academic detailing") personal visits by a trained, credible person to health professionals in their own settings in which evidence-based, tailored information is provided for the purposes of influencing specific practice behaviours

effect size a descriptive statistic that conveys the estimated magnitude of a relationship without making any statement about whether the apparent relationship in the data reflects a true relationship in the population

(statistical) efficiency (see also *sampling error*) a relative measure that indicates how a given sampling strategy will be more or less costly than a competing sampling strategy for the same expected precision or, conversely, how more or less precise a sampling strategy will be for a given cost (i.e. sample size)

end-aversion bias the tendency of a participant to avoid the extreme categories of a response

epidemiology the study of the distribution and patterns of health-related conditions and the factors that affect them in a population

epistemology the branch of philosophy concerned with the nature and breadth of knowledge and truth

equal variances the notion that the variances of a measure calculated from two groups or more groups are considered to be close enough to be equal

error variations in a scale's score due to unknown factors (see *random error* and *systematic theory*); mistakes in data that can be sensibly set aside when calculating descriptive and inferential statistics in a study, though they should always be reported in the findings

ethics a branch of philosophy that is concerned with systematic investigation of right and wrong conduct

ethnography a form of qualitative inquiry that is both a process and a product; aims to investigate and uncover cultural systems of meaning and knowledge; as a process, ethnography consists of in-depth, first hand fieldwork where the researcher is immersed in the day-to-day life of the cultural group through participant observation; as a product, ethnography is a written, detailed text that describes and interprets the everyday life and practices (including the language, behaviour and beliefs) of the culture from an insider perspective

evidence-based behavioural practice decisions about how to promote health or provide care by integrating the best available evidence with practitioner expertise and other resources

with the characteristics, state, needs, values, and preferences of those who will be affected

evidence-based medicine the conscientious, explicit, and judicious use of current best evidence in making decisions about the care of individual patients; requires the integration of individual clinical expertise with the best available external clinical evidence from systematic research and the patient's or client's unique values and circumstances

evidence-based practice an interdisciplinary approach to clinical practice that evolved from *evidence-based medicine*

exclusion criteria the standards or conditions that are used to determine whether or not an individual is eligible to participate in a study

exhaustive a set of categories that encompass all the observed data for a variable

experimental study a study design in which the researcher controls allocation of the exposure of interest to assess the effect on a particular outcome

explicit knowledge the form of knowledge that follows logic, can be codified, written down and effectively communicated to others

exploratory data analysis techniques used to find and summarize patterns in the data

exposure the measure in a study that reflects the factor or characteristic that is being assessed as a determinant of the health outcome of interest

fabrication deliberately made up data, methodology, or findings that are recorded or reported

factor analysis a statistical procedure used to determine whether many items can be grouped into subsets of items that are correlated with one another

falsification a manipulation, misrepresentation or alteration in data or equipment without acknowledgment and which results in research findings that are not accurately represented

fixed response range a type of response option often used in questionnaires where participants are given limited choices through which to express their answers; may take the form of *Likert* or Likert-type scales

focus groups a qualitative research technique that consists of an interview involving more than two participants, usually six to ten, where data is collected through group interaction on a topic determined by the researcher

frequency a count of how often something happens over a particular time period or within a particular population

generalize, generalizability the ability to extend the results obtained from a sample to the whole population without bias; sometimes called "representativity" or "representativeness"

graph a visual display of data

grounded theory a research methodology used to generate meaningful theory about social phenomena from systematically collected data

group(s) a distinct set of data considered to be homogeneous

  one a single group of data that has the same trait or characteristic

  two two distinct groups of data where each group has a different trait or characteristic

haphazard sampling a non-probability based method of selecting individuals from a population for study participation where individuals are identified in a random, arbitrary manner

Harter scale a variation of a *Likert scale*

health literacy the degree to which individuals have the capacity to obtain, process, and understand health information and services needed to make appropriate health decisions

hypothesis a tentative, testable statement or explanation for a phenomenon; a prediction of outcomes

hypothesis testing an inferential procedure that uses sample data to evaluate the credibility of a premise about a population; used to prove or disprove a research question

hypothetical construct an intangible factor that cannot be directly observed; can be useful in explaining effects drawn from observable phenomena

implementation considered the most active process in mobilizing knowledge; generally requires persistent and multi-faceted efforts that may be directed through various routes, yet undertaken primarily at a local level, where barriers to the use of new knowledge can be effectively addressed and overcome

implementation science the study of strategies to promote, adopt and integrate evidence-based health interventions into health care policy and change practice patterns within specific settings

IMRaD the acronym for *Introduction, Methods, Results* and *Discussion*; the sections of a typical research report or manuscript

incidence density the number of new cases of disease during a given time divided by the total person-time of observation among those at risk; considered to be a measure of the rate of development of a particular health condition within the population of interest

incidence rate the number of new cases of disease among those at risk during a given time period

inclusion criteria the standards or conditions that are used to determine whether an individual is eligible to participate in a study

independent raters members of the research team that individually assess a particular component of a study without knowledge of how other team members assessed the same component

independent sample a sample where observations are selected from separate units in a population, such as distinct people

independent variable the exposure variable of interest that affects, or is presumed to affect, the dependent variable under study

in-depth interview a qualitative research approach where open-ended questions are asked with the goal of obtaining a detailed perspective from the respondent

induction a form of reasoning in research where generalizations are made following empirical observation, leading to new theoretical assertions and the generation of new knowledge

institutional ethnography a type of ethnography which focuses on institutional practices and culture as the target of inquiry

instructions to authors a set of statements made by a journal that advises authors on how to prepare a manuscript for publication in their pages

integrated knowledge translation signifies that potential knowledge users have been meaningfully engaged in the entire research process, involved from the outset and instrumental in shaping, refining and optimizing research development and implementation

intention to treat analysis an analysis based on the initial treatment assignment and not on the treatment eventually received; performed to avoid the effects of cross-over and drop-out

intercept the numerical value of the y axis where a model, such as a straight line, intersects the axis

internal consistency the degree to which the items in a scale are correlated with each other (see *Cronbach's alpha*)

interpretive description a research methodology that is used to investigate or increase understanding of clinical health practices

interpretive research research that seeks to make sense of or interpret the meanings of our social world or actions; emphasis is on the understanding of the complexity of human social life which is influenced by the contexts of time and place

interpretivism an epistemological position that emphasizes the subjective understanding of social phenomena; in contrast to positivism, interpretivism does not seek to measure outcomes, but rather, to understand phenomena from the perspective of those involved

interquartile range (IQR) a measure of the variability of a set of data; it is the length of the middle 50 per cent of the ordered data in a sample, and is a single number computed as the difference between the *upper quartile* and the *lower quartile*; the index of *dispersion* for *ordinal* or ranked data

inter-rater reliability the degree to which two or more independent evaluators of the same phenomenon agree with one another

intersectionality a sociological theory and methodology that examines various systems of oppression and their interconnections

interval scale the third level of measurement where scale responses have meaningful intervals and are categorized by type and order

interval variable a variable consisting of equally spaced responses with an arbitrary zero point (e.g., Celsius or Fahrenheit scales)

intervention an interference, intrusion, or involvement of interest; usually compared against another intervention; a test intervention is often compared against an alternative intervention

intra-class correlation (ICC) a descriptive statistic that provides a measure of relatedness; a measure of rater agreement, based on an analysis of variance

introduction the beginning section of a report or manuscript that puts the study into context;

often states the objectives and hypotheses of a study

invertible a term describing a measure that can be changed or turned in the opposite direction; a measure is invertible if results drawing from a positive outcome are equivalent to those drawing from the negative outcome

judgement sampling a non-probability based method of selecting individuals from a population for study participation where an expert decides which individuals in the population should be selected

knowledge brokers individuals who are trained to bridge the gap between groups in which there is a need to exchange and communicate knowledge, such as scientists who produce knowledge about certain health care practices and government decision-makers who are implementing policies

knowledge translation an interactive process in which knowledge, such as scientific findings or patient experience, is exchanged, disseminated, transmitted or moved into action through various means and modalities, including publication, education, campaigns, and policy development

leaf the smaller digit of a two-digit number, e.g., the 1 in 21 would be the leaf (see *stem*)

LGBTQ an acronym that refers collectively to lesbian, gay, bisexual, transgender, and queer persons

Likert scale a bipolar categorical scale that measures a response using statements which reflect extremes at each end

line of no effect the line, often used in meta-analysis graphs, indicating that there is no difference between the exposure or intervention of interest and the unexposed or control group

linkage and exchange concerted activities to bridge research and practice or policy environments; often aimed at building long-term relationships and collaborative work through various means such as the establishment of programs and networks, regular joint education sessions, and funding mechanisms

longitudinal survey a study in which data is gathered from the same participants repeatedly over time

mass media campaigns determined efforts used to promote health behaviour across large populations through television, radio, the internet and print or other media

maximum the largest value observed in a set of data

mean the "average" of a set of values; the sum of a set of values divided by the number of values; the measure of *central tendency* for *interval* and *ratio* data

measure of variation a measure that describes the spread or scatter of data; (see *range*)

median the middle value of an ordered set of values; bisects the data into two equally frequent parts; the measure of *central tendency* for *ordinal* data

MeSH (Medical Subject Headings) a comprehensive controlled vocabulary for the purpose of indexing journal articles and books in the life sciences; it can also serve as a thesaurus that facilitates searching

meta-analysis a systematic method of integrating and analyzing data from independent studies

methodology a body of practices or set of methods that underlie research

methods the section of a report or manuscript that describes all the procedures and processes in a study including recruitment of participants, data collection, measurement, and analytical approach

methodological quality an assessment of how well a study adheres to the principles of high quality research; can be assessed at multiple levels including: individual studies, systematic reviews, or practice guidelines

middle 50 per cent (see *interquartile range*)

minimal risk the probability and magnitude of possible harms associated with the research that are no greater than those encountered by the participants in those aspects of their everyday life that relate to the research

minimum the smallest value observed in a set of data

Minitab a statistical software package that facilitates analysis of data

mode the number or category that occurs most frequently in a set of data; the measure of *central tendency* for *nominal* data

modifiable risk factor a factor that is causally related to an outcome, and where a change can affect the outcome

modified probability sampling a multi-stage approach of selecting individuals from a population for study participation that combines both probability and non-probability based methods; often the first stage of selection is based on probability based methods and the second stage is based on non-probability based methods

morals principles or standard ways in which individuals or groups behave

mortality rate the number of individuals who die in a population of interest, during a given time period, per population size, usually expressed as per 1000

multi-stage sampling a probability based method of selecting individuals or units from a population for study participation in two or more successive stages in increasing order of refinement

mutually exclusive a term to describe two or more classifications of data where no elements or measurements are in common

narrative inquiry a qualitative methodology used to gain an understanding of how people make meaning of their experiences through the stories that they tell

naturalistic inquiry observational research that emphasizes the understanding of social phenomena that can only be understood from first hand observation of the phenomena as it occurs naturally in the environment

network sampling (see *snowball sampling*)

NOIR an acronym for the scales of measurement: Nominal, Ordinal, Interval, Ratio

nominal scale the lowest scale of measurement where the scale responses are categorized by type, yet have none of the other measurement properties of the higher levels of measurement, such as order

nominal variable a variable consisting of unordered categories (e.g., gender, diagnosis)

non-invertible a term describing a measure that cannot be changed or turned in the opposite direction; a measure is non-invertible if results drawing from a positive outcome are not equivalent to those drawing from the negative outcome

non-parametric statistics a family of statistical tests that do not make any assumptions about the underlying distribution of the data (see *parametric statistics*)

non-probability/non-probabilistic sampling a non-random, subjective method of selecting individuals in the population for study participation

non-response a phenomenon where data is not collected from some individuals selected in the sample; can lead to bias if selected groups are over or under represented in the sample and the groups operate differently with respect to study variables of interest

normal distribution a bell-shaped, symmetrical distribution of data where most of the data cluster near the *mean* and the further a value is from the mean, the less likely it will appear

null hypothesis a tentative, testable statement proposing that there is no relationship between two variables; in typical health related studies, researchers attempt to demonstrate that the null hypothesis is false

number needed to harm the number of people who must be treated for there to be one additional person with an adverse outcome

number needed to treat the number of people who must be treated for there to be one additional positive outcome

number summary a set of *summary statistics* that describe a sample of data

    three number summary using exactly three summary statistics such as sample size, mean and standard deviation to describe a sample of data

    five number summary using exactly five summary statistics such as *minimum*, *lower quartile*, *median*, *upper quartile*, *maximum* to describe a sample of data

Nuremberg Code a set of principles for human experimentation; considered to be one of the most seminal documents on research ethics

objectivism an ontological position that emphasizes the fixed and independent reality of subjects under study

observational study a study design in which the exposure factor of interest has been self-administered or was administered by accident; exposure of interest is outside of the control of the researcher

odds ratio the ratio of the odds of an event occurring in one group relative to the odds of the same event occurring in another group; also called the *relative odds*

ontology the branch of philosophy concerned with the nature of reality

operational definition the clear, concise and detailed description of a measure

opinion leaders influential members of a community or field of practice, whom other health care providers often turn to for advice, opinions and clinical direction

optimizing a response approach that gives the optimal answer to an item (see *satisficing*)

ordinal (scale) the second scale of measurement where the scale responses can be categorized in an ordered manner yet have none of the other measurement properties of the higher levels of measurement

ordinal variable a variable consisting of ordered categories or ranks (e.g., Unsatisfactory/ Satisfactory/Above Average)

other-deception bias a form of *social desirability* bias where the person intends to present him- or herself in a favourable light (see *self-deception bias*)

outcome the measure in a study that reflects the impact of the exposure or intervention

Ownership, Control, Access, and Possession (OCAP) an ethical framework for research in Canadian First Nation, Métis, and Inuit communities that allows these communities to own, protect, and control how their information is used

parallel forms reliability the degree to which two versions of the same scale yield comparable results

parameter a characteristic of the distribution of a variable in a population and is not another name for a variable in a sample of data

parametric statistics a family of statistical tests that assume that the underlying distribution has certain parameters (e.g., a mean and standard deviation)

Pareto chart a graphical display of data, usually nominal, where measure categories are ranked in decreasing order with counts displayed on the left y axis and cumulative frequencies displayed on the right y axis

parsimonious a term used to describe simplicity and succinctness in explanations

participant observation/observer a qualitative research approach to data collection where the researcher takes on a role in the social situation under observation by sharing and participating in activities

participants an individual who is studied in research

phenomenolog(y/ism) a research method that aims to identify, describe, analyze and interpret the subjective experience of participants by studying the everyday, lived experience from the point of view of the participant

phenomenological nod a concept that is used to describe the rigour and merits of phenomenological research findings; speaks to the resonance that audiences experience upon hearing or reading research results: the findings ring true

photovoice a visual qualitative research method in which participants are asked to use cameras to take pictures relating to the research question

PICO(T) the acronym for an approach used to develop well-designed research questions where P = patient or population, I = intervention, C = comparison, O = outcomes, T = time

pilot or feasibility study a small preliminary study which gathers information to help improve the design of a planned larger comprehensive study or to see if such a study is plausible

placebo an inactive treatment or procedure

plagiarism appropriation of another person's ideas, data, or words without giving appropriate credit

plots graphical displays of data (e.g., box, *pareto, scatter, stem leaf*)

population the (actual or virtual) set of all individuals or units of interest

target population the population for which estimates are sought, e.g., Canadian adults living in private dwellings in 2012

survey population the population that can be reasonably, economically reached; typically the survey population is the one for which the researcher can find a sampling frame

population attributable risk the proportion of the health problem or disease that is related to a given exposure of interest; the reduction in the incidence of an outcome in the population that would result from elimination of the exposure of interest or risk factor

positivism an epistemological position which asserts that valid knowledge is generated through a scientific process of observation, measurement, and generalization

precision refers to how close estimates from repeated occurrences of the same sample design are to each other; inversely related to *sampling error*

prevalence the proportion of the population who have a specific condition at a specific time or during a specific time period

lifetime prevalence the proportion of people in a population who have ever had a disorder at any time in their lives

period prevalence the proportion of the population who have a specific condition during a given time period; usually expressed as a percentage of the population

point prevalence the proportion of the population who have a specific condition at a specific time; usually expressed as a percentage of the population

privacy the right of an individual to control and limit access to their personal data and information

probability-proportional-to-size sampling a probability based method of selecting individuals or units in the population for study participation where the probability of being selected is based on a proportional measure of size; draws on auxiliary data and yields unequal probabilities of inclusion; most useful when the sampling units vary considerably in size

probability/probabilistic sampling a method of selecting individuals in the population for study participation where individuals are randomly selected and every individual in the population has a known probability of being included; allows inferences to be made about the population based on observations from the sample

proportional mortality rate the proportion of people who die from a specific disorder in a given time span in comparison to people who die from all causes

proportional review the concept that the level of ethical scrutiny and review that a research study undergoes should reflect the magnitude and probability of harm to the participants

prospective refers to the collection of follow-up data into the future

pull the effort to enhance the movement of knowledge that is instigated by consumer requests

push the effort to enhance the movement of knowledge from those who generate knowledge outward to those who may be able to benefit from its utilization

qualitative description a research methodology that is useful when the purpose of the study is to provide a comprehensive and valid description or summary of a phenomenon where the phenomenon in question is studied in its natural setting

qualitative research a method of inquiry widely used in the social sciences that encompasses a diverse range of methodological tools and strategies (e.g., case study, discourse analysis, ethnography, narrative analysis); concerned with generating an understanding of how the social world is interpreted, understood, experienced, produced or constituted

quantitative research a method of inquiry where data collection includes measurements and groups are compared making possible statistical testing of hypotheses

quartile one of three cut points that separate an ordered sample of observations onto equally frequent parts

> **lower** the number that cuts the bottom 25 per cent from the top 75 per cent
>
> **middle** the number that cuts the bottom 50 per cent from the top 50 per cent; bisects the data; also called the *median*
>
> **upper** the number that cuts the top 25 per cent from the bottom 75 per cent

quota sampling a common non-probability based method of selecting individuals from a population for study participation where the researcher selects individuals based on a characteristic of the population such that the total sample has the same distribution of the characteristic assumed to be present in the population; often used as a means for satisfying sample size objectives for study subpopulations

random assignment the process of allocating individuals or groups to different treatment or exposure conditions where no human choice is involved; a defining feature in RCTs

randomized controlled trial (RCT) a study design where different interventions or exposures are allocated to participants through random assignment and participants are followed to assess the outcome(s) of interest; often used to test the efficacy and/or effectiveness of various types of interventions

random error *errors* that have a mean of zero; that is, over time, they will cancel each other out and not bias the *true score* (see *systematic error*)

range the length of the interval from the minimum to the maximum of the observations in a sample, expressed as a single number

ratio (scale) the highest scale of measurement where the scale responses can be categorized as to type, order, equality of intervals, equality of ratios and meaningful zero

ratio variable a variable consisting of equally spaced responses with a fixed zero point (e.g., height, weight, temperature measured in Kelvins)

reference list the set of all writings, manuscripts, studies or other sources that have been referred to in the write-up of a study; a bibliography

referent distribution the distribution of a test statistic when all assumptions are satisfied; can be used to generate valid p-values

regression a form of statistical analysis where an outcome (or *dependent variable*) is predicted/associated with one or more exposures (or *independent variables*) of interest

relative odds the ratio of the odds of an event occurring in one group relative to the odds of the same event occurring in another group; also called the *odds ratio*

relative risk the ratio of the probability of an outcome or disease occurring in an exposed group to the probability of the same outcome or disease occurring in an unexposed group

relative risk reduction the proportional change in outcome in the treatment group as a percentage relative to the control group; speaks to how much the exposure/treatment reduced

the risk of disease relative to the unexposed/control group

reliability (reliable) the ability of a scale to produce consistent results under varying conditions, such as time; reflects the amount of variance in a set of observed scores due to *true score* variation

reliability coefficient a number between 0 and 1 that reflects how consistent the scores on a scale are from one administration to another

replicated sampling a random subset of the sample; often used in complex survey research to estimate sampling errors

Research Ethics Boards (REBs) a group of independent, multi-disciplinary researchers, community members, and others with expertise in research ethics, study designs, and the relevant discipline related knowledge established by an institution to review the acceptability of proposed research involving human subjects that is conducted under the auspices of the institution

research paradigm a set of beliefs and practices regarding what constitutes knowledge and how that knowledge is to be generated

responsiveness the ability of a measure to change when indeed there is real change in the patient or unit being measured; a reaction to a given stimulus

results the section of a report or manuscript that summarizes the findings of a given study or analysis

right-censored data collected over time that has been terminated because the study has ended before the outcome occurred or the participant dropped out of the study before the outcome occurred

RIN the acronym for random, independent and normally distributed

risk the probability that an event will occur

risk determinant a factor that is associated with the likelihood of a particular health problem or disease

risk factor an attribute associated with a particular health problem, disease or outcome

risk marker a factor that is associated with a particular health problem, disease or outcome, and may or may not be causally related

risk of bias a process for assessing the extent to which a study was conducted well

sample a subset of a population

    sample size the number of participant, individuals or units under study; sometimes referred to with a lower case n

sampling error a measure that indicates by how much one can expect estimates of a given parameter (e.g. mean, proportion) to change from one sample to the next; depends on the sampling strategy implemented; used to build *confidence* intervals and margins of error; is inversely related to precision

sampling frame a list of all the individuals or units in the population of interest; provides a means of access to individuals in a population for recruitment into the study

satisficing a response approach where participants settle with "good enough" answers or provide suboptimal responses to an item; (see *optimizing*)

saturation the point in the qualitative research collection process where new cases do not bring any new information

scatter plot a visual diagram that displays the relationship between the variables

screening the investigation of a great number of studies assessing them for those with a particular feature

search strategy a systematic process used to identify studies most relevant to a particular question or topic of interest

selected at random a statement surrounding the method of identifying individuals for participation in a study where identification of participants is devoid of human choice

selection bias an error in identifying individuals for participation in a study where some individuals have no chance of being identified for recruitment into the sample; can result in a distortion in statistical analyses

self-deception bias an error introduced to data collection where respondents deny or rationalize their response based on an illogical truth; a form of *social desirability bias* that the respondent is unaware of (see *other-deception bias*)

self-management an approach to enhance an individual's ability to manage the symptoms, treatment, physical, and psychological consequences and life style changes associated with a health condition

semi-structured interview an interviewing practice in which the researcher develops and asks a set of open-ended questions about the topics of interest prior to the interview

shared decision-making an approach to clinical care that involves an interaction between clinicians about the scientific evidence and patients who bring information about their personal preferences and attributes in order to come to a joint plan about the best actions for an individual or group facing health care issues

simple random sampling a probability based method of selecting individuals or units from a population of interest for study participation that ensures that every individual in the population has an equal probability of being selected

situational variable (see *control variable*)

skewed an asymmetric distribution or tails in a data display

    left the long tail is to the left of the display; also referred to as a negative skew

right the long tail is to the right of the display; also referred to as a positive skew

slope a measure of the steepness of a line; the amount a straight line changes its y axis per unit of change on the x axis

snowball sampling a non-probability based method of selecting individuals from a population for study participation where the researcher identifies a small number individuals from the population of interest and seeks to obtain contact information for other members of the same population from those who have already participated; an approach that is often used for hard to locate populations of interest

social desirability bias the tendency to distort a response on a scale in order to create a more favourable impression (see *other-deception bias, self-deception bias*)

social epidemiology an approach to epidemiological research closely tied to sociological ideas regarding the social determinants of health; emphasizes the role of contextual, social-structural factors

social marketing strategies that apply commercial marketing technologies and techniques to initiatives that seek to improve the welfare of individuals and society

standard deviation a measure of the degree of spread or dispersion in a set of data; an indicator of the variation in the data; the index of *dispersion* of data for *interval* and *ratio* data

standard error the variation measure usually associated with a specific statistic or effect measure

standardized mortality rate the number of observed deaths in a study population to the number of deaths expected based on the age and sex specific rates in the general population

statistical efficiency (see also *sampling error*) a relative measure that indicates how a given sampling strategy will be more or less costly than a competing sampling strategy for the same expected precision or, conversely, how more or less precise a sampling strategy will be for a given cost (i.e., sample size)

statistics summary measures that are computed from samples of data; also a name for the discipline of studying how these measures function and are properly used

descriptive the measures used to describe the data's key features such as location, variation and effect

order the set of observed data that are sorted from smallest to largest in magnitude; can be done for all scales except nominal

statistical inference the judgement or conclusions made about a population drawn from a sample of data selected from that population

statistically significant the probability that the observed data would occur by chance in a given population; a p value from a test statistic that is less than the alpha value

stem the larger digit of a two digit number, e.g., the 2 in 21 would be the stem (see *leaf*)

stem leaf plot (SLP) a summary display of data where the data is ordered by place value with stems ordered from smallest to largest listed downwards and the leaves associated with that stem listed horizontally to the right of the stem from smallest on the left to largest on the right and the depths listed to the left of the stems

straight line a functional relationship between two variables that contains an intercept and a slope to describe the line

relationship the nature of the function between two variables

stratified sampling an approach to selecting individuals or units from a population of interest for study participation where the members of the population are divided into mutually exclusive, homogeneous groups (or strata) and selection of individuals or units from the population occurs within each group

structured interview an interviewing practice in which the interviewer adheres to a formal interview schedule of questions where the wording and sequence of the questions is prescribed; typically draws on close-ended questions

structured observation a systematic method of data collection where observation of pre-coded behaviour(s) takes place in the form of recording when, how often, or for how long the behaviour(s) occurs; researchers seek to avoid influencing the environment and behaviour they are observing

summary statistic quantitative measure used to summarize a set of data; communicates the largest amount as simply as possible

supported self-management (also known as "guided self-management") signifies the involvement of a health care provider in translating knowledge to patients for the purpose of self-management, or coaching patients to support their efforts at self-management, either in individual or group formats

symmetric a shape of a distribution that is a mirror image of itself, such as a *normal distribution*

systematic error *errors* that occur when results differ in a systematic way from the truth; may inflate or deflate the *true score* (see *random error*)

systematic review a literature review focused on a clearly formulated question that seeks to identify, select, and critically appraise relevant research, and to synthesize and analyze the evidence as it relates to the question of interest

systematic sampling a probability based method of selecting individuals from a population of interest for study participation where indi-

viduals are selected from the population at regular intervals; involves a random start with selection of every kth individual

tacit knowledge a form of knowledge that is developed from direct experience and action; is highly pragmatic and situation-specific and is often understood and applied subconsciously; is often difficult to articulate or codify, but is usually learned through interactive conversation and shared experience

test-retest reliability the degree to which two or more administrations of the same scale yield the same result

test of heterogeneity a test that determines whether the results of studies included in a meta-analysis are similar or not

thematic analysis a method for identifying, analyzing and reporting patterns within data; a theme or pattern captures something important pertaining to the research question and ideally occurs a number of times across the data; a common form of analysis in qualitative research studies

theoretical sampling a form of sampling that does not take place at a single point in the inquiry process but is a recurrent feature where participants are recruited to participate at various times throughout the study as the researcher develops aspects of an emerging theory; a central feature of grounded theory research

therapeutic misconception an ethical problem that describes a phenomenon where study participants have difficulty in differentiating between the goals of clinical research and clinical treatment

transcription a form of data entry where audio-recordings are converted to written form; often used in qualitative research studies

treatment group individuals in a study who receive the independent variable or exposure that is being assessed

true score the hypothetical score that would be obtained if the scale contained no *random error*, or were administered an infinite number of times

trustworthiness a term that refers to the truthfulness or validity of the qualitative research findings; consists of four constructs:

    (1) credibility

    (2) transferability

    (3) dependability

    (4) confirmability

two-tailed test a statistical test in which values of a sample statistic are assessed as being either greater than or less than a certain range of values.

unipolar scale an item response format where the scores go from the least amount to the most (contrast with *bipolar scale*)

unpublished study a study that has not been published in the peer-reviewed literature; a study that has not undergone assessment by one's peers or deemed suitable for publication

unstructured/open-ended interview an interviewing practice in which the researcher engages with the participant to elicit their stories with minimal interruption; an interview guide which outlines the topics to be covered may be developed prior to the interview and usually draws from open-ended questions

utilitarianism a theory in ethics that holds that the proper course of action is one that maximizes happiness and reduces suffering

valid study results drawn from a sample that represents the true value for a population

validity the degree to which scores on a scale give meaningful information about the participant; the degree to which a measure captures what it is intended to reflect

variables factors in a study that have data associated with them

    input variables that can be measured or controlled by the designer of the study; sometimes called independent or exposure variables

    response variables that are not intended to be input but are intended to be output from the study; sometimes called dependent or disease variables

variance a numerical indicator of how widely a measure in the data varies

visual analogue scale a type of continuous judgement scale consisting of a line with extreme adjectives at each end

volunteer sampling a non-probability based method of selecting individuals from a population for study participation where individuals in the population volunteer or select themselves for participation

weight the average number of individuals or units in the survey population that the sample represents; the inverse of the inclusion probability

whiskers the lines sticking out of a box plot

x axis the horizontal axis in a graphical display

y axis the vertical axis in a graphical display

yea-saying bias a tendency to agree with items on a scale, irrespective of their content (also called *acquiescence bias*)

Index